Exercise and Respiratory Diseases in Paediatrics

It is commonly accepted that 'exercise is good for children' but, considering the number of children worldwide exercising, we know comparatively little, compared to adults, about how specific mechanisms influence health and sports performance. There are considerable obstacles that challenge the progress of paediatric research, not least in relation to ethical and methodological considerations. Therefore, advances in the science and clinical application of paediatric exercise physiology, psychology, and biomechanics have not reached their potential.

Paediatric clinical exercise physiology has application to the role of exercise in the assessment and treatment of paediatric chronic diseases, the utilisation of physical activity in preventing illness and enhancing wellbeing and can enhance our understanding of how sports can be made safer and more enjoyable for our young athletes.

Exercise and Respiratory Diseases in Paediatrics highlights research by various methodologies, including literature reviews, experimental research and innovations, applied to children and adolescents with respiratory diseases. Chronic conditions such as asthma, bronchiectasis (e.g., cystic fibrosis), and those associated with prematurity and medical complexity are worldwide health problems for young people and although management includes pharmaceutical medications, physiotherapy, nutritional and psychological support, exercise has a role in optimising multidisciplinary care. There has been unprecedented acceleration in new technologies and methodologies that promise to facilitate paediatric research and these are explained and discussed as future research directions.

This is reading for post graduate students, researchers, academics, and policy makers within the field of paediatric healthcare, physical activity, physiology, and the related disciplines.

Craig A. Williams is Director of the Children's Health and Exercise Research Centre (CHERC). As a Fellow of the American College of Sports Medicine and the British Association of Sport and Exercise Sciences, he is a passionate advocate for the health and well-being of young people. He has lectured in Higher Education for the last 30 years and is currently based at University of Exeter, UK.

Patrick J. Oades has been a Consultant Paediatrician at the Royal Devon and Exeter Foundation NHS Trust for over 25 years, providing care in neonatal, acute and community settings. He has a specialist interest in paediatric pulmonology and was Clinical Director of the Exeter Cystic Fibrosis Centre and the SW Peninsula Cystic Fibrosis Services in the UK for nearly two decades. As an advocate for the role of exercise in medicine, he has collaborated with the University of Exeter CHERC, to promote joint working and innovation.

Routledge Research in Paediatric Sport and Exercise Science
Series Editor: Craig Williams, University of Exeter, UK

The *Routledge Research in Paediatric Sport and Exercise Science* series provides a multi-disciplinary platform for established and emerging academics and practitioners to showcase cutting-edge research in all aspects of sport and exercise science in children and adolescents. Edited by Professor Craig Williams, director of the world-leading Children's Health and Exercise Research Centre at the University of Exeter, UK (http://sshs.exeter.ac.uk/research/centres/cherc/), the series includes contributions from applied sport performance monographs to clinical studies in exercise and chronic disease. The series makes a profound contribution to paediatric exercise science scholarship, and provides a vital well of resources for sport scientists and clinicians working with children of all ages.

Elite Youth Cycling
Edited by Alfred Nimmerichter

High Performance Youth Swimming
Edited by Jeanne Dekerle

Exercise and Respiratory Diseases in Paediatrics
Edited by Craig A. Williams and Patrick J. Oades

For more information about this series, please visit: https://www.routledge.com/sport/series/RRPSES

Exercise and Respiratory Diseases in Paediatrics

Edited by Craig A. Williams
and Patrick J. Oades

Routledge
Taylor & Francis Group
NEW YORK AND LONDON

UNIVERSITY OF EXETER | Children's Health and Exercise Research Centre

First published 2022
by Routledge
605 Third Avenue, New York, NY 10158

and by Routledge
2 Park Square, Milton Park, Abingdon, Oxon, OX14 4RN

Routledge is an imprint of the Taylor & Francis Group, an informa business

Library of Congress Cataloging-in-Publication Data
A catalog record for this title has been requested

ISBN: 978-0-367-89617-1 (hbk)
ISBN: 978-1-032-07111-4 (pbk)
ISBN: 978-1-003-02046-2 (ebk)

DOI: 10.4324/9781003020462

Typeset in Bembo
by KnowledgeWorks Global Ltd.

Contents

List of Figures ix
List of Tables xiv
List of Contributors xv
The Children's Health and Exercise Research Centre (CHERC) xvii
Foreword xviii
Preface xx
Acknowledgements xxiii

1 The Role of Physical Activity, Exercise, and Fitness in Medicine **1**
CRAIG ANTHONY WILLIAMS AND ALAN ROBERT BARKER

2 Tests of Respiratory Function to Monitor Health and Exercise Tests to Assess Physical Function **21**
OWEN WILLIAM TOMLINSON, EMILY BELL, AND SIMON LANGTON HEWER

3 The Physiology and Psychological Consequence of Breathlessness in Children **48**
JAYNE TROTT, HOLLY JONES, AND PATRICK J. OADES

4 Towards a Comprehensive Assessment of Physical Function in Young People with Cystic Fibrosis and Non-cystic Fibrosis Bronchiectasis **72**
ZOE SAYNOR, DONALD URQUHART, THOMAS RADTKE, MELITTA MCNARRY, AND MATHIEU GRUET

5 Using Behaviour Change Theory and Evidence to Understand and Support Physical Activity among People with Cystic Fibrosis **96**
SARAH DENFORD AND PAUL O'HALLORAN

6 **Exercise in Children and Adolescents with Asthma** **111**
MARIETTA NÚÑEZ CÁMARA AND GUILLERMO ZEPEDA

7 **Competitive Sports and Respiratory Illness** **128**
GUILLERMO ZEPEDA AND MARIETTA NÚÑEZ CAMARA

8 **Tailoring Physical Activity and Exercise Prescription in Children with Respiratory Diseases** **149**
DANIEL STEVENS

9 **Exercise in Children with Medical Complexity: A Need for Individualised Training** **174**
CLAUDIA ASTUDILLO MAGGIO AND GREGORY VILLARROEL SILVA

10 **Exercise Capacity in Children Born Early** **204**
E MARK WILLIAMS AND SAILESH KOTECHA

Index 220

List of Figures

1.1 Model of definition of generic or non-categorical chronic health conditions according to Stein et al. (1993). 4
1.2 Conceptual framework outlining the pathways through which physical activity in a child and young person can lead to improved health. See the main text for a description of the pathways (i.e., A, B…) linking childhood physical activity to health. 5
1.3 Framework outlining the (in)direct causes of reduced physical inactivity in a child or young person with a chronic disease. The solid straight arrow indicates a reduction in physical activity caused directly by the chronic condition. The dashed straight arrows outline indirect factors that may cause a reduction in physical activity. A reduction in physical activity is proposed to have a deconditioning effect, leading to a reduction in fitness and functional capacity, which may lead to further reductions in physical activity. See the main text for further details. 10
2.1 Schematic displaying the integrated function of key organ systems in the transport and utilisation of oxygen, from atmosphere to mitochondria (and subsequent return of carbon dioxide as a waste product), alongside potential diseases that affect each organ system. 24
2.2 (A) The normal resting maximal flow-volume loop. (B) Flow volume loops during moderate and intensive exercise. **A: The normal resting maximal flow-volume loop**. y-axis: flow (L/min); x-axis: volume (L). Following a maximal inspiration to total lung capacity (TLC), the normal expiratory portion of the flow-volume curve is characterized by a rapid rise to the peak flow rate, followed by a nearly linear fall in flow as the patient exhales toward residual volume (RV), the amount of air remaining in the lungs after maximal exhalation. FRC = functional residual capacity, the amount of air remaining in the

lungs at the end of expiration during normal tidal breathing at rest. **B: Flow volume loops during moderate and intensive exercise**. On exercising at low and moderate levels there is a reduction in end expiratory volume and an increase in end inspiratory volume to increase tidal volume (TV, the amount of air moved in/out of lungs in one breath) to approximately 50% of vital capacity (VC, maximum amount of air that can be exhaled in one breath) before respiratory rate increases to assist in the increase in minute ventilation (VE) to meet the metabolic demands of increasing levels of exercise. Flow increases with exercise in health, but only approaches maximum resting expiratory levels at low lung volumes, while inspiratory flows do not usually reach those attained at rest. There is a balance to be struck between rate and depth of respiration during exercise in order to achieve maximum efficiency (work of breathing). At maximum exercise in health, VE is typically only 60% of an individual's ventilatory capacity, which is why in health ventilation does not normally limit exercise. Where there is airway obstruction or volume restriction, (see figure 2.3), VE during exercise may become the limiting factor 28

2.3 Abnormal spirometry flow-volume loops. (A) Mild obstruction (e.g., asthma, cystic fibrosis, bronchiectasis). (B) Severe obstruction (e.g., obliterative bronchiolitis, more severe cystic fibrosis and bronchiectasis). (C) Variable intrathoracic upper airway obstruction (UAO), (e.g., tracheomalacia). (D) Variable extrathoracic upper airway obstruction (e.g., unilateral vocal cord paralysis, exercised induced and other causes of inducible laryngeal obstruction). (E) Fixed intrathoracic or extrathoracic upper airway obstruction (e.g., tracheal stenosis, compression from extra-tracheal mass). (F) Restriction - parenchymal restrictive lung disease (e.g., pulmonary fibrosis or interstitial lung disease causing 'stiff,' non-compliant lungs, pulmonary hypoplasia and post-lung resection). (G) Obstruction pre- and post-bronchodilator (e.g., in reversible obstruction such as in asthma) Improvement of FEV_1 and FEV_1/FVC by ≥12% following the administration of a bronchodilator confirms the diagnosis of asthma or airway hyper-responsiveness. (H) Restriction - chest wall deformity and/or respiratory muscle weakness (e.g., kyphoscoliosis, the physical constraint of obesity, and neuromuscular disease, NMD). 29

2.4 Schematic displaying the difference between ramp and step tests, as used in cycle ergometry tests. Both retain fundamental similarities in a warm-up phase (A), incremental phase (B1) and cool-down phase (C), although it is the manner in which the increments occur that provides the difference. A supra-maximal (Smax) phase is shown as an optional extra, displaying a warm-up (A), a singular square-wave phase (B2) and a cool-down phase (C). 37

3.1 Clinical signs of respiratory distress in children. The flexible cartilage rib-cage in children increases chest wall compliance allowing paradoxical costal and sternal recession during inspiration when the diaphragm contracts, pushing the abdomen out, causing characteristic '*see-sawing*' of the abdomen and thorax. Such deformations undermine the efficiency of breathing as effort increases. Respiratory muscles in young children are relatively underdeveloped and prone to fatigue and the accessory muscles are less well anchored, '*head bobbing*' is a feature of this. Obstruction of smaller airways in children causes air trapping and chest hyperinflation. '*Nasal flaring*', on inspiration is a sign of increased effort and audible expiratory '*grunting*' in infants generates positive airway pressure, splinting them and helping prevent alveolar collapse. 56

3.2 Positioning to reduce work of breathing and relieve breathlessness in respiratory distress. A child will naturally fix their upper limbs to anchor the accessory muscles, reversing the origin and insertion of muscles such as latissimus dorsi to assist in lifting the rib cage during inspiration. Additional muscle work to fix the shoulder girdle can increase thoracic volume and ventilation, but positioning a child's upper limbs as illustrated, achieves the same effect without increasing oxygen demands (Bott et al., 2009). 62

3.3 A Cognitive Behaviour Therapy construct of psychological considerations in managing breathlessness in a child with asthma. 63

4.1 An illustration of children with cystic fibrosis performing cycle-based cardiopulmonary exercise testing using electrocardiography (A) or thoracic impedance cardiography (B) to assess cardiac function during exercise. 74

4.2 Schematic overview of how to determine whether a maximal effort has been given during a cardiopulmonary exercise testing and the cause(s) of any exercise limitation. 75

4.3 An illustration of a child with cystic fibrosis performing swimming-based cardiopulmonary exercise testing. 81

4.4 Schematic illustration of peripheral and respiratory muscle testing. (A) Isometric knee extensors strength testing using a chair with a fixed strain gauge; adapted and modified from Gruet (2020). (B) Standard evaluation of neuromuscular function using volitional and magnetically-evoked contractions. Strength is recorded using a fixed strain gauge and electrical activity of the muscles is recorded using surface electromyography. This set-up can be used to assess the peripheral and central factors associated with muscle fatigability during endurance testing, see Gruet *et al.*, (2016a) for the use of such methodology in people with CF; adapted from Gruet (2018). (C) Inspiratory resistive breathing endurance test using the PrO2® device. Such device permits the realisation of intermittent incremental inspiratory tests (e.g. Larribaut *et al.*, 2020) with participants inspiring through a mouthpiece attached to the device and expiring outside the device. The device can be connected to a smartphone or a digital tablet, allowing continuous visual feedback of the inspiratory pressures produced during the test. (D) Isocapnic hyperpnea endurance test using the Spirotiger® device. Such device permits partial CO_2 rebreathing, ensuring to maintain normocapnic ventilation throughout the test. Participants are asked to breathe at a given frequency through a mouthpiece attached to a tube connected by a bi-directional valve to a rebreathing bag and ambient air. Such set-up allows the realization of incremental endurance test, using progressive increments of breathing frequency (e.g. Larribaut *et al.*, 2020). The device provides continuous audio and visual feedbacks to control for breathing frequency and tidal volume throughout the test. 84

6.1 Diagnostic pathway for respiratory symptoms associated with exercise. 116

9.1 Playful stimuli and incentives combined with verbal encouragement are utilised to ensure collaboration and motivate children in order to achieve maximal effort. These need to be age appropriate and individualised. Pre-test familiarisation with the test environment and process helps to prepare children to do their best. The exercise area needs to be free from hazards and obstructions and any medical equipment that the child is attached must be supported and moved so as not to impede progress. 193

9.2 Diagramatic outline of a typical aerobic interval training protocol. Following initial familiarisation and calibration testing of the subjects' fitness and ability, regular training sessions are scheduled with a pre-determined duration. The intensity of work is increased incrementally as shown in the step-ups. Variable to increase workload will include speed (level walking or treadmill), incline gradient (treadmill) or resistance (cycle ergometer). At the JMH, training sessions are

typically 20 minutes in duration, conducted 2–3 times per week over 8–12 weeks. 194
9.3 Measurement of inspiratory pressure in children with tracheostomies who cannot tolerate breathing through their mouths when their tracheostomy is obstructed. The tube cuff is inflated to prevent breathing around the tube via the upper airway. The non-rebreathing valve obstructs any airflow so that inspiratory effort generates negative pressure which is measured via an enclosed tube circuit connected to a manometer. The procedure can be uncomfortable and so needs to be explained and the subject familiarised with the procedure. 196
9.4 Protocol of inspiratory muscle training in tracheostomised children. Bouts of work to generate inspiratory pressure (IP), by breathing through inspiratory valves are regularly scheduled. The target IP is tailored to the individual as a percentage fraction of their MIP and then as training progresses, the valve resistance and so the IP can be incrementally increased. 197
10.1 Normal values for forced vital capacity (FVC), forced expiratory volume in 1 second (FEV_1), and forced expiratory flow 25–75% (FEF 25–75%). Y-axis is expressed in litres for FVC and FEV_1, and in L sec^{-1} for FEF 25–75%. 206
10.2 Age-specific predictions of height (A), forced expiratory volume in second (FEV_1) (B), forced vital capacity (FVC) (C), and FEV_1/FVC ratio (D), for males (solid line) and females (dashed line), respectively. 207
10.3 A Forest plot comparison of 14 studies reporting VO_{2max} ($mL \cdot kg^{-1} \cdot min^{-1}$) between children born early and born at term. 1. Cycle ergometry, 2. Treadmill. Mean, mean value of VO_{2max} for participants studied; SD, standard deviation of mean; Total, total number of subjects; Weight, overall weight for a study towards total mean difference; 95% CI, 95% confidence interval. 212
10.4 A Forest plot comparison of eight studies reporting VO_{2max} ($mL \cdot kg^{-1} \cdot min^{-1}$) between children born early with BPD, and term. 1. Cycle ergometry, 2. Treadmill. Mean, mean value of VO_{2max} for participants studied; SD, standard deviation of mean; Total, total number of subjects; Weight, overall weight for a study towards total mean difference; 95% CI, 95% confidence interval. 213
10.5 Swedish cohort study of male military conscripts (median age 18 years, range 18–26 years). Maximal exercise capacity by gestational age. Mean ± SD shown, ANOVA, overall $p < 0.001$. GA (weeks): ≤27, $n = 56$; 28–31, $n = 726$; 32–36, $n = 9,930$; 37–41, $n = 182,490$; >42, $n = 25,618$. 214

List of Tables

1.1	Classification System of Complex Chronic Conditions According to Feudtner et al. (2000)	3
2.1	Pulmonary Function Tests in Paediatrics	25
2.2	Investigations That May Be Indicated to Complete a Comprehensive Assessment	32
2.3	Characteristics of Field, and Lab-Based Exercise Tests	34
3.1	Paediatric Respiratory Diseases Associated with Breathlessness	52
7.1	The Treatment Goals for Exercise-Induced Asthma (EIA) and Exercise-Induced Bronchoconstriction (EIB)	135
7.2	Pharmacological Treatment of EIB and EIA	136
7.3	Common Drugs Used in Respiratory Medicine and WADA Status (WADA 2020; Global DRO 2020)	141
8.1	Randomised Controlled Exercise Interventions in Paediatric Cystic Fibrosis	154
8.2	The '5 As'	159
8.3	Ongoing Studies Using Digital Technologies to Promote Physical Activity in Paediatric Respiratory Disease	161
9.1	Clinical Features That May Raise Concern about Respiratory Function in Children with Medical Complexity	178
9.2	Investigations and Interventions in Children with Medical Complexity Who Have Compromised Respiratory and Physical Function (Hull *et al.*, 2012)	179
9.3	A Framework for Constructing a Physical Activity and Exercise Plan for Children with Medical Complexity	187
9.4	Set-up, Monitoring, and Safety Precautions Undertaken When Conducting Exercise Testing and Training for Children Who Require Respiratory Support at the Josefina Martinez Hospital, Chile	189
9.5	Measurement of Maximal Inspiratory or Expiratory Muscle Strength	195
10.1	Phases of Prenatal Lung Development (Cousins *et al.*, 2018)	205

List of Contributors

Claudia Astudillo Maggio, MD
Hospital Josefina Martinez and Catholic University, Chile

Alan Robert Barker, PhD
Children's Health and Exercise Research Centre, College of Life and Environmental Sciences, University of Exeter, UK

Emily Bell, MRCPH
Royal Devon and Exeter Foundation NHS Trust Hospital, UK

Marietta Núñez Cámara, MD
Hospital Roberto del Rio, Chile

Sarah Denford, PhD
University of Bristol, Bristol Medical School, UK

Mathieu Gruet, PhD
LAMHESS, Université de Toulon, France

Holly Jones, DClin
Children and Family Health Devon, UK

Sailesh Kotecha, FRCPCH, PhD
Cardiff University, UK

Simon Langton Hewer, MD, FRCP, FRCPH
University Hospitals Bristol and Weston Foundation NHS Trust, UK

Melitta McNarry, PhD
Sports Science, College of Engineering, University of Swansea, UK

Paul O'Halloran, PhD
Technology and Engineering, La Trobe University, Australia

Patrick J Oades, MA, MRCP, FRCPH
Royal Devon and Exeter Foundation NHS Trust Hospital, UK

Thomas Radtke, PhD
Division of Occupational and Environmental Medicine and the Division of Chronic Disease Epidemiology, University of Zurich, Switzerland

Zoe Saynor, PhD
School of Sport, Health and Exercise Science, University of Portsmouth, UK

Daniel Stevens, PhD
Department of Pediatrics, Division of Respirology, Dalhousie University, Canada

Owen William Tomlinson, PhD
Children's Health and Exercise Research Centre, College of Life and Environmental Sciences, University of Exeter, UK

Jayne Trott, BSc
Royal Devon and Exeter Foundation NHS Trust Hospital, UK

Donald Urquhart, BSc, MSc, MD, FRCPCH
Paediatric Respiratory Medicine at the Royal Hospital for Sick Children and University of Edinburgh, UK

Gregory Villarroel Silva, BSc
Hospital Josefina Martinez and Catholic University, Chile

Craig Anthony Williams, PhD
Children's Health and Exercise Research Centre, College of Life and Environmental Sciences, University of Exeter, UK

E. Mark Williams, PhD
University of South Wales, UK

Guillermo Zepeda, MD
Hospital Roberto del Rio, Chile

The Children's Health and Exercise Research Centre (CHERC)

The Children's Health and Exercise Research Centre (CHERC) was established in 1987 and is based in Sport and Health Sciences at the University of Exeter. The Centre consists of a critical mass of researchers working within an experienced support structure and has as one of its core aims the promotion of paediatric exercise science as a worldwide academic field of study. CHERC is one of the world's leading centres in the scientific study of children's fitness, physical activity, and health. Its international eminence in paediatric exercise science was recognised by the award of a Queen's Anniversary Prize for Higher Education. The Prize, the first to be awarded in the exercise and sport sciences was presented by HM The Queen. The Centre has established Children's Health and Exercise research as a major academic field internationally and was the first to provide PhD training, as well as the first taught programme in paediatric exercise science in the UK. To date, over 55 postgraduates of the Centre are now promoting the subject from academic posts in the UK and international universities in Austria, Canada, France, Holland, Hong Kong, Mexico, Malaysia, Portugal, Singapore, and the United States. CHERCs collaboration through this Routledge Research in Paediatric Sport & Exercise Science series is an exciting venture and we hope it will continue to advance the cause worldwide.

Professor Craig A. Williams
Director of CHERC

Foreword

"*Exercise – I take plenty, I never use the lift in the Club*" said Swithin Forsyte in The Forsyte Saga. Today he might say instead "*I never use the TV remote*". Lockdown in its various forms has meant exercise time has dropped, as we rely more and more on internet resources; will exercise join the Bakelite telephone and the Telegram as relics of a bygone age?

This book gives an emphatic '*no*' to such nihilism. Exercise as a diagnostic and therapeutic procedure needs to be more not less embedded in paediatric respiratory practice. Breathlessness on exercise is common and all too often leads to the uncritical prescription of asthma inhalers, but the commonest cause, and not just in the obese, is simple deconditioning, which can and should be documented in the physiology laboratory. The benefits of exercise on respiratory function and general well-being are well documented. Exercise as an adjunct to sputum clearance and an independent predictor of prognosis is well described in cystic fibrosis, for example, as is the beneficial effect of weight-bearing exercise on bone mineral density. Looking beyond the respiratory system, we know that impaired spirometry is a marker for premature cardiovascular and metabolic mortality and morbidity. The obesity pandemic is killing more than COVID. These are other areas highly relevant to paediatric respiratory medicine where exercise is beneficial.

But will children actually exercise if left to their own devices? Almost certainly not; the lure of warmth and the screen will almost certainly trump sweating around in the cold. If we left a few pots of random pills in the bathroom saying that they would help and swallow some when the mood takes you, nothing would happen. Medication prescription is purposeful; why not exercise prescription as well? This book challenges us to use this powerful tool more effectively. There is an international perspective, highlighting what is known and what needs to be found out with future research. It will challenge the practice of all of us in Paediatric Respiratory Medicine; and may even stir the elderly couch-potatoes in the profession into much needed physical training!

Andy Bush MD FHEA FRCP FRCPCH FERS FAPSR ATSF
Professor of Paediatrics and Paediatric Respirology, National Heart and Lung Institute, London, UK.
Consultant Paediatric Chest Physician, Royal Brompton & Harefield NHS Foundation Trust, UK.
Director, Imperial Centre for Paediatrics and Child Health
NIHR Senior Investigator Emeritus

Preface

Whilst the term Exercise is Medicine (EIM) has become popular since the turn of the 21st century, the link between exercise and improved physical and mental health outcomes has a venerable historical basis and can be traced as far back as 2600 Before the Common Era (BCE) when, in China, breathing exercises were advised for the sick. Later, around 1500 BCE, more traditional whole-body exercises were used for people experiencing '*chills or paralysis*' and in 600 BCE the Indian physician Susruta recommended moderate physical exercise to his patients. These EIM initiatives predate those advocated by the polymaths of ancient Greece; Homer, Hippocrates and Galen.

Although the benefits of exercise are especially pertinent to diseases that we now recognise as being non-communicable, e.g., atherosclerosis, the importance of exercise for rehabilitation after surgery was cited by Clement Tissot, a French physician, in the latter part of the 1700s. Since that time, exercise has formed an important framework for rehabilitation of patients, young and old, with chronic diseases; pulmonary and stroke rehabilitation being most prominent. With increasing survival of children with chronic diseases progressing into adulthood, lifestyle choices that have their roots in childhood contribute to poor fitness and comorbidities such as obesity, type 2 diabetes and cardiovascular diseases that are at least as prevalent as in the general population. Consequently, from outset, the promotion of activity and exercise as a component of routine care in chronic illness is important in optimising health outcomes.

Paediatric Respiratory Disease and Exercise provides an overview of the utility and value of physical activity and exercise in paediatric respiratory clinical practice. It aims to encompass how respiratory disease in children impacts on exercise performance and physical activity levels, how performance can be objectively assessed and how health benefits from participation in regular exercise or training programmes. Children with chronic illness suffer the physiological impairments of their disease and treatment burden whilst their physical, psychological, social and educational development is in progress. Maintaining self-esteem and peer group integration is paramount in order to ensure that individual potential is achieved. The challenges in promoting lifestyle change, motivating participation and the design of physical training interventions are critically reviewed. Gaps in knowledge are highlighted and the desirability of disease specific, standardised, physical training guidelines are promoted as they will enable prospective refinement in longitudinal research. Extrapolated from adult research is included where deemed appropriate.

In **Chapter 1, Williams and Barker** set the scene for the role of physical activity and its sub-component exercise, as discussed in the context of people with chronic medical conditions, such as cystic fibrosis and asthma. The role of exercise testing and its prescription is examined in relation to physical and mental health benefits. Following on in **Chapter 2, Tomlinson, Bell and Langton Hewer** describe the scope of pulmonary function and exercise tests as a toolkit that may be utilised in paediatric respiratory clinical practice, highlighting their place, feasibility and technical considerations. The added value of exercise testing and how performance can vary independent of static pulmonary function measures is emphasised. In **Chapter 3, Trott, Jones and Oades** provide an overview of breathlessness in children, a universal experience contributing to physiological limitation in health, but also an important consequence of respiratory disease that is not usually the focus of attention in research. Discordance between subjective and objective measures of breathlessness is explored and how perception and tolerance can vary in individuals. Practical guidance is presented to help in the assessment and management of breathlessness in children, which can be important in maintaining physical activity levels. In **Chapter 4, Saynor, Urquhart, Radtke, McNarry and Gruet** provide a comprehensive contemporary review of physiological impairment and exercise testing in children with Cystic Fibrosis and bronchiectasis. Strategies to improve fitness and functional abilities are discussed. The chapter concludes with the presentation of current best practice recommendations to comprehensively assess physical function in young people with cystic fibrosis and, by association, bronchiectasis.

Denford and O'Halloran in Chapter 5 discuss the all-important topic of bringing about behaviour change in relation to physical activity and exercise garnered from work in people with cystic fibrosis. Of course, knowing '*why and what should be done*' from a physical activity perspective is very different from the '*how do we do it*' and more importantly how to sustain physical activity. Theoretical frameworks are described and information about barriers and facilitators to physical activity are detailed, as well as the use of technologies, which have become topical during the current COVID pandemic. In **Chapter 6, Núñez Cámara and Zepeda** turn their attention to the most common chronic respiratory disease in children; asthma. Although a heterogeneous disease in diagnosis, the research data base is extensive and utilising their clinical experience the authors outline the negative consequences of asthma on physical activity levels in youth. Exercise induced bronchoconstriction is distinguished from exercise induced asthma and the association between asthma and obesity is reviewed.

Respiratory disorders encountered by young competitive athletes are reviewed in **Chapter 7** by **Zepeda and Núñez Cámara**. Recognising that sporting careers start young, the authors review the pathophysiology, prevalence, assessment and management of conditions. Restrictions on drug usage enforced by anti-doping agencies are outlined and the importance of both athlete and coach being appraised of the physiological, environmental and intrinsic medical mechanisms behind the respiratory disease are emphasised.

Stevens, in **Chapter 8**, reviews physical activity interventions from around the world. Even in healthy individuals, these initiatives are inherently complex and fraught with challenges. The importance of identifying barriers and facilitators for physical activity participation and the role of counselling are discussed. Digital technologies and the potential use of telehealth/medicine to promote a healthy lifestyle are given focus in delivering physical activity programs and formalising exercise prescriptions in young people with health problems.

Children suffering from medically complex conditions may develop comorbidities through inactivity but may also gain health benefit when supported in increasing physical activity or participating in exercise. In **Chapter 9 Astudillo and Villarroel** review the relatively sparse literature that encompasses a wide range of complex disorders that share physical and respiratory impairments which impact on ability to engage in and sustain physical activity. Initial incremental increases in physical activity are rewarded with proportionally more health benefit than increments at higher activity levels. However, at an individual level, training benefits by being bespoke, guided by patient centered goals and physical limitations. They conclude by describing the package of care they provide, in a limited resource setting, for a heterogeneous group of children at the severe end of the spectrum, many with tracheostomies requiring respiratory support. The model serves as an exemplar of innovation and enthusiasm that illustrates how patient and medical goals can be achieved despite such medical complexity.

The concluding **Chapter 10** by **Williams and Kotecha** is left to the large cohort of children born prematurely, many of whom have impaired lung function and exercise capacity. Furthermore, it is recognised that children born prematurely are habitually less active. Factors related to exercise capacity and physical activity levels are critiqued, including the need for more longitudinal studies to examine long-term effects on the biological, neurodevelopmental and psychological aspects of physical activity throughout life.

We hope that this book will be of interest to paediatric clinicians, sports scientists, psychologists and physiotherapists alike, whether in training or established in their field of work. As such, the promotion of exercise and physical activity for children with chronic disease is recognised as a role and responsibility of multidisciplinary care teams in delivering optimal routine care.

Craig A. Williams and Patrick J. Oades

Acknowledgements

We acknowledge the valued support of our employing institutions, our families and the support of the UK Cystic Fibrosis Trust in our work.

Professor Craig A. Williams and Dr Patrick J. Oades

1 The Role of Physical Activity, Exercise, and Fitness in Medicine

Craig Anthony Williams and Alan Robert Barker

Introduction

Most chronic medical conditions of childhood including congenital heart disease, respiratory diseases, such as cystic fibrosis (CF) or asthma, and neuromuscular diseases, such as muscular dystrophy, are not preventable by lifestyle changes. However, these diseases have a considerable impact on lifestyle, particularly when it involves physical activity or its sub-components exercise, sports, and recreation. Changes to modifiable lifestyle choices during childhood and adolescence, e.g., increased physical activity, prevention of smoking, avoidance of alcohol consumption, and improved dietary habits, can minimise disease processes such as cardiovascular disease that are known to develop early in childhood and are now accepted health strategies and policies for healthy living and ageing. However, a particular focus on the role of physical activity for promoting health and wellbeing in children and young people with chronic medical conditions has been remarkably neglected. For two important reasons, this prior focus on *healthy* children and young people now needs to shift to the specific needs of children and young people with chronic medical conditions. Firstly, the number of children and young people with chronic medical conditions have increased over the last three decades and will continue to increase over the next decade. Secondly, because of the increased survival rate, more children and young people will be transitioning through adult services and with an ageing patient population will become susceptible to non-communicable diseases, i.e., obesity, diabetes, as currently experienced by healthy adults (Sawyer et al., 2007; Riner and Sellhorst, 2013).

Over the last 20 years, there has been a significant worldwide accumulation of evidence to support the importance of physical activity participation for early years (Jones et al., 2020), primary school aged children (Hesketh et al., 2017), young people of secondary school age (Farooq et al., 2020), adults (Warburton et al., 2010), and older adults (Zubala et al., 2017). However, there is one group of people where evidence is noticeably lacking and that is individuals with chronic medical conditions. Currently, there are globally national physical activity guidelines for healthy individuals, whilst any guidelines for those with a chronic medical condition, if they exist at all,

DOI: 10.4324/9781003020462-1

are often left to medical organisations or societies recommendations. This observation is surprising given that advances in medicine have resulted in more children and young people surviving into adulthood. For example, in the United Kingdom, CF was once considered a paediatric disease with a survival rate into the second decade of life in the 1980s. Since 2019, there are more adults with CF than in paediatrics, resulting in new and different challenges for the clinical teams, such as how the individuals can safely engage in physical activity and the potential health-related benefits that this may bring (UK Cystic Fibrosis Registry, 2019).

What Is a Chronic Medical Condition?

There are numerous terms used to describe children and young people who have a long-term illness, i.e., chronic medical condition, medically complex conditions, and long-term condition. The U.S. Maternal and Child Health Bureau defines this cohort as "those with increased risk of chronic physical, developmental, behavioural or emotional conditions, requiring healthcare and related services of a type or amount beyond that required by children generally" (McPherson et al., 1998, p. 137). Cohen et al. (2011) state that these children "require extra time, expertise and resource to achieve optimal health outcomes" (p. 529). An internationally recognised classification and diagnoses system (Table 1.1) has been devised that allows for a unified approach to paediatric care (Feudtner, Christakis, and Connell, 2000). This was updated and its performance evaluated in 2014 to accommodate the International Classification of Disease 10th Revision (ICD-10), (Feudtner et al, 2014). A similar non-categorical approach has also been used to define children and young people with special healthcare needs as those who "have or are at increased risk for a chronic physical, developmental, behavioural or emotional condition and who also require health and related services of a type or amount beyond that required by children generally" (McPherson et al 1998, p. 137). Irrespective of the nuances of the definitions used, it is agreed by all practitioners and researchers that a child or young person will possess complex health needs (Figure 1.1).

Prevalence

Besides asthma and allergy, most individual chronic medical conditions are uncommon, but when summated, they comprise a substantial proportion of the total child and young person population. In the U.S., it is estimated that 31% of children report a chronic medical condition (Newacheck and Taylor, 1992). In another U.S.-based study, the 2007 National Survey of Children's Health reported 13.6% of children aged 0–17 years had at least one current chronic condition (excluding obesity), while 8.7% had two or more chronic conditions (U.S. Department of Health and Human Services, 2019). Accurate worldwide numbers on the prevalence of chronic medical conditions can be difficult to assimilate due to differences in definitions, recording and counting procedures and interpretations of complex health needs by clinicians. In one

Table 1.1 Classification System of Complex Chronic Conditions According to Feudtner et al. (2000)

CCC Category and Included Diagnoses	*ICD-9 Code*
Neuromuscular malformation	
Brain and spinal cord	740.0–742.9
Mental retardation	318.0–318.2
Central nervous system degeneration and disease	330.0–330.9, 334.0–334.2, 335.0–335.9
Infantile CP	343.0–343.9
Muscular dystrophies and myopathies	359.0–359.3
Cardiovascular malformation	
Heart and great vessel	745.0–747.4
Cardiomyopathies	425.0–425.5, 429.1
Conduction disorders	426.0–427.4
Dysrhythmias	427.6–427.9
Respiratory	
Respiratory malformations	748.0–748.9
Chronic respiratory disease	770.7
Cystic fibrosis	277.0
Renal	
Congenital anomalies	753.0–753.9
Chronic renal failure	585
Gastrointestinal	
Congenital anomalies	750.3, 751.1–751.3 751.6–751.9
Chronic liver disease and cirrhosis	571.4–571.9
Inflammatory bowel disease	555.0–556.9
Hematologic or immunologic	
Sickle cell disease	282.5–282.6
Hereditary anaemias	282.0–282.4
Hereditary immunodeficiency	279.00–279.9, 288.1–288.2, 466.1
Acquired immunodeficiency	042
Metabolic	
Amino acid metabolism	270.0–270.9
Carbohydrate metabolism	271.0–271.9
Lipid metabolism	272.0–272.9
Storage disorders	277.3–277.5
Other metabolic disorders	275.0–275.3, 277.2, 277.4, 277.6, 277.8–277.9
Other congenital or genetic defect	
Chromosomal anomalies	758.0–758.9
Bone and joint anomalies	259.4, 737.3, 756.0–756.5
Diaphragm and abdominal wall	553.3, 756.6–756.7
Other congenital anomalies	759.7–759.9
Malignancy	
Malignant neoplasms	140.0–208.9, 235.0–239.9

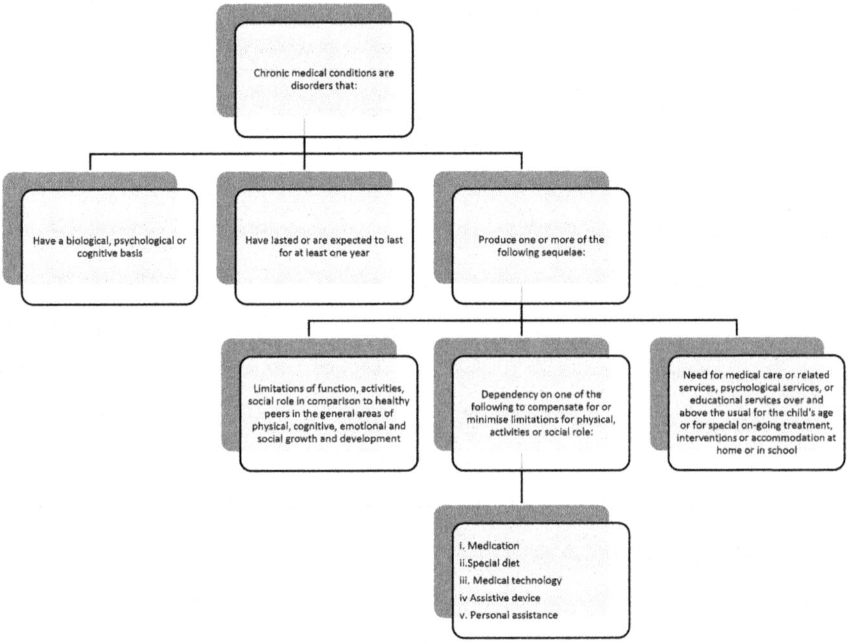

Figure 1.1 Model of definition of generic or non-categorical chronic health conditions according to Stein et al. (1993).

U.K. study in an inner-city general practice clinic of North West London, it was found that most of the children and young people were healthy (77% or 1,188 patients), but over three times more children with complex health needs (17.2%, 266 patients) compared to those with a single long-term condition (5.6%, 87 patients) were identified, which highlights that children with complexity are not always clinically apparent (Aitchison et al., 2020). Irrespective of the accuracy of the numbers, prevalence numbers will continue to increase over time either because of their increasing incidence, e.g., diabetes or the improving survival rates in CF, or the better detection of cancer. Due to improving survival rates, to ensure these individuals have the best life chances transitioning into adulthood, it is important to understand the role of physical activity and its consequences on the physical, psychological, social, and emotional wellbeing of young people with a chronic disease. In seeking to improve these outcomes, clinicians and their support teams will be better able to support young people's development for autonomy.

Physical Activity and Exercise in Healthy Children and Young People

Physical activity is defined as any bodily movement resulting in energy expenditure over and above the resting basal state, whilst exercise is a subcomponent of physical activity that is planned, structured, and whose goal is to maintain or enhance a specific fitness trait (Caspersen, Powell, and Christenson, 1985). Describing or reporting physical activity in terms of frequency and mode presents few problems for definitions, but the same cannot be stated for defining the intensity of activity. Physical activity is often categorised according to descriptors such as low, moderate, vigorous, and care is needed in interpretation, as there is no consensus or standardisation, and intensity categories can differ across studies. This is important to note, as for example in early physical activity studies, children reported as exhibiting low activity were often classified as sedentary. However, more recent evidence shows that even low levels of physical activity may contribute to health status (Marshall et al., 2002).

Figure 1.2 illustrates a conceptual model or framework outlining how the physical activity status of a child can lead to an improved health status (Blair et al., 1989). This model proposes that physical activity in children and young people may either have a direct impact on future adult health (path A), or that the pathway to adult heath is indirect, through improving childhood health status (path B), which can either lead to improved adult health (path C), or influence the physical activity status of an adult (path D). Alternatively, another indirect pathway to improving adult health is through childhood physical activity status influencing the physical activity status in adulthood (path E), which then leads to improved adult health (path F). The indirect pathways by which the status of a child can lead to improved adult health are based on the concept of tracking; that is, to what extent the relative rank

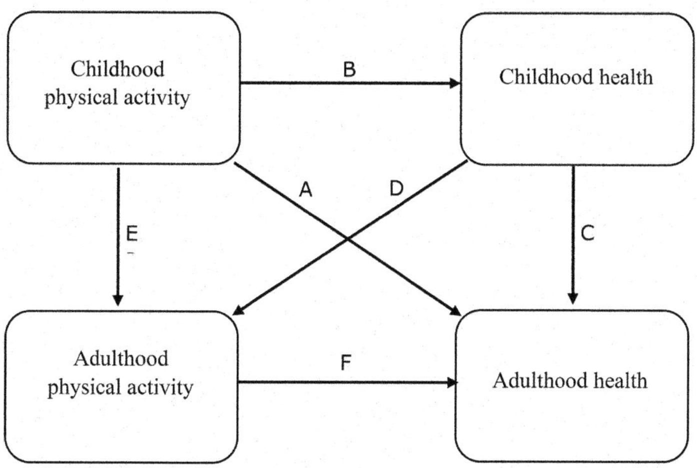

Figure 1.2 Conceptual framework outlining the pathways through which physical activity in a child and young person can lead to improved health. See the main text for a description of the pathways (i.e., A, B…) linking childhood physical activity to health.

Source: Adapted from Blair et al. (1989).

or position of a child's level of physical activity or health status tracks into adulthood.

Currently, there is very limited evidence in support of a direct long-term effect on future adult health (path A), mostly because these studies are few in number due to the requirement of a prospective approach. In addition, the evidence provides limited support that the physical activity status of a child and young person is related to future adult health, but it should be noted that the research methodology is mostly limited to indirect self-report measures of physical activity (Twisk et al., 2002). By contrast, there is strong evidence indicating the physical activity status of a child and young person can lead to improvements in health status (path B), and this forms the scientific basis for current national and worldwide physical activity recommendations for health (U.S. Department of Health and Human Services, 2018, 2019; WHO, 2020).

A number of studies have explored the tracking of physical activity from childhood to adulthood and are supportive of this concept (path E), although the area is complex and dependent on many factors including the age of the individual, e.g., tracking is likely stronger in adolescents than children due to their closer proximity to adulthood, and intensity of physical activity, e.g., tracking may be stronger for lower intensity physical activity and sedentary behaviours (Jones et al., 2013; Telama, 2009). As physical activity is a behaviour, there is also evidence to suggest that the tracking of a child's health into adulthood may be stronger (path C). For example, Herman et al. (2009) studied the tracking of physical activity and body mass index (BMI) over a 22-year period in 7–18 year olds, and found moderate to strong evidence for the tracking of BMI, but not for physical activity.

The concept of tracking is attractive from a public health perspective, as it forms the basis that healthy lifestyle behaviours that are established in childhood transfer into adulthood and lead to improved health outcomes. Indeed, this underscores the life-course perspective of physical activity for the promotion of health across the lifespan. In the context of a healthy child or young person, physical activity is viewed as having a positive impact on growth, maturation, and development. In terms of contributing to health status, physical activity in children and young people focuses on the primary prevention of disease through the modification of risk factors, e.g., cardiovascular disease factors, such as body composition, that we know are related to the development of disease, e.g., type 2 diabetes, cardiovascular disease, in later adult life.

It is widely accepted that physical activity is beneficial for children and young people who do not have a chronic disease. Indeed, physical activity has been positively associated with enhanced physical and psychosocial health in children and adults, and there is emerging evidence that this may extend to cognitive and academic achievement outcomes (Norris et al., 2015). More recent research has tended to focus on sedentary behaviour, defined as sitting or lying during the waking hours and resulting in less than 1.5 metabolic equivalents (METs). It has been shown that high levels of sedentary behaviour are a risk factor for poor childhood and adolescent health status (Tremblay et al., 2011; Mitchell and Byun, 2014). However, evidence also shows that the relationship between sedentary behaviours and health may be modified by the physical activity status of the individual (Ekelund et al., 2012). These observations have important consequences regarding conceptual thinking about physical activity initiatives and whether policies should try to break up and reduce or displace sedentary behaviour as opposed to trying to increase physical activity. Indeed, national and international guidelines highlight the importance of increasing levels of physical activity, reducing time spent pursuing sedentary behaviours, and breaking-up sedentary activity with periods of light intensity activity (Bull et al., 2020). Thus, it should not be assumed that physical inactivity or sedentary behaviours are just the flip side of the physical activity coin.

The strongest association of intensity of physical activity to health outcomes appears to be in relation to moderate to vigorous levels, especially for cardiometabolic health. Whilst this observation has undoubtedly influenced national physical activity guidelines that typically and broadly advocate 60 minutes of moderate to vigorous physical activity per day for children and young people (Bull et al., 2020; Department of Health and Social Care, 2019; Pate et al., 2006), there are many unresolved questions to the issue of the total volume of physical activity.

These unresolved questions are partly a reflection of the complexity of the phenomenon and the numerous confounders such as environmental, social, and political factors. Whilst definitions for physical activity and sedentary behaviour are broadly accepted, instruments to capture these variables are numerous from self-report questionnaires, direct observations, pedometers, accelerometers, and global positioning systems (GPS), all of which have different reliability and validity issues. The outcome of these problems results in inconsistent measurement agreement and thus an increased likelihood of misclassification of participants' physical activity (Armstrong and Welsman, 2006).

Despite some of the inherent difficulties in measuring and interpreting physical activity and sedentary behaviour, there are several worldwide observations that appear consistent (Steene-Johannessen et al., 2020; Tremblay et al., 2014). Firstly, is the finding that physical activity decreases with age, an observation also found in animal studies, and that boys are usually more active and less sedentary than girls throughout childhood and adolescence. Interestingly, differences in pubertal status may account for the gender-related differences in physical activity during the transition from childhood to adolescence (Sherar et al., 2007), highlighting the importance of considering both chronological and biological age of an individual in physical activity research. Secondly, that most children and young people fail to meet the recommended national physical activity guidelines, and the proportion meeting the guidelines falls with advancing age (Cale and Almond, 1992; Cooper et al., 2015; Voss 2014). Lastly, when comparing studies of physical activity levels both within countries and between countries, there is considerable variability that reflects different environmental, societal, cultural, and political influences (Voss, 2014).

Physical Activity in Children and Young People with Chronic Health Conditions

Whilst the evidence base for children without chronic diseases being physically active has been extensively demonstrated, the case for those with chronic diseases is still being amassed but has shown that physical activity also enhances the quality of life and benefits for children with various chronic diseases (Dwyer et al., 2011; Gates et al., 2012; Morris, 2008). One of the leading proponents of physical activity, sport, and exercise for children with chronic diseases was Professor Oded Bar-Or, who as a paediatrician produced several seminal pieces of research across a variety of paediatric diseases including exercise-induced asthma and cerebral palsy. He particularly espoused the importance of involvement in physical activity, sport, and exercise as an inclusive activity for children so as not to miss out on opportunities that their normal healthy aged peers were also participating in. From this positive and 'can do' attitude to one standing up for equity and equality rights, Bar-Or was able to argue for 'normalising' physical activity participation, albeit modified according to the chronic health condition and how it affected physical function. Bar-Or along with another leading proponent of physical activity, Professor Thomas Rowland, a paediatric cardiologist, proposed several fundamental questions to be asked when viewing physical activity in a clinical context (Bar-Or and Rowland, 2004), including:

- Is the child or young person sufficiently active?
- Will increasing physical activity lead to improved health and wellbeing?
- Is physical activity detrimental to health?
- What are the underlying causes of physical inactivity?

Currently, paediatric physical activity guidelines for those with chronic diseases have not been developed in the same guise as for healthy children. Most organisations or societies responsible for children with chronic conditions tend to broadly support the physical activity guidelines for 5–18-year olds of moderate-to-vigorous activity for 60 minutes per day (Department of Health and Social Care, 2019). However, these have not been clinically verified in terms of their safety and efficacy in paediatric clinical groups. Consequently, authors in the field have adopted a narrative approach to summarise the evidence base for the safe and effective prescription of physical activity across paediatric clinical groups (respiratory, congenital, metabolic, inflammatory/autoimmune, and cancer) (West et al., 2019). Clearly, there is a requirement for more high-quality research into physical activity prevalence, variability of intensity, and frequency in order to develop bespoke disease specific advice, which can be captured though systematic reviews.

One of the challenges to determining physical activity levels is the establishment of cut-points. These cut-points classify physical activity into light, moderate, vigorous categories, based on the METs classification system assuming 1 MET is equivalent to a resting energy expenditure of 3.5 $mL \cdot kg^{-1} \cdot min^{-1}$ of oxygen uptake. One issue this raises is that resting energy expenditure is not only known to change during childhood and adolescence but also be altered in relation to the child's disease status. In addition, these cut-points vary according to the make of the accelerometer, the calibration procedures, the analytical technique used to establish cut-points, whilst other factors such demographic and physiological variations are yet to be factored in. This has resulted in an array of different cut-points. For example, in one type of accelerometer, the MVPA cut-point in healthy youth ranges from 400 to 3,600 $counts.min^{-1}$ (Cain et al., 2013). Based on these challenges alone, it is obvious that in a clinical population, the chances of over- or under predicting physical activity levels are high. In a systematic review, Bianchim et al. (2020) found only 5 out of 619 full text eligibility screening that had calibrated and validated accelerometry-derived MVPA cut-points in children and adolescents with clinical conditions. The chronic diseases covered were cerebral palsy, intellectual disabilities, CF, congenital heart diseases, haemophilia, inherited muscle disease, and juvenile idiopathic arthritis. The main finding found little consensus to MVPA cut-points, due to, at least in part, the low number of calibration studies and broad range of protocol designs and accelerometer settings used in the studies. This observation limited inter-study comparisons. A key recommendation from the authors was that if practitioners wish to develop disease-specific paediatric cut-points, the pathophysiology of the disease needs to be considered. An important aspect would include a measure of energy expenditure, as most children with chronic diseases will likely have a higher expenditure during that activity, an accurate assessment of resting metabolic rate, as most children would likely have a higher resting rate due to medication and the disease process, and the inclusion of a healthy comparison group. On development, cut-points should also be cross-validated.

A key clinical question posed by Bar-Or and Rowland (2004) relates to the underlying causes of physical inactivity in children and young people with chronic diseases. This is important to consider, as physical inactivity may be viewed as a direct consequence of the disease, e.g., a child with cerebral palsy with limited locomotor movements, or an indirect consequence of the disease, such as a child with type 1 diabetes who fears taking part in physical activity due to the increase in risk of hypoglycaemia either during or following exercise. Indeed, fear of hypoglycaemia is one of the key barriers for young people with type 1 diabetes and their caregivers, which may result in low levels of physical activity in a child with type 1 diabetes. The consequence of this will be that the child may not reap the potential health-related benefits, e.g., improvements in glycaemic control, of engaging in physical

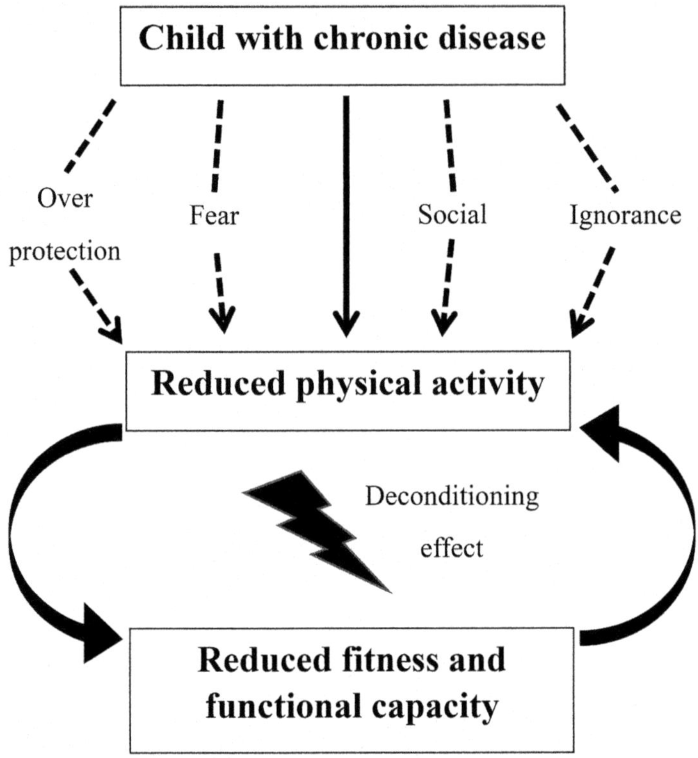

Figure 1.3 Framework outlining the (in)direct causes of reduced physical inactivity in a child or young person with a chronic disease. The solid straight arrow indicates a reduction in physical activity caused directly by the chronic condition. The dashed straight arrows outline indirect factors that may cause a reduction in physical activity. A reduction in physical activity is proposed to have a deconditioning effect, leading to a reduction in fitness and functional capacity, which may lead to further reductions in physical activity. See the main text for further details.

Source: Adapted from Bar-Or and Rowland (2004).

activity and exercise. In addition, as noted by Bar-or and Rowland, this may lead to a vicious circle of deconditioning, a reduction in functional capacity and physical fitness, and a further decline in physical activity (Figure 1.3).

Physical Fitness in Children and Young People with Chronic Health Conditions

It is important to consider the role of physical fitness in children and young people with chronic diseases. Physical fitness can be defined as a set of attributes that a person has, which relates to their ability to undertake daily tasks and is considered to have components that are important for health

(Caspersen et al., 1985). Health-related components include cardiorespiratory and muscular fitness for example, and in children and young people without chronic conditions, these outcomes have been shown to be positively related to current and future health status (Barker et al., 2018; García-Hermoso et al., 2019). For example, there is evidence that a high cardiorespiratory and muscular fitness in young people are independent predictors of morbidity and mortality in later adult life (Högström et al., 2016; Ortega et al., 2012). This underscores the potential value in measuring and understanding the potential clinical relevance (i.e., prognostic value) of physical fitness in children and young people with chronic conditions.

A number of studies have sought to quantify the physical fitness status of children or young people with chronic diseases, with a particular focus on the aerobic fitness status of the individual. Quantification of aerobic fitness may be undertaken for several reasons, including to:

- Quantify the degree of aerobic fitness impairment
- Explore the potential causes of reduced fitness
- Inform exercise training prescription (i.e., percentage of heart rate maximum)
- Quantify the effect of exercise training programme
- Examine prognostic value

The gold standard measurement of aerobic fitness is maximal oxygen uptake (VO_{2max}), which is typically determined during a graded cycling or treadmill exercise tests to exhaustion and is often termed cardiopulmonary exercise testing (CPET). It should be noted, like their healthy peers, children and young people with chronic disease, seldom reach a VO_2 'plateau' during exercise to the limit of tolerance, meaning the term peak VO_2 is often used in the literature. As peak VO_2 is dependent on the integrated response of the pulmonary, cardiovascular, and muscular systems during exercise, there is a clear potential for chronic disease to impair peak VO_2 in children and young people. For example, in a child with congenital heart disease, changes in cardiac structure and function will be characterised though impaired stroke volume, which will lead to a reduction in cardiac output and an impaired peak VO_2, as predicted by the Fick equation (Budts et al., 2013). Thus, exercise testing has the potential not only to identify any potential impairments in aerobic fitness, but also to identify the mechanistic basis of exercise limitation, which may become a target for modification through exercise training. In addition to peak $VO_{2,}$ there are many additional variables that can be gleaned during a CPET, such as the oxygen cost of exercise, which may be important in children with locomotor impairment such as cerebral palsy, or various sub-maximal thresholds related to blood acid–base status (i.e., ventilatory threshold). Interestingly, there are data showing such sub-maximal measures of aerobic fitness, such as the ventilatory threshold, is positively correlated with peak VO_2 in children (Hebestreit, Staschen, and Hebestreit, 2000). This may be an attractive solution to measuring aerobic fitness in children and young people with chronic disease who are either unable or unwilling to exercise to exhaustion.

Although physical fitness is likely to hold important health benefits in children and young people with chronic diseases, it may have added value in term of providing additional prognostic insight beyond traditional clinical measures. For example, in CF, it has been shown that CPET-derived outcomes such as peak VO_2 (expressed as a percentage of predicted VO_2) and peak power output (a marker of cycling performance) are predictors of time to death and lung transplantation (Hebestreit et al., 2019). Importantly, these outcomes were independent of traditional prognostic indicators, including sex, lung function, and BMI. This finding underscores the powerful potential of measuring physical fitness outcomes in children and young people with chronic disease and has contributed to establishing guidelines on exercise testing in specific chronic conditions (e.g., Hebestreit et al., 2015). However, despite seeing the value in exercise testing, it is important to acknowledge that many healthcare settings may not have the capacity to undertake regular exercise testing using direct approaches, such as a CPET. Therefore, there is great interest in exploring the utility, validity, and clinical significance of indirect fitness measures, such as tests based on performance (i.e., 6-minute walk test, bench step test) alongside measures of a physiological responses (i.e., heart rate, oxygen saturation). For further information on the utility of testing including fitness parameters, see Chapters 2 and 4.

Interventions: A Medical or Holistic Approach?

It is obvious that if physical activity and exercise promotion and adoption of programmes are to be championed within a hospital, clinical, or community setting, then clinicians and their associated healthcare teams will play a vital role in its success. Whilst worldwide medical programmes contain little formal training in exercise physiology and psychology, initiatives like *Exercise is Medicine©* and *ExerciseWorks©* are ensuring medical and health professions, i.e., physicians, physiotherapists, and nursing, are exposed to information about physical activity promotion. Having clinicians and their colleagues in associated healthcare professions promoting physical activity to patients recognises several important factors. Firstly, any child or young person with a chronic medical condition will be seen regularly by their healthcare team and form important relationships. Secondly, as a result of clinical meetings and working relationship, the teams will get to know the individual patient and their disease condition well. Lastly, there is logical assumption that if a patient is ill, partaking in 'medicine' that might make them better, would be valued as good outcome.

The *Exercise is Medicine©* (EIM) initiative was launched in 2007 by the American College and Sports Medicine Association. Although initiated at that time to promote physical activity in the context of public health, EIM draws interesting and parallel issues for children and young people with chronic medical conditions. EIM has three broad aims. Firstly, to ensure exercise is considered as a medication to be prescribed to patients. One way it can try to achieve this aim is to ensure all physicians engage in a conversation about physical activity at every opportunity with their patients, Additionally, activity assessments and prescription become a standard part of the treatment and prevention model. Lastly, it aims to assist in merging the fitness industry into the healthcare industry (Sallis, 2009).

The EIM is not without its critics, not least because it pertains to a reductionist perspective that emphasises physiological over social or psychological effects, presupposes knowledge and motivation that determines the health-related behaviour (Neville, 2013; Smith, 2016). Opponents of EIM reflect that whilst physical inactivity is viewed as a cause of ill-health, it does not necessarily make exercise promotion the cure. It is argued that an over-emphasis, particularly of a physiological nature, places too many foci on the individual and less on social institutions and practices (Busfield, 2017). Another aspect not commonly acknowledged within the literature is the view that if patients foresee exercise as a medicine, then it might be perceived as another form of therapy to be tolerated at best, or ignored at worst, like all the other medications patients consume. By default, the patient will then not accept the wider benefits of exercise such as having fun, being with one's friends or learning a new skill. Despite the criticisms of the EIM, Sallis (2009) was correct in pointing out that the three major factors influencing health and longevity are genetics, the environment, and behaviour. For people with chronic medical conditions, there is little control over genetic factors, but the focus on the environmental and behavioural factors is just as relevant to this group as to their healthy peers to improve health. Whilst important advancements have been made in reducing the environmental factors influencing diseases, e.g., vaccinations, hygiene, and safety regulations, factors influencing behaviour remain elusive.

There is surprisingly little research conducted on the efficacy of clinicians, paediatric or adults and their support teams in how, this message of being more physically active, is implemented and its benefits to a chronic medical condition. Some recent studies have identified barriers to promoting physical activity by clinicians and other health professionals in congenital heart disease (Williams et al., 2017), CF (Denford et al., 2019), and type 1 diabetes (Dash et al., 2020) relating to time, knowledge, and lack of resources. For further discussion of this polarised perspective of exercise as another 'pill' for children and young people, see Chapter 5.

Implications

The most recent call to arms for direct action to promote and invest in physical activity is the publication by the International Society of Physical Activity and Health (ISPAH, 2020) that outlines the best evidence to be used to advocate, inform, and lead physical activity policy and discussion.

In this document that provides eight different categories for investments in physical activity, healthcare is referenced as one of those investments. The importance of the investment is predicated on healthcare professionals' regular contact with large proportions of the population and with chronic disease and their widely held respect and trust, which allows for positions of public and individual influence (van Doorslaer et al., 2006; Weiler et al., 2012). This position of influence can be observed when providing advice or referral of patients to physical activity opportunities for patients (WHO, 2013). Finally, the authors propose that health professionals need more continuing professional development to increase their knowledge and skills in the assessment, counselling, and prescription of physical activity. This latter point is important as it has been shown that doctors and medical students possess poor knowledge and skills when it comes to prescribing and advising about physical activity and those that do have adequate knowledge, are in the minority (Lobelo, Duperly, and Frank, 2009).

Therefore, if there is to be more investment in the healthcare system for physical activity research, more research, as highlighted in this textbook, is required. There is certainly a need for more high quality longitudinal studies and randomised control trials using appropriate measurements of physical activity and exercise. As important is the coordination and communication between hospital caregivers, primary care providers, and specialists in delivering interventions that are either hospital or home based, or even a combination of the two. Importantly, an appreciation of the similarities and differences between specific diseases and groups of disorders should help inform practice and policy. However, the current separation of healthcare research, practice, and policy as demonstrated by individual compartmentalising of physical diseases prevents a more holistic approach. For example, to the best of the authors' knowledge, we are not aware of any paediatric research that has combined respiratory diseases, e.g., CF, asthma, bronchiectasis, to explore commonalities and share best practice regarding exercise rehabilitation. It is hoped that the research highlighted in the ensuing chapters show what can be achieved between different organisational groups to advance the course of better advice and prescription of physical activity and exercise for our vulnerable young people.

Conclusion

Children and young people with medical complexities have been shown to be experiencing increased hospitalisation, which are likely to have a significant physical, psychological, emotional, and social effects upon them. Hospitals that care for this group of patients need to consider clinical training programmes, not just for clinical staff but patients, parents/carers, and support workers focused on this increasing proportion of this inpatient population. Children with complex medical conditions should be encouraged to participate in physical activity. Although there will be some serious conditions that might restrict opportunities to be involved in physical activity, for most young people the benefits will outweigh the risks. Whilst such organisations as the American Academy of Paediatricians recommend physical activity participation for most chronic conditions, subject to minimising injury risk and exacerbation of existing medical condition, a stronger advocacy by professional organisations worldwide would provide better support for patients, parents, and healthcare teams.

Key Points

- There is a greater need for self-care of children and young people with complex chronic medical conditions inclusive of physical activity rehabilitation.
- Physical activity and health status are complex behaviours and need to be determined from a holistic perspective as opposed to a single or unidimensional approach.
- There is a greater need specific for child and youth health policies that incorporate physical activity for patients.
- Physical activity promotion needs to be better nuanced for those with chronic and complex medical conditions and must consider age, sex, and developmental factors, as well as known influences of geographical and cultural differences.
- For physical activity interventions to be effective, there must be a recognition of any concurrent co-morbidities and services to deliver the intervention needed to be established in conjunction with the young patients.
- Physical activity and fitness are not interchangeable and should be assessed separately.
- Physical fitness is an important diagnostic and prognostic characteristic that should be implemented more systematically into clinical care.
- The measurement of physical fitness needs within clinical sciences needs more longitudinal studies and investigation of the numerous confounders before it can be incorporated into clinical practice.
- Healthcare professionals must be educated to provide better pre- and in-service training to increase their knowledge and skills in physical activity promotion.
- Healthcare professionals should support the integration of physical activity provision into routine care and engage with other physical activity/exercise professionals to be able to deliver the individualised patient plan.

References

Aitchison, K., McGeown, H., Holden, B., Watson, M., Klaber, R.E., and Hargreaves, D. (2020). Population child health: understanding and addressing complex health needs. *Archives of Disease in Childhood Published.* Online First: 13 May 2020. doi: 10.1136/archdischild-2019-317373.

Armstrong, N. and Welsman, J.R. (2006). The physical activity patterns of European youth with reference to methods of assessment. *Sports Medicine, 36*(12), 1067–1086. doi: 10.2165/00007256-200636120-00005.

Bar-Or, O., and Rowland, T.W. (2004). *Pediatric exercise medicine: from physiologic principles to health care application*. Human Kinetics.

Barker, A.R., Gracia-Marco, L., Ruiz, J.R., Castillo, M.J., Aparicio-Ugarriza, R., González-Gross, M. … and Moreno, LA. (2018). Physical activity, sedentary time, TV viewing, physical fitness and cardiovascular disease risk in adolescents: the HELENA study. *International Journal of Cardiology, 1*(254), 303–309. doi: 10.1016/j.ijcard.2017.11.080.

Bianchim, M.S., McNarry, M.A., Larun, L., Barker, A.R., Williams, C.A. and Mackintosh, K.A. (2020). Calibration and validation of accelerometry using cut-points to assess physical activity in paediatric clinical groups: A systematic review. *Preventive Medicine Reports, 19*, 101142. doi: 10.1016/j.pmedr.2020.101142.

Blair, S.N., Clark, D.G., Cureton, K.J. and Powell, K.E. (1989). Exercise and fitness in childhood: implications for a lifetime of health. C.V. Gisolfi, D.R Lamb, (Eds), *Perspectives in Exercise Science and Sports Medicine*. Indianapolis: Indianapolis Benchmark Press.

Budts, W., Börjesson, M., Chessa, M., Van Buuren, F., Trigo Trindade, P., Corrado, D. … and Papadakis, M. (2013). Physical activity in adolescents and adults with congenital heart defects: individualized exercise prescription. *European Heart Journal, 34*(47): 3669–3674. doi: 10.1093/eurheartj/eht433.

Bull, F.C., Al-Ansari, S.S., Biddle, S., Borodulin, K., Buman, M., Cardon, G. … and Dempsey, P. C. (2020). World Health Organization 2020 guidelines on physical activity and sedentary behaviour. *British Journal of Sports Medicine, 54*(24), 1451–1462. doi: 10.1136/bjsports-2020-102955.

Busfield, J. (2017). The concept of medicalisation reassessed. *Sociology of Health and Illness, 39*(5), 759–774. doi: 10.1111/1467-9566.12538.

Cain, K.L., Sallis, J.F., Conway, T.L., Van Dyck, D. and Calhoon, L. (2013). Using accelerometers in youth physical activity studies: a review of methods. *Journal of Physical Activity and Health, 10*, 437–450. doi: 10.1123/jpah.10.3.437.

Cale, L.A. and Almond, L. (1992). Children's activity levels: a review of studies conducted on British children. *Physical Education Review, 15*(2), 111–118.

Caspersen, C.J., Powell, K.E. and Christenson, G.M. (1985). Physical activity, exercise, and physical fitness: definitions and distinctions for health-related research. *Public Health Report, 100*(2): 126–131. PMCID: PMC1424733.

Cohen, E., Kuo, D.Z., Agrawal, R., Berry, J.G., Bhagat, S.K.M., Simon, T.D. and Srivastava, R. (2011). Children with medical complexity: an emerging population for clinical and research initiatives. *Pediatrics, 127*, 529–538. doi: 10.1542/peds.2010-0910.

Cooper, A.R., Goodman, A., Page, A.S., Sherar, L.B., Esliger, D.W., van Sluijs, E.M. … and Froberg, K. (2015). Objectively measured physical activity and sedentary time in youth: the International children's accelerometry database (ICAD). *International Journal of Behavioral Nutrition and Physical Activity, 12*(1), 1–10. doi: 10.1186/s12966-015-0274-5.

Dash, K., Goyder, E. C., and Quirk, H. (2020). A qualitative synthesis of the perceived factors that affect participation in physical activity among children and adolescents with type 1 diabetes. *Diabetic Medicine, 37*, 934–944. doi: 10.1111/dme.14299.

Department of Health and Social Care (2019). *Physical Activity Guidelines: UK Chief Medical Officers' Report*. Department of Health and Social Care; London, UK. [Accessed on 16 July 2020]. Available online: https://www.gov.uk/government/publications/physical-activity-guidelines-uk-chief-medical-officers-report.

Denford, S., Mackintosh, K., McNarry, M., Barker, A. and Williams, C. (2019). Enhancing intrinsic motivation for physical activity among adolescents with cystic fibrosis: a qualitative study of the views of healthcare professionals. *British Medical Journal Open*, *9*(6). doi: 10.1136/bmjopen-2019-028996.

Dwyer, T.J., Elkins, M.R. and Bye, P.T. (2011). The role of exercise in maintaining health in cystic fibrosis. *Current Opinion in Pulmonary Medicine*, *17*, 455e60. doi: 10.1097/MCP.0b013e32834b6af4.

Ekelund, U., Luan, J., Sherar, L.B., Esliger, D.W., Griew, P., Cooper, A., for the International Children's Accelerometry Database (ICAD) Collaborators. (2012). Moderate to vigorous physical activity and sedentary time and cardiometabolic risk factors in children and adolescents. *JAMA*. *307*(7), 704–712. doi:10.1001/jama.2012.156.

Farooq, A., Martin, A., Janssen, X., Wilson, M.G., Gibson, A.M., Hughes, A. and Reilly, J.J. (2020). Longitudinal changes in moderate-to-vigorous-intensity physical activity in children and adolescents: a systematic review and meta-analysis. *Obesity Reviews*, *21*(1), e12953. doi: 10.1111/obr.12953.

Feudtner C., Christakis, D.A., Connell, F.A. (2000). Pediatric deaths attributable to complex chronic conditions: a population-based study of Washington state, 1980-1997. *Pediatrics*, *106*, 205–209. ISSN 0031 4005.

Feudtner, C., Feinstein, J.A., Zhong, W., Hall, M. and Dai, D., 2014. Pediatric complex chronic conditions classification system version 2: updated for ICD-10 and complex medical technology dependence and transplantation. BMC pediatrics, 14(1), 1-7. Doi 10.1186/1471-2431-14-199

García-Hermoso A., Ramírez-Campillo R. and Izquierdo M. (2019). Is muscular fitness associated with future health benefits in children and adolescents? A systematic review and meta-analysis of longitudinal studies. *Sports Medicine*, *49*(7):1079–1094. doi: 10.1007/s40279-019-01098-6.

Gates, P.E., Banks, D., Johnston, T.E., Campbell, S.R., Gaughan, J.P., Ross, S.A., Engsberg, J.R. and Tucker, C. (2012). Randomized controlled trial assessing participation and quality of life in a supported speed treadmill training exercise program vs. a strengthening program for children with cerebral palsy. *Journal of Pediatric Rehabilitation Medicine*, *5*(2), 75e88. doi: 10.3233/PRM-2012-0199.

Hebestreit H., Staschen B. and Hebestreit A. (2000). Ventilatory threshold: a useful method to determine aerobic fitness in children? *Medicine and Science in Sports and Exercise*, *32*(11), 1964–1969. doi: 10.1097/00005768-200011000-00022.

Hebestreit, H., Arets, H.G.M., Aurora, P., Boas, S., Cerny, F., Hulzebos, E.H.J. ... and Urquhart, D.S. (2015). Statement on exercise testing in cystic fibrosis. *Respiration*, 90, 332–351. doi: 10.1159/000439057.

Hebestreit, H., Hulzebos, E.H.J., Schneiderman, J.E., Karila, C., Boas, S.R, Kriemler, S. ... and Radtke, T., Prognostic Value of CPET in CF Study Group. (2019). Cardiopulmonary exercise testing provides additional prognostic information in cystic fibrosis. *American Journal of Respiratory and Critical Care Medicine*, 15, *199*(8), 987–995. doi: 10.1164/rccm.201806-1110OC. Erratum in: American Journal of Respiratory and Critical Care Medicine. 2020 Sep 1;202(5):780.

Herman, K.M., Craig, C.L., Gauvin, L. and Katzmarzyk, P.T. (2009). Tracking of obesity and physical activity from childhood to adulthood: the physical activity longitudinal study. *International Journal of Pediatric Obesity*, *4*(4):281–288. doi: 10.3109/17477160802596171.

Hesketh, K.R., Lakshman, R. and van Sluijs, E.M. (2017). Barriers and facilitators to young children's physical activity and sedentary behaviour: a systematic review and synthesis of qualitative literature. *Obesity Reviews*, *18*(9), 987–1017. doi: 10.1111/obr.12562.

Högström G., Nordström A. and Nordström P. (2016). Aerobic fitness in late adolescence and the risk of early death: a prospective cohort study of 1.3 million Swedish men. *International Journal of Epidemiology*, 45(4):1159–1168. doi: 10.1093/ije/dyv321.

International Society for Physical Activity and Health (ISPAH). (2020). ISPAH's Eight Investments That Work for Physical Activity. Available from: www.ISPAH.org/Resources.

Jones, R.A., Hinkley, T., Okely, A.D. and Salmon, J. (2013). Tracking physical activity and sedentary behavior in childhood: a systematic review. *American Journal of Preventive Medicine*, *44*(6), 651–658. doi: 10.1016/j.amepre.2013.03.001.

Jones, D., Innerd, A., Giles, E.L. and Azevedo, L.B. (2020). Association between fundamental motor skills and physical activity in the early years: a systematic review and meta-analysis. *Journal of Sport and Health Science.* doi: 10.1016/j.jshs.2020.03.001.

Lobelo, F., Duperly, J. and Frank, E. (2009). Physical activity habits of doctors and medical students influence their counselling practices. *British Journal of Sports Medicine*, *43*(2), 89–92. doi: 10.1136/bjsm.2008.055426.

Marshall, S.J., Biddle, S.J., Sallis, J.F., McKenzie, T.L. and Conway, T.L. (2002). Clustering of sedentary behaviors and physical activity among youth: a cross-national study. *Pediatric Exercise Science*, *14*(4), 401–417. doi: 10.1123/pes.14.4.401.

McPherson, M., Arango, P., Fox, H., Lauver, C., McManus, M., Newacheck, P.W. … and Strickland, B. (1998). A new definition of children with special health care needs. *Pediatrics*, *102*, 137–139. doi: 10.1542/peds.102.1.137.

Mitchell, J.A. and Byun, W. (2014). Sedentary behavior and health outcomes in children and adolescents. *American Journal of Lifestyle Medicine*, *8*(3), 173–199. doi: 10.1177/1559827613498700.

Morris, P.J. (2008). Physical activity recommendations for children and adolescents with chronic disease. *Current Sports Medicine Reports*, 7, 353e8. doi: 10.1249/JSR.0b013e31818f0795.

Neville, R.D. (2013). Exercise is medicine: some cautionary remarks in principle as well as in practice. *Medicine, Health Care and Philosophy*, *16*(3), 615–622. doi: 10.1007/s11019-012-9383-y.

Newacheck, P.W. and Taylor, W.R. (1992). Childhood chronic illness: prevalence, severity, and impact. *American Journal of Public Health*, *82*, 364–371. doi: 10.2105/AJPH.82.3.364.

Norris, E., Shelton, N., Dunsmuir, S., Duke-Williams, O. and Stamatakis, E. (2015). Physically active lessons as physical activity and educational interventions: a systematic review of methods and results. *Preventive Medicine*, 72, 116–125. doi:/10.1016/j.ypmed.2014.12.027.

Ortega, F.B., Silventoinen, K., Tynelius, P. and Rasmussen, F. (2012). Muscular strength in male adolescents and premature death: cohort study of one million participants. *BMJ (Clinical Research Ed.)*, *345*, e7279. doi: 10.1136/bmj.e7279.

Pate, R.R., Davis, M.G., Robinson, T.N., Stone, E.J., McKenzie, T.L. and Young, J.C. (2006). Promoting physical activity in children and youth: a leadership role for schools: a scientific statement from the American Heart Association Council on Nutrition, Physical Activity, and Metabolism (Physical Activity Committee) in collaboration with the Councils on Cardiovascular Disease in the Young and Cardiovascular Nursing. *Circulation, 114*(11), 1214–1224. doi: 10.1161/CIRCULATIONAHA.106.177052.

Riner, W.F. and Sellhorst, S.H., (2013). Physical activity and exercise in children with chronic health conditions. *Journal of Sport and Health Science, 2*(1), 12–20. doi: 10.1016/j.jshs.2012.11.00.

Sallis, R.E. (2009). Exercise is medicine and physicians need to prescribe it! *British Journal of Sports Medicine, 43*(1), 3–4. doi: 10.1136/bjsm.2008.054825.

Sawyer, S.M., Drew, S., Yeo, M.S. and Britto, M.T. (2007). Adolescents with a chronic condition: challenges living, challenges treating. *The Lancet, 369*(9571), 1481–1489. doi: 10.1016/S0140-6736(07)60370-5.

Smith, A. (2016). Exercise is recreation not medicine. *Journal of Sport and Health Science, 5*(2), 129–134. doi: 10.1016/j.jshs.2016.03.002.

Sherar, L.B, Esliger, D.W., Baxter-Jones, A.D. and Tremblay, M.S. (2007). Age and gender differences in youth physical activity: does physical maturity matter? *Medicine and Science in Sports and Exercise, 39*(5):830–835. doi: 10.1249/mss.0b013e3180335c3c.

Steene-Johannessen, J., Hansen, B.H., Dalene, K.E., Kolle, E., Northstone, K., Møller, N.C. … and Puder, J.J. (2020). Variations in accelerometry measured physical activity and sedentary time across Europe–harmonized analyses of 47,497 children and adolescents. *International Journal of Behavioral Nutrition and Physical Activity, 17*(1), 1–14. doi: 10.1186/s12966-020-00930-x.

Stein, R.E.K., Bauman, L.J., Westbrook, L.E., Coupey, S.M. and Ireys, H.T. (1993). Framework for identifying children who have chronic conditions: the case for a new definition. *Journal of Pediatrics*, 122, 342–347. doi: 10.1016/s0022-3476(05)83414-6.

Telama R. (2009). Tracking of physical activity from childhood to adulthood: a review. *Obesity Facts, 2*(3), 187–195. doi: 10.1159/000222244.

Tremblay, M.S., LeBlanc, A.G., Kho, M.E., Saunders, T.J., Larouche, R., Colley, R.C. … and Gorber, S.C. (2011). Systematic review of sedentary behaviour and health indicators in school-aged children and youth. *International Journal of Behavioral Nutrition and Physical Activity, 8*(1), 98. doi: 10.1186/1479-5868-8-98.

Tremblay, M.S., Gray, C.E., Akinroye, K., Harrington, D.M., Katzmarzyk, P.T., Lambert, E.V. … and Prista, A. (2014). Physical activity of children: a global matrix of grades comparing 15 countries. *Journal of Physical Activity and Health, 11*(s1), S113–S125. doi: 10.1123/jpah.2014-0177.

Twisk, J. W. R., Kemper H. C. G., and W. Van Mechelen. (2002). Prediction of cardiovascular disease risk factors later in life by physical activity and physical fitness in youth: general comments and conclusions. *International Journal of Sports Medicine, 23*(S1), 44–50. doi: 10.1055/s-2002-28461.

UK Cystic Fibrosis Registry. (2019). Annual Data Report. Cystic Fibrosis Trust, London, UK. Available from: https://www.cysticfibrosis.org.uk/registryreports/. Retrieved November 2020.

U.S. Department of Health and Human Services. (2018). Physical Activity Guidelines for Americans, 2nd edition. Washington, DC.

U.S. Department of Health and Human Services. (2019). Health Resources and Services Administration, Maternal and Child Health Bureau. The National Survey of Children's Health (2007). Rockville, MD. https://mchb.hrsa.gov/data/national-surveys.

van Doorslaer E., Masseria C., Koolman X. and Group OECD Health Equity Research Group. (2006). Inequalities in access to medical care by income in developed countries. *Canadian Medical Association Journal, 174*(2):177–183. doi: 10.1503/cmaj.050584.

Voss, C. British Journal of Sports medicine Blog. A Global fail? International Comparison of Physical Activity of Children and Youth Report cards. 24 June, 2014. Available from: http://blogs.bjsm.com/bjsm/2014/06/24/a-global-fail-international-comparisons-of–physical-activity-of-children-and-youth-report-cards/. [cited 2020].

Warburton, D.E., Charlesworth, S., Ivey, A., Nettlefold, L. and Bredin, S.S.D. (2010). A systematic review of the evidence for Canada's Physical Activity Guidelines for Adults. *International Journal of Behavioural Nutrition and Physical Activity*, *7*, 39. doi.:10.1186/1479-5868-7-39.

Weiler R., Chew, S., Coombs, N., Hamer M. and Stamatakis E. (2012). Physical activity education in the undergraduate curricula of all UK medical schools. Are tomorrow's doctors equipped to follow clinical guidelines? *British Journal of Sports Medicine*, *46*(14):1024–1026. doi: 10.1136/bjsports-2012-091380.

West, S.L., Banks, L., Schneiderman, J.E., Caterini, J.E., Stephens, S., White, G., Dogra, S. and Wells, G.D. (2019). Physical activity for children with chronic disease; a narrative review and practical applications. *BMC Pediatrics*, *19*, 12. doi:10.1186/s12887-018-1377-3.

Williams, C.A., Gowing, L., Horn, R. and Stuart, A.G. (2017). A survey of exercise advice and recommendations in UK paediatric cardiac clinics. *Cardiology in the Young*, *27*(5): 951–956. doi: 10.1017/S1047951116002729.

World Health Organization. (2013). Global action plan for the prevention and control of noncommunicable diseases 2013–2020. Geneva, Switzerland [Available from: https://www.who.int/nmh/events/ncd_action_plan/en/].

Zubala, A., MacGillivray, S., Frost, H., Kroll, T., Skelton, D.A., Gavine, A., Gray, N.M., Toma, M. and Morris, J. (2017). Promotion of physical activity interventions for community dwelling older adults: a systematic review of reviews. *PloS ONE*, *12*(7), e0180902. doi: 10.1371/journal.pone.0180902.

2 Tests of Respiratory Function to Monitor Health and Exercise Tests to Assess Physical Function

Owen William Tomlinson, Emily Bell, and Simon Langton Hewer

Introduction

For children with chronic respiratory disease, achieving favourable outcomes is dependent upon comprehensive effective management. To achieve this requires an early correct diagnosis, meaningful and sensitive monitoring, appropriate and timely intervention with an evaluation of response. Obtaining accurate and physiologically pertinent measures to guide management is essential. Changes in symptoms, pulmonary function measures (relative to a child's predicted values), as well as exercise tolerance, can indicate changing disease status prompting further investigation and changes in management. Knowing when to perform the different tests available and how to interpret results requires experience and understanding of test limitations and feasibility in the young, ensuring that optimal clinical management is delivered and that resources are utilised effectively. This chapter aims to provide an overview of current pulmonary function and exercise testing in children and adolescents with respiratory disease.

Foundations of Pulmonary and Exercise Function

Growth, Maturation, and Changing Lungs

In order to recognise clinically significant changes in pulmonary function and exercise tolerance in children with respiratory disease, appreciation of normal lung development and physiological change is necessary. Early childhood (birth–8 years) and adolescence (11–16 years) are both associated with periods of rapid physical growth, with stature increasing particularly rapidly (Baxter-Jones, 2017). This growth has an impact on pulmonary volumes, whereby total lung capacity (TLC) increases, reflecting growth of the thoracic cage in both sexes (Kivastik and Kingisepp, 1997). However, there is a lag between change in stature and subsequent change in lung volumes, which is affected by the timing and tempo of pubertal maturation (Neve *et al.*, 2002). Therefore, seated stature which reflects trunk growth is more indicative of thoracic size and is preferred over total stature as a reference

DOI: 10.4324/9781003020462-2

value during growth spurts. There is also a sex influence, whereby boys present with greater thoracic dimension than girls of the same stature (Kivastik and Kingisepp, 1997). Consequently, age, stature, and sex need consideration when expressing pulmonary function in relation to normative values (Quanjer *et al.*, 2012).

These rapid changes in stature and weight in childhood can also directly impact exercise capacity. This is predominantly driven through increases in lean mass that become more pronounced between boys and girls during adolescence (Baxter-Jones, 2017). Fat-free mass (FFM) in particular influences exercise capacity, whereby adolescent boys present with greater FFM values and therefore exercise capacity than female counterparts. This difference between sexes increases with age (Armstrong and Welsman, 2019) and therefore, much like pulmonary function, both age and sex are incorporated into reference values for exercise capacity (Bongers *et al.*, 2014).

Monitoring in Clinical Practice

Children with chronic respiratory disease, such as cystic fibrosis (CF), benefit most by being reviewed regularly and cared for by experienced multidisciplinary teams who monitor clinical progress and adjust treatment plans accordingly. Assessments include anthropometric measures of growth (height, weight, and body mass index (BMI) centiles), a review of symptoms and clinical examination findings, pulse oximetry, radiological imaging, respiratory microbiological surveillance, and relevant blood investigations. Objective measures of pulmonary function are desirable but in routine hospital clinics, these are challenged by the level of understanding, cooperation, and coordination of children. Usually it becomes possible to perform spirometry in developmentally normal children from about 5 years of age. Physiotherapists are often adept at training young children to perform forced expiratory manoeuvres by using play and tools such as windmills or blowing bubbles to focus their interest. Spirometers equipped with images of candles can be used to incentivise children to blow harder as this is something with which many young children will be familiar. The assessment of pulmonary function in preschool children presents even more of a challenge as they are unable to perform voluntarily many of the physiological manoeuvres required for testing. Furthermore, the interpretation of results is complicated by the fact that respiratory mechanics change and lung growth is rapid in this age group, with significant developmental changes to lung structure that continue from foetal development into infancy and early preschool life, see Chapter 10. Sedation is used in infants, allowing the application of flow-measuring equipment and compression jackets to simulate forced expiration, but physiology may change with sedation and certainly with anaesthesia. There are international consensus guidelines to guide investigation in this age group (Beydon *et al.*, 2007).

Spirometry is a cornerstone in the monitoring of children and adults with respiratory disease. Longitudinal spirometric data is valuable in helping to detect fluctuations in disease activity, such as infective exacerbations in bronchiectasis, assess response to therapeutic interventions, and also identify progressive decline in lung function when serial recordings are made during periods of apparent clinical stability. Spirometry is routinely performed in hospital clinics but is increasingly being done remotely using a home spirometer that transmits values to the patient's care centre (Shakkottai *et al.*, 2018; Logie, Welsh and Ranganathan, 2019), this can increase the frequency of monitoring whilst reducing the number of hospital visits saving time and the travel burden for families.

Other measurements of lung function are also available for more limited numbers of children, and within the context of randomised clinical trials. These will be discussed later in the chapter, but of particular interest is the lung clearance index (LCI), a measure of ventilation inhomogeneity derived from the multiple breath inert gas washout (MBW), that can detect abnormal lung function earlier than spirometry. It takes over an hour to perform by a careful and skilled technician.

Children and adolescents suffering from respiratory disorders or their carers are prompted to seek medical attention when symptoms such as cough or excessive breathlessness on exertion arise. It is apparent that pulmonary function alone does not necessarily predict exercise performance and yet this is what has a direct impact on the quality, opportunities in a young person's daily life. Furthermore, there are instances where exercise-based parameters predict mortality (Hulzebos *et al.*, 2014) and risk of hospitalisation (Pérez *et al.*, 2014) to a greater extent than when using spirometry alone. Hence for the physician, the objective clarification of exercise and physical activity limitation is helpful in understanding the consequences of disease processes. The range of exercise tests available are discussed later in this chapter.

Why Measure Both?

Good pulmonary and exercise function are associated with better clinical outcomes including an enhanced quality of life (QoL) (Hebestreit *et al.*, 2014), lower overall treatment burden (Vandekerckhove *et al.*, 2017), and a lower risk of mortality or major morbidity, such as lung transplantation (Hebestreit *et al.*, 2019).

In contrast to spirometry, whereby measures are usually done at rest, exercise testing facilitates the simultaneous integrated assessment of pulmonary, cardiovascular, and musculoskeletal function during physical and metabolically demanding activity. Each system plays a necessary role in transporting oxygen from the atmosphere to mitochondria in working muscles for use in energy transfer (Figure 2.1), the functional limits and efficiency of each system to transfer oxygen determine an individual's exercise capacity and the oxygen cost of their physical work. Whilst the function of the respiratory system is clearly linked to exercise performance, it is only a single component

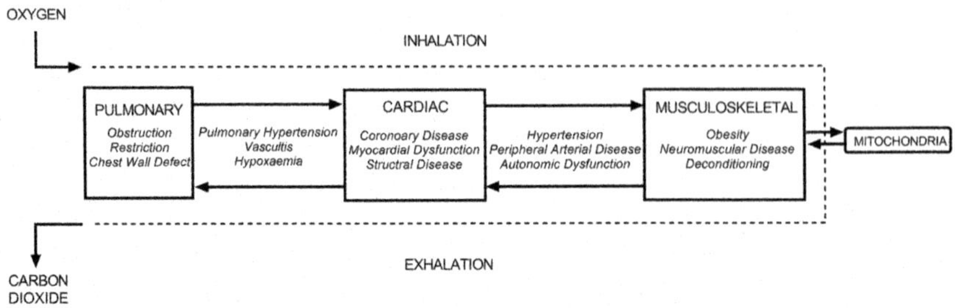

Figure 2.1 Schematic displaying the integrated function of key organ systems in the transport and utilisation of oxygen, from atmosphere to mitochondria (and subsequent return of carbon dioxide as a waste product), alongside potential diseases that affect each organ system.

of this multi-faceted process. Therefore, objective measures of exercise performance provide alternative insight into the consequences and capabilities of those with respiratory disease (Teoh *et al.*, 2009).

Although a primary disease process may arise within the respiratory system, there is scope for cardiovascular and musculoskeletal compensation or conversely additional decompensation if disease processes have other negative systemic effects (e.g., inflammatory or nutritional). Hence, relationships between pulmonary function and exercise performance can be variable or even absent and both may independently predict morbidity. Longitudinal studies evidence differing directions and magnitudes of change in pulmonary function (forced expiratory volume in one second, FEV_1) and exercise capacity (peak oxygen uptake, VO_{2peak}), that occur independent of one another in children. However, this variability may depend on disease severity, whereby a critical threshold of ~80%$_{predicted}$ exists in children. When FEV_1 drops below this, declines in VO_{2peak} occur faster in patients than in those with FEV_1 above the threshold (Pianosi, LeBlanc and Almudevar, 2005b). A similar moderating effect of disease severity is observed in adults (Pastre *et al.*, 2014). In addition, the independence of pulmonary function and exercise parameters provides a larger catalogue of outcomes that may be appropriate for assessing interventions in clinical practice (Burghard *et al.*, 2020).

Pulmonary Function Testing

Objective measures of lung function characterise impairments within the respiratory system, quantify the severity of impairment, prompt further investigation, and ascertain the efficacy of therapeutic interventions (Ranu, Wilde and Madden, 2011). Whilst multiple pulmonary function investigations are available (Table 2.1), this chapter focuses on the tests commonly used in clinical practice.

Table 2.1 Pulmonary Function Tests in Paediatrics

			Gas diffusion techniques		
	Spirometry	*Plethysmography*	*Inert gas dilution*	*Multiple breath washout (MBW)*	*Gas transfer*
Outline methodology	Best of at least three quality assured forced ventilatory manoeuvres from maximal inspiration, via a mouthpiece without leakage. Flow and time are measured. Flow determined by the rotation of a turbine or pressure gradients across resistance in a pneumotachograph.	Subject is tested in a pressure monitored whole body rigid box while breathing into a circuit that measures flow and pressure. Boyle's law utilised with shuttered interruptions or panting breathing patterns to derive parameters.	Dilution of inert gas (He) either by single breath hold or rebreathing to steady state in a closed circuit starting at FRC, adding O_2 and removing CO_2 to keep volume constant.	Measures the decline in the expired concentration of an inert tracer gas (SF_6, He or indirectly N_2) to 1/40th of the equilibrated starting value. Circuit includes a spirometer.	A gas mixture with a known concentration of CO is inhaled and held. CO diffuses across the alveolar-capillary membrane and is bound by red blood cells, while an inert tracer (He) determines V_A.
What is measured?	Dynamic lung volumes and flow rates. In health, flow is maximal with modest effort, giving good reproducibility. Normally flow rates fall as lung volumes decrease, which is augmented in obstruction caused by disease. Abnormal flow–volume loops are shown in Figure 2.3.	Static lung volumes. Effort independent measures of airway resistance, derived from flow and volume changes becoming out of phase with airways obstruction.	Static lung volumes. Circuit includes spirometer to allow derivation of parameters.	Relative ventilation required to clear tracer gas from the lungs. Small airway disease causes ventilation inhomogeneity and so a prolonged clearance time.	Efficiency of pulmonary gas exchange. Abnormal if surface area for gas exchange reduced, abnormal pulmonary vasculature, or interstitial lung disease impairing diffusion.

(continued)

Table 2.1 (Continued)

			Gas diffusion techniques		
	Spirometry	*Plethysmography*	*Inert gas dilution*	*Multiple breath washout (MBW)*	*Gas transfer*
Parameters derived and reference values	VC (slow non-forced expiration), FVC, FEV_1, FEV_1/FVC ratio, FEF_{25-75}, PEFR, PIFR. Former predictive equations largely superseded by GLI, taking account of age, sex, height, and ethnicity.	TLC, FRC, RV sR_{AW}, $sG_{AW,}$ R_{INT} Normative data available for both preschool and school aged children.	TLC, FRC, RV GLI reference data now available.	LCI - (CEV/FRC sometimes referred to as 'turnovers' to clear tracer gas). Normal range differs with gas used, but is usually 6–7 in healthy children.	T_{LCO} or D_{LCO} kCO (adjusted for V_A) allows assessment of well-ventilated lung tissue. GLI reference data now available.
Technical considerations and feasibility in children.	Widely available and central to respiratory management. Calibration before use. Home devices for remote monitoring. Requires cooperation and effort, from ~5 years of age.	Error due to non-pulmonary body gas. Overestimation if there is airway obstruction. Possible at any age if compliant, may need sedation/nose clip/ prevention of cheek inflation in younger children. (R_{INT}) difficult to standardise.	Requires airtight circuit. Difficult in the young, requires breath hold of 10s for single breath technique. VC > 1.5 L. Under-estimates volumes if there is airway obstruction.	Expensive and requires experienced skilled technicians. Comparisons must use the same methodology. Can be done on pre-school children, including sleeping infants	Requires 10–15 seconds breath hold, so cooperative school age children only. VC >1.0 L. Correction for Hb as anaemia lowers value. A low kCO is associated with exercise-related hypoxaemia.

Abbreviations: Boyle's Law (Pressure × Volume = constant at constant temperature); CEV = cumulative expired volume, corrected for apparatus dead-space); CO = carbon monoxide; D_{LCO} = diffusing capacity of the lung for CO; FEF_{25-75} = forced expiratory flow at 25–75% of forced vital capacity; FEV_1 = forced expiratory volume in one second; FRC = functional residual capacity; FVC = forced vital capacity; sG_{AW} = specific airway conductance, the reciprocal of sR_{AW}; GLI = Global Lung Initiative; He = Helium, inert gas; kCO = carbon monoxide transfer coefficient; PEFR = peak expiratory flow rate; PIFR = peak inspiratory flow rate; sR_{AW} = specific airway resistance; R_{INT} = interrupter technique; RV = residual volume; SF_6 = sulphur hexafluoride; TLC = total lung capacity; T_{LCO} = transfer factor of the lung for CO; VC = vital capacity.

Spirometry, Plethysmography, and Gas Dilution Techniques

Peak Expiratory Flow

Portable, hand-held devices, such as peak-flow meters, have applicability in determining measures, such as peak expiratory flow (PEF), (i.e., speed) of air that can be forcefully exhaled from the lungs following a full inhalation. Some evidence suggests that such portable devices can both over- and under-estimate true PEF values (Miller, Dickinson and Hitchings, 1992; Sly *et al.*, 1994; Choi, Koh and Lim, 2002) when compared to conventional spirometry and therefore results should be interpreted with caution. There is, however, a place for PEF monitoring in the long-term, outpatient surveillance of patients with asthma, using multiple measurements over two or more weeks. British Thoracic Society (BTS) guidelines suggest PEF should be used for children over 12 years old, but could be used in younger patients if able to perform forced exhalation reliably (BTS, 2019).

Spirometry

Spirometry is the process of simultaneously measuring flow and volume of air during inspiration and expiration in relation to time. When done properly, spirometry is reproducible and can be performed reliably in most children aged five years upwards. Established guidelines that have been evaluated help ensure standardisation across clinics and give consideration to pre-school children, for whom compliance or ability to follow instructions may be sub-optimal (Gaffin *et al.*, 2010). Spirometer equipment produces and records flow-volume loops, and volume-time curves. A typical flow-volume curve is generated on a maximal forced ventilatory manoeuvre at rest (Figure 2.2), the volumes and flow rates generated are significantly larger than those during exercise where there is a playoff between the rate and depth of respiration to achieve the most energy efficient pattern of breathing.

Equipment must be well maintained and quality-assured spirometry requires pre-use calibration, then a minimum of three acceptable vital capacity (VC) manoeuvres are followed by three forced vital capacity (FVC) manoeuvres. Good repeatability demands that there are no leaks, ideally a nose clip is worn, the mouthpiece must not be obstructed, expiration must follow maximal inspiration, and the subject must exhale fully with good effort. Visual incentives such as cartoon games and blowing candles are helpful in children to encourage cooperation and effort. Spirometry is a safe technique for measuring peak flow, FEV_1, FVC, and flows at low lung volumes (e.g., FEF_{25-75}). There are a number of cautions to consider prior to performing spirometry; such as current infection, haemoptysis, or a history of recent pneumothorax (Graham *et al.*, 2019). In-depth guidelines on spirometry, developed by clinical physiologists and supported by national societies, are available and are utilised by clinicians and academics alike to ensure standardised processes

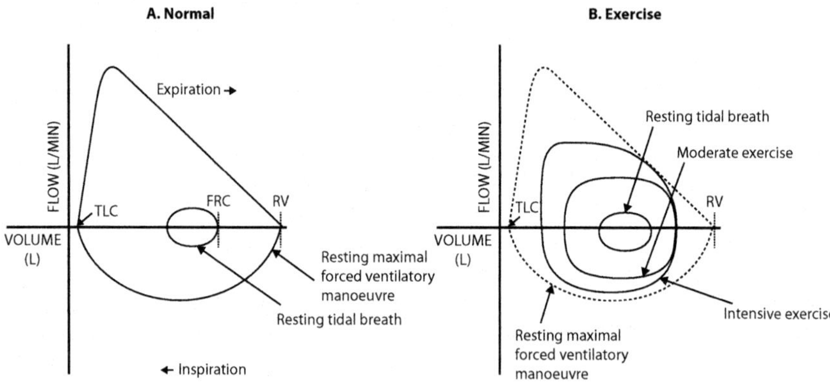

Figure 2.2 (A) The normal resting maximal flow-volume loop. (B) Flow volume loops during moderate and intensive exercise. **A: The normal resting maximal flow-volume loop**. y-axis: flow (L/min); x-axis: volume (L). Following a maximal inspiration to total lung capacity (TLC), the normal expiratory portion of the flow-volume curve is characterized by a rapid rise to the peak flow rate, followed by a nearly linear fall in flow as the patient exhales toward residual volume (RV), the amount of air remaining in the lungs after maximal exhalation. FRC = functional residual capacity, the amount of air remaining in the lungs at the end of expiration during normal tidal breathing at rest. **B: Flow volume loops during moderate and intensive exercise**. On exercising at low and moderate levels there is a reduction in end expiratory volume and an increase in end inspiratory volume to increase tidal volume (TV, the amount of air moved in/out of lungs in one breath) to approximately 50% of vital capacity (VC, maximum amount of air that can be exhaled in one breath) before respiratory rate increases to assist in the increase in minute ventilation (VE) to meet the metabolic demands of increasing levels of exercise. Flow increases with exercise in health, but only approaches maximum resting expiratory levels at low lung volumes, while inspiratory flows do not usually reach those attained at rest. There is a balance to be struck between rate and depth of respiration during exercise in order to achieve maximum efficiency (work of breathing). At maximum exercise in health, VE is typically only 60% of an individual's ventilatory capacity, which is why in health ventilation does not normally limit exercise. Where there is airway obstruction or volume restriction, (see figure 2.3), VE during exercise may become the limiting factor

are followed (Sylvester *et al.*, 2020). The patterns generated (Figure 2.3) are then utilised to support diagnoses, assess severity and then serial measures can track disease progression and determine therapeutic responses.

Children will mature at differing rates and lung function can increase as much as 20-fold in the first decade of life, (Stanojevic *et al.*, 2009) before peaking in early adulthood. Therefore, reference data is required to interpret PFT data in relation to age, sex, maturity, and ethnicity and extensive variability has been observed in young children (<11 years) (Stanojevic *et al.*, 2008). Measured parameters increase at different rates during growth and maturation in childhood and so relationships between them also change.

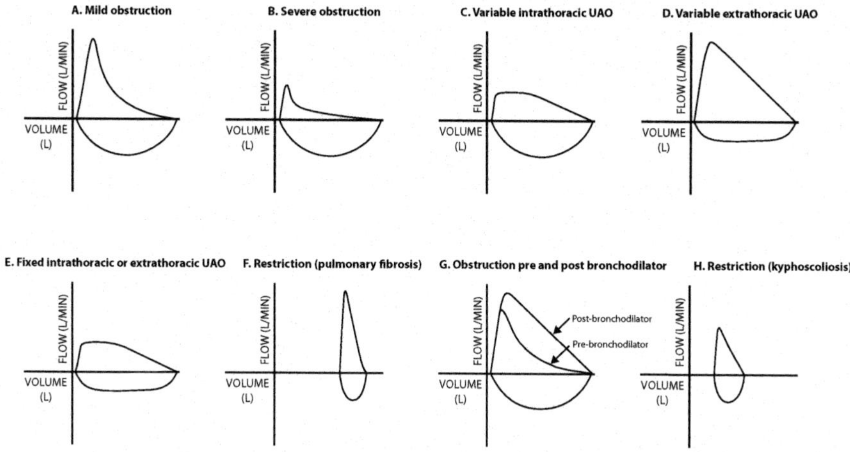

Figure 2.3 Abnormal spirometry flow-volume loops. (A) Mild obstruction (e.g., asthma, cystic fibrosis, bronchiectasis). (B) Severe obstruction (e.g., obliterative bronchiolitis, more severe cystic fibrosis and bronchiectasis). (C) Variable intrathoracic upper airway obstruction (UAO), (e.g., tracheomalacia). (D) Variable extrathoracic upper airway obstruction (e.g., unilateral vocal cord paralysis, exercised induced and other causes of inducible laryngeal obstruction). (E) Fixed intrathoracic or extrathoracic upper airway obstruction (e.g., tracheal stenosis, compression from extra-tracheal mass). (F) Restriction – parenchymal restrictive lung disease (e.g., pulmonary fibrosis or interstitial lung disease causing 'stiff,' non-compliant lungs, pulmonary hypoplasia and post-lung resection). (G) Obstruction pre- and post-bronchodilator (e.g., in reversible obstruction such as in asthma) Improvement of FEV_1 and FEV_1/FVC by ≥12% following the administration of a bronchodilator confirms the diagnosis of asthma or airway hyper-responsiveness. (H) Restriction – chest wall deformity and/or respiratory muscle weakness (e.g., kyphoscoliosis, the physical constraint of obesity, and neuromuscular disease, NMD).

Vital capacity increases relatively faster following birth than FEV_1 then this difference temporarily reverses during the adolescent pubertal growth spurt. As such the predicted FEV_1/FVC ratio falls, i.e., from around 0.95 at age 3 to 0.89 at age 10 (in white Caucasians; being higher in SE Asians), followed by a small increase up to 16 before a non-linear decline in adults. Awareness of these patterns is attributed to the collaborative work from the Global Lung Function Initiative (GLI) (Cooper *et al.*, 2017) that has pooled over 150,000 lung function data points. This has yielded the limits of normality for parameters which are adjusted for the heterogeneity of between-subject variability and take account of age, sex, and ethnicity (Quanjer *et al.*, 2012) and has enabled data to be presented as a 'percentage of predicted'; a format that can be easily understood by clinicians and patients alike. Compared to the numerous former predictive equations, GLI has refined the cut-offs for 'lower limits of normal' (LLN), thresholds used to delineate between health and disease. These are now recognised to change with age, sex, and ethnicity such that the historical arbitrary cut-off of 80% of predicted, being the lower limit of normal, is not valid. The LLN for FEV_1 in 3-year-olds is 74% predicted, but is 80% at 20 years then declines with advancing age. A benefit to this unique dataset is that it allows for continual monitoring of children, through adolescence, and into adulthood, without an abrupt transition between reference datasets (i.e., from paediatric data, to adult data). Therefore, these GLI data provide an excellent resource, ensuring consistency between centres and countries in the interpretation of PFT data. Pictograms in which z-scores of spirometry measures can display results relative to a normal range and help those with less understanding of pulmonary physiology interpret them.

Current reproducibility limits for FEV_1 were initially derived from adult data and suggest a relative change in FEV_1 of greater than 12% from baseline and an absolute change of 200 mL as clinically significant (Pellegrino *et al.*, 2005). More recent studies have tried to address the issue of defining FEV_1 annual reproducibility in the paediatric population, with some difficulty (Kirkby *et al.*, 2016). In practice, at present, a change in the FEV_1 of 10% from baseline is used clinically as a threshold in patients with CF to help identify a pulmonary exacerbation (Flume *et al.*, 2009; Bilton *et al.*, 2011).

Research into the possibility of using a change score to aid interpretation of repeated lung function measurements has been recently undertaken and may be useful to interpret inter-measurement variability seen in healthy children (Stanojevic, Filipow and Ratjen, 2020).

FEV_1 is the spirometry parameter most commonly used as an outcome measure in clinical trials and longitudinal evaluation of respiratory health (Szczesniak *et al.*, 2017). Lower FEV_1 values are associated with higher morbidity and mortality in CF (Emerson *et al.*, 2002). FEV_1 is reduced in obstructive small airways disease and the flow–volume loop has a 'scooped-out' appearance, see Figure 2.2. This is usually expressed as the ratio of FEV_1/FVC% because in severe obstructive disease, the FVC can be low too, but the ratio is always reduced (i.e., FEV_1 is most affected). The FVC is reduced in restrictive lung defects due to either poorly compliant lungs; as in pulmonary hypoplasia and interstitial lung disease (ILD), or thoracic cage restriction due to deformity and/or respiratory muscle weakness. Instead of FEV_1/FVC%, the average forced expiratory flow rate between 25% and 75% of the lung capacity (FEF_{25-75}) may be a more sensitive way of demonstrating small airways disease, as it reflects flow rates in the smaller airways.

FEV_1, FVC, and FEF_{25-75} can be expressed as raw values but are of greatest value in clinical practice and as a research tool when expressed as a percentage of the predicted value or in terms of the number of standard deviations from the mean (the Z-score).

Spirometry plays a central role in the diagnosis and management of paediatric asthma and exercise-related respiratory illnesses. This is discussed in more detail in Chapters 6 and 7. On the whole, patients with CF no longer present late and with reduced in lung function, but are diagnosed via newborn screening and will therefore have normal lung function at diagnosis (Linnane *et al.*, 2008). Over time, however, without intervention their lung function will decline – inevitably this is variable between individuals (Ranganathan *et al.*, 2004). Individuals with primary ciliary dyskinesia and other forms of bronchiectasis can present with reduced lung function (Halbeisen *et al.*, 2019); however, baseline lung function is not necessarily indicative of future disease progression (Marthin *et al.*, 2010).

An FEV_1, of below 40% of predicted value, represents a significant risk factor for death in children with CF (Zolin *et al.*, 2018), even in children as young as six years of age (Vandenbroucke, Zampoli and Morrow, 2020), highlighting the importance of accurately assessing and improving lung function in young children.

Whilst there are clear benefits to the use of spirometry in identifying changes in pulmonary function, there is a lack of sensitivity in it detecting the progression of peripheral airway disease (de Jong *et al.*, 2006), and therefore alternative methods of assessing respiratory function are needed and LCI offers some hope in this respect. Spirometry is not a tool that should be used in isolation of other clinically important parameters of pulmonary function, and it should be used in conjunction with other investigations (Table 2.2).

Gas Dilution and Diffusion Techniques

Gas dilution techniques can be used to measure static lung volumes and to determine efficiency of gaseous exchange. This can be single-breath wash out (e.g., using helium), multiple breath washout (MBW) technique (using helium or nitrogen to measure the lung clearance index (LCI)), or carbon monoxide transfer tests. They are not used routinely in most clinical practice unless there are specific indications due to time and resource limitations as well as lack of reliability in testing children (Table 2.1).

Recently, LCI – the primary outcome from MBW – has emerged as a novel way of assessing peripheral airway function. Primarily this has been utilised in research studies and is yet to be established as a routine measure in clinical practice. The technique records the clearance of inert tracer gases from the lung during normal tidal breathing (i.e., a passive manoeuvre), and is therefore classified as an effort-independent measure, highlighting its suitability for use in children in whom it has been shown to be reproducible (Fuchs *et al.*, 2009, 2012); sensitive to change (Gustafsson *et al.*, 2008) and correlates with structural lung changes over time (Fuchs *et al.*, 2014). It can discriminate between healthy and diseased lungs (Stahl *et al.*, 2014); is more predictive than FEV_1 in identifying risk of pulmonary infection exacerbations (Vermeulen *et al.*, 2014), and is responsive to pharmacological intervention (Aurora *et al.*, 2004; Amin *et al.*, 2011; Davies *et al.*, 2013).

Table 2.2 Investigations That May Be Indicated to Complete a Comprehensive Assessment

Test	*Details*	*Indications*
Blood tests	Full blood count, Ferritin Blood gas	Concern re: anaemia – breathlessness, pallor Assessment of ventilation – e.g., chronic lung disease, CO_2 retention
Pulse oximetry	Normal levels 96–100%	Routinely checked in all respiratory patients
Transcutaneous or end-tidal CO_2	Non-invasive, continuous measure of CO_2 levels	Useful in ventilated patients or in context of sleep studies where trends of CO_2 will be analysed
Skin prick testing	Targeted testing dependent on allergy history	History of possible reaction to allergen – can help confirm allergy
Exhaled nitric oxide (FeNO)	<18 ppb = normal	High in asthma, CF exacerbation Low in PCD and CF (when stable)
Nasal nitric oxide (nNO)	Normal range = 150–1,000 ppb Usually, <100 ppb in PCD	Low in PCD and CF Used in older, co-operative children (>5 years)
Chest X-ray	Anterior-posterior film	Investigating acute or chronic symptoms, to look for changes such as collapse, consolidation, bronchiectasis, thoracic cage deformity
CT Thorax	CT with contrast or in some centres 4D CT to construct 3D dynamic images of lung structure	Detailed assessment of the airways, bloods vessels, lungs and surrounding tissues
Bronchoscopy	With BAL	To look at anatomy of airways, to obtain BAL samples Sometimes trans bronchial lung biopsies.
Ambulatory and sleep oximetry/ Polysomnography	Can have problems with interpretation Caution due to movement artefact or faulty probe positioning	Can measure multiple parameters – selected depending on indication for study, e.g., EEG, ECG, end-tidal CO_2
Ciliary brush biopsy	To be analysed via TEM and assess CBF and CBP	To identify ciliary abnormalities (as in Primary Ciliary Dyskinesia).

Abbreviations: BAL = bronchoalveolar lavage; CO_2 = carbon dioxide; CT = computerised tomography; CXR = chest X-ray; CBF = ciliary beat frequency; CBP = ciliary beat pattern; ECG = electrocardiograph; EEG = electroencephalogram; FENO = exhaled nitric oxide; nNO = nasal nitric oxide; PCD = primary ciliary dyskinesia; ppb = parts per billion; TEM = transmission electron microscopy.

The MBW is a two-phase process, whereby a 'wash-in' phase, the inhalation of an inert gas, such as sulphur hexafluoride (SF6), or less polluting nitrogen (N_2, which is a more complex indirect measure), is followed by a 'wash-out' phase, the passive inhalation and exhalation of room air, until the concentration of inert gas reaches 1/40th of the initial level. The ratio of the cumulative expired volume of gas (required to reach 1/40th of baseline), to FRC, is the LCI. A higher value is indicative of worse pulmonary function (Saunders *et al.*, 2017). Given that FRC (and therefore LCI) is influenced by age and stature (Lum *et al.*, 2013), changes in LCI *z*-score are recommended, particularly for young children and infants. However, normative data for LCI have yet to be established, as reference values to date are specific to the age-group studied, as well as the apparatus and gas used (Kent *et al.*, 2014).

Therefore, whilst there is evidence that LCI is a useful measure, there are many technical considerations that must be made prior to it becoming routine, and it should not be considered as an outcome measure in isolation. Furthermore, whilst LCI is collected in a passive manner, it is unclear how useful a parameter it is in indicating the functional health status of the lungs during everyday activity and exercise.

Plethysmography

Plethysmography interrogates air flow, mouth, and external 'box' pressure to measure static lung volumes, in particular the functional residual capacity (FRC), TLC, and residual volume (RV). Some effort-independent measurements can also be performed to ascertain readings such as specific airways resistance and airway conductance. However, these are time-consuming measurements and do not form a part of routine monitoring for most children or adults.

Exercise Testing

Exercise testing has clinical value beyond pulmonary function testing alone and affords differential diagnoses of exertional dyspnoea (Milani, Lavie and Mehra, 2004), evaluation of disability (Pianosi, LeBlanc and Almudevar, 2005b), prognostic value (Hebestreit *et al.*, 2019), and alternative outcomes following intervention (Burghard *et al.*, 2020).

Exercise tests are broadly split into 'field tests,' functional assessments that have discrete limitations in terms of either time or distance, measuring a limited number of parameters, but using fewer resources; and 'laboratory tests' which can simultaneously assess multiple facets of physiological function in controlled, albeit resource-intensive settings. The gold standard laboratory test is cardiopulmonary exercise testing (CPET), which seeks to measure aerobic fitness (VO_{2peak}). A brief breakdown of tests is provided in Table 2.3, outlining characteristics and required resources. Further discussion of multi-modal tests of function are discussed in Chapter 4, including tests of anaerobic fitness and localised muscle function.

The advantage of field tests is that they follow simple protocols with minimal equipment although need experienced supervision, careful recording, and sometimes space or facility (Stevens *et al.*, 2010). Despite a number of

Table 2.3 Characteristics of Field, and Lab-Based Exercise Tests

	Field test	*Lab test (CPET)*
Equipment needed and costs	Minimal equipment needed, although most will include a pulse oximeter and/or heart rate monitor Test-specific equipment includes cones, measuring tape, timer (6MWT); step, metronome, time (step test); cones, measuring tape, CD and CD player (shuttle test) Cost <£500 (GBP)[a]	Metabolic cart (with gas analyser), cycle ergometer or treadmill, pulse oximeter, heart rate monitor or ECG Cost >£15,000 (GBP)[a]
Maximal	Most tests only produce a maximal effort in the most unwell patients, as healthier patients will exceed the permitted time allowed on tests	Maximal for all patients
Outcome measures	Distance (6MWT, shuttle test), repetitions (step test); HR, SpO_2, RPE, RPD	Primary outcome is predominantly VO_{2peak} Secondary outcomes can include WR_{peak}, HR, SpO_2, V_{Epeak}, RER, RPE, RPD
Staffing and space	Minimum of one person, with minimal training necessary, required to administer test	Minimum of one person, although higher level of education/training required (likely to postgraduate degree in clinical physiology or similar). Presence of two people enhances safety
Space	Space is test dependent: 6MWT test is 30 m (therefore >30 m required); step test ~4 m^2; shuttle test is 10–20 m (therefore >20 m required)	Space required ~10 m^2
Suitability for population	Suitable for all, but may fail to elicit a maximal response in healthier individuals	Suitable for all, although pre-test evaluation must consider risk of (rare) adverse events (e.g. rapid desaturation, haemoptysis) Consider use of field tests for patients with advanced disease.
Age restrictions	Suitable for children ≥6 years Reference data available for ISWT (≥6 years) (Lanza *et al.*, 2015) and 6MWT (≥7 years) (Li *et al.*, 2007)	Recommended for children aged ≥10 years, although possible in some younger children if they will physically fit ergometer and cognitively understand remits of protocol. Paediatric ergometers are available to facilitate implementation of CPET in children. Reference data available for children ≥8 years.(Bongers *et al.*, 2014)

Source: Information adapted from Hebestreit *et al.* (2015).

[a]Costs are for equipment only, and are exclusive of any financial requirements for staff.

Abbreviations: 6MWT = six-minute walk test; CPET = cardiopulmonary exercise test; ECG = electrocardiogram; HR = heart rate; ISWT = incremental shuttle walk test; RER = respiratory exchange ratio; RPE = rating of perceived effort; RPD = rating of perceived dyspnoea; SpO_2 = peripheral oxygen saturation; V_{Epeak} = peak minute ventilation; VO_{2peak} = peak oxygen uptake; WR_{peak} = peak work rate.

field tests being incremental in nature, many children will not be sufficiently stressed to elicit maximal responses during field tests (Urquhart and Saynor, 2018), although maximal responses may be obtained in severely deconditioned patients. Regardless, field tests are frequently used, and provide a platform with which to undertake assessments of exercise tolerance in clinical settings. Numerous formats are available, traditionally consisting of a walking and/or running challenge within a fixed time frame or distance, although alternatives such as step-ups or sit-to-stand sequences are popular when less space is available.

In contrast, CPET makes a direct measurement of exhaled oxygen and carbon dioxide, alongside measures of cardiac function, workload, and perceived effort, to diagnose causes of dyspnoea and exercise dysfunction in a controlled, systematic manner (Hebestreit *et al.*, 2015). VO_{2peak}, the primary parameter derived from CPET represents the highest volume of oxygen the body can transport and utilise during exercise, thus characterising the functional integration of the pulmonary, cardiovascular, and musculoskeletal systems. Alongside VO_{2peak} (Pianosi, LeBlanc and Almudevar, 2005a), the ventilatory equivalent for oxygen (Hulzebos *et al.*, 2014) has prognostic significance in people with CF. However, long-term prediction of mortality may not be appropriate for young children, especially as therapies and life-expectancy show consistent improvement. Therefore, it is appropriate to consider that results from CPET also predict risk of hospitalisation (Pérez *et al.*, 2014) and are associated with QoL (Hebestreit *et al.*, 2014), parameters that have far greater bearing on day-to-day lives of young patients.

Field Tests

The modified shuttle walk test (MSWT) is an externally paced, progressive walking test over a straight-line course of 10 m, with each 'shuttle' undertaken in time to an audio signal of increasing frequency, which reduces time available to complete each shuttle (Singh *et al.*, 1992). Typically, the 15-level MSWT is easily completed by children aged 13 years and over and an extended incremental SWT (ISWT) has been used to test fitter or younger subjects to exhaustion and generate reference data (Lanza *et al.*, 2015). Another 25-level extension has also been developed (Elkins, Dentice and Bye, 2009) in order to elicit maximal responses. The MSWT is apparently valid in children with CF, due to high correlations observed between MSWT performance and VO_{2peak}, although a mean bias of up to 5 $mL \cdot kg^{-1} \cdot min^{-1}$ is present when compared against treadmill-derived fitness, an error that could reach significance in deconditioned individuals (Selvadurai *et al.*, 2003). Reproducibility and minimal clinically important differences have also been established, whereby a change in distance covered of >97 m has been proposed as the minimal clinically significant change in adolescents with CF (del Corral *et al.*, 2019). The MSWT has also been validated in children with asthma, although body mass and sex significantly interact with distance when predicting VO_{2peak} and must be accounted for when utilising estimation equations (Lanza *et al.*, 2018).

The six-minute walk test (6MWT), another common test, requires patients to walk as far as possible in a six-minute window, over a flat 30–40 m course such as a hospital corridor. Unlike the MSWT, this is not externally paced, but patients are encouraged throughout (Holland *et al.*, 2014). Much like the MSWT, the 6MWT is apparently valid and reliable in young people with CF, due to high correlations between walking distance and CPET-derived VO_{2peak}, as well as high correlations between tests when performed one-week apart (Gulmans *et al.*, 1996). The 6MWT will not elicit maximal responses in most children (Lang *et al.*, 2020), as typically maximal heart rates of only 150–160 beats·min^{-1} are achieved even with encouragement; far below theoretical age predicted maximums >200 beats·min^{-1}. Reference data is available for the 6MWT (Li *et al.*, 2007), it retains utility in patients with advanced disease, whereby transplant clinics stratify patients using distance covered (Ramos *et al.,* 2019), and this is despite there being no association between 6MWT distance and disease severity in CF (Andrade *et al.*, 2018) and asthma (Andrade *et al.*, 2014).

Shorter tests, requiring less space such as the one-minute sit-to-stand (Gruet *et al.*, 2016) and three-minute step test (Narang *et al.*, 2003) have been developed, but these still fail to reliably elicit maximal physiological responses and apparent ceiling effects are present in children with mild-to-moderate lung disease (Balfour-Lynn *et al.*, 1998), likely due to relatively short time frames involved. Moreover, the iStep test, developed for children with CF, is reported to achieve maximal responses in >60% of patients (Rand, Prasad and Main, 2015). Other tests such as the Bratteby Walk Test and two-minute walk test lack sufficient data on validity to know how they can be utilised (Lang *et al.*, 2020).

Validity and repeatability of the MSWT and 6MWT have largely been established on the basis of high correlation coefficients, an erroneous approach that fails to account for any systematic bias that may occur between measures (Bland and Altman, 1986), such as learning and/or training effects. However, despite these issues, field tests hold relevance within clinics because they are straight forward to administer, have some objectivity and are low cost so should not be discounted from use. In a survey of UK-based adult and paediatric CF clinics, 43% of adult and 30% of paediatric patients had performed an exercise test in the previous 12 months; although 48% of clinics did not respond to the questionnaire, so these data are likely an overestimate. 37% of clinics were utilising the MSWT, and 25% the 6MWT to assess exercise capacity, citing time and resource availability as barriers to undertaking comprehensive, gold-standard CPET (Stevens *et al.*, 2010). Even for clinics where access to CPET is available, annual testing may not be feasible, as clinical and logistical reasons may interfere with individual ability and willingness to undergo testing (Tomlinson *et al.*, 2020).

Cardiopulmonary Exercise Testing (CPET)

The purpose of CPET is to elicit a maximal, exhaustive, response to exercise, and therefore different modalities such as cycling and treadmill running are available, alongside differing test protocols. For both modalities, testing is typically undertaken in children when they reach ~10 years of age and this is the age from which annual exercise testing has been recommended in those with CF (Hebestreit *et al.*, 2015). In younger children cooperation with CPET has been reported to be lower (Weir *et al.*, 2017), although field tests may be feasible until they have the physical and cognitive ability to perform CPET (Tomlinson *et al.*, 2020).

The Bruce protocol (Bruce, Kusumi and Hosmer, 1973) is acknowledged as the most popular treadmill testing protocol, and has been used longitudinally to monitor exercise capacity (Klijn *et al.*, 2003), as well as responses to training (Selvadurai *et al.*, 2002) in children with CF. When analysis of pulmonary gas exchange is not available for directly determining VO_{2peak}, equations for estimation have been proposed (Foster *et al.*, 1984), although their validity in respiratory disease is unknown. Furthermore, in the absence of VO_{2peak}, calculation of peak work-rate (WR_{peak}) is possible, but requires measures of body mass, the gravitational constant, final velocity, incline gradient, and exercise duration (Hebestreit *et al.*, 2015).

In relation to cycle ergometry, the Godfrey protocol (Godfrey *et al.*, 1971) has been endorsed by the European Respiratory Society and the European CF Society (Hebestreit *et al.*, 2015), where work increments increase in a 'step-wise' fashion, and participants cycle at a set work-rate for successive periods of time before the next increase, see Figure 2.4. However, a number of methodological issues are associated with this protocol, notably a lack of validity and reliability data, particularly with reference as to how a maximal effort is defined (Saynor *et al.*, 2016). An alternative is the 'ramp-incremental' protocol, whereby work-rate continually increases (e.g., 10–30 $W \cdot min^{-1}$), avoiding the periodic steps and plateaus of a step-wise protocol (Figure 2.4). Limitation during a plateau phase may mean that peak values obtained may fall short of that achieved on a ramp protocol, especially in children. Additionally, step tests exclusively use stature to identify work rate increments that can result in very short tests. Linear ramp tests provide a smoother profile and thus allow greater opportunity for children to hit a 'true' maximum.

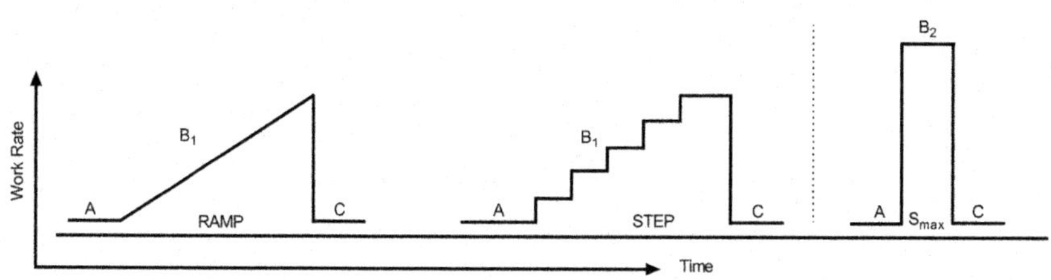

Figure 2.4 Schematic displaying the difference between ramp and step tests, as used in cycle ergometry tests. Both retain fundamental similarities in a warm-up phase (A), incremental phase (B1) and cool-down phase (C), although it is the manner in which the increments occur that provides the difference. A supra-maximal (Smax) phase is shown as an optional extra, displaying a warm-up (A), a singular square-wave phase (B2) and a cool-down phase (C).

Moreover, a supramaximal verification (S_{max}), consisting of a 'square-wave' bout of work set at 110% of the peak power attained following a short rest during initial testing, can be used to verify VO_{2peak} as being maximal, regardless of whether a step-wise, or ramp-incremental, protocol is used. These verification bouts of exercise are performed in the severe exercise intensity domain, and if the VO_{2peak} obtained during verification is equal to, or less than the VO_{2peak} from initial tests, then clinicians can be assured that a 'true' VO_{2max} has been identified (Barker *et al.*, 2011). This protocol has been found to be valid and reliable in young people with CF (Saynor *et al.*, 2013b, 2013a). Consequently, the American Physiological Society has published a statement advocating the use of S_{max} within CPET as a 'gold standard' (Poole and Jones, 2017), albeit in healthy individuals. However, a recent statement from the European Respiratory Society has recognised the potential value of S_{max} in respiratory patients, and suggests further investigation is needed into optimising work-rate increments when performing CPET in this population (Radtke *et al.*, 2019).

Unlike pulmonary function testing, where large-scale reference data is available (Quanjer *et al.*, 2012), the same for exercise testing is relatively sparse. For field testing, reference data for healthy children has been generated for the 6MWT (Lammers *et al.*, 2008), although for CPET, there are conflicting reference equations available (Jones *et al.*, 1985; Orenstein, 1993; Werkman *et al.*, 2014). These produce significantly conflicting values for 'percentage of predicted' when applied to children with respiratory disease (Tomlinson *et al.*, 2019). Therefore, until more robust reference data is available, clinicians should ensure that any reference equations used are applicable to the population being examined, and match (where possible) testing modality, such as paediatric data obtained via cycle ergometry (Bongers *et al.*, 2014). In spite of this, an individual's longitudinal data has important clinical value.

Technical Considerations in Exercise Testing

As shown in Table 2.3, multiple functional and clinical factors must be considered when implementing exercise testing. For example, costs associated with field testing are negligible when considered relative to CPET, but the physical space they demand (up to 40m for the 6MWT) can be difficult to identify in a hospital or clinic environment. In addition, staffing requirements for all tests must be acknowledged and CPET requires expertise in the interpretation of physiological data, whereas field tests can be implemented by allied health professionals.

Safety must be considered, whereby the dynamic nature of exercise testing is inherently associated with risk of desaturation, dizziness, and musculoskeletal discomfort. A number of absolute (e.g., uncontrolled asthma, pneumothorax) and relative (e.g., severe hypertension) contraindications to exercise testing have been established (Hebestreit *et al.*, 2015) and infection control measures must always be considered. In relation to specific modalities, cycle ergometry poses fewer risks, as deconditioned patients have minimal risk of injury due to falling, unlike intense exercise on a treadmill, noting that harnesses may constrict breathing. Overall, however, it is well documented that exercise testing is safe in people with respiratory disease, and adverse events are rare (Ruf *et al.*, 2010).

Conclusion

Measures of lung function, and exercise testing, are essential components of successful disease management for children with respiratory disease. Together, their use contributes to a multidisciplinary and holistic approach, from diagnosis through to monitoring of disease progression and response to intervention. Their use must be combined with clinical assessments from other disciplines, imaging, blood tests, and anthropometric data in order to shape and inform therapeutic interventions. Exercise testing is safe, valid, and reliable, and is of clear benefit to clinicians and researchers working within paediatric respiratory medicine. Whilst the outcomes associated with exercise testing have prognostic value (Hebestreit *et al.*, 2019), it is the association of poor fitness with lower QoL (Hebestreit *et al.*, 2014) and increased treatment burden (Pérez *et al.*, 2014) that impacts directly on the lives of patients and their families.

Key Points

- Pulmonary and exercise function are key in diagnosing, assessing progression and determining intervention efficacy in young people with respiratory disease, providing complementary and independent information.
- Spirometry is an established investigation in paediatric respiratory medicine, which is now being extended from the clinic into the home.
- Pulmonary function in preschool children is more challenging but new methodology, such as LCI offers promise in this age group and may detect abnormalities in advance of spirometric abnormality.
- A variety of both field and laboratory-based exercise tests can be performed and add important additional information to the assessment of respiratory disease in children and exercise parameters may vary independent of spirometry.
- Discussions around the importance of health, fitness, and strength form a necessary part of health promotion for children who are healthy as well as those with respiratory disease.

Future Research

- With evolving treatments in respiratory disease, the intendent nature of pulmonary and exercise function must be further evidenced, and the utility of both modalities of testing be emphasised for monitoring disease progression.

- Home-based pulmonary function and its value in determining disease status and trajectory warrants further investigation along with its potential to reduce the burden of hospital visits and promote self-management.
- Development of field tests that elicit a maximal response in all patients is needed to provide viable, cost-effective alternatives to CPET.
- Adequately developed and validated reference data is needed for exercise testing in paediatric respiratory disease.

References

Amin, R., Subbarao, P., Lou, W., Jabar, A., Balkovec, S., Jensen, R., Kerrigan, S., Gustafsson, P. and Ratjen, F. (2011) 'The effect of dornase alfa on ventilation inhomogeneity in patients with cystic fibrosis', *European Respiratory Journal*, 37(4), pp. 806–812. doi: 10.1183/09031936.00072510.

Andrade, L.B., Silva, D.A., Salgado, T.L., Figueroa, J.N., Lucena-Silva, N. and Britto, M.C. (2014) 'Comparison of six-minute walk test in children with moderate/severe asthma with reference values for healthy children', *Jornal de Pediatria*, 90(3), pp. 250–257. doi: 10.1016/j.jped.2013.08.006.

Andrade Lima, C., Dornelas de Andrade, A., Campos, S.L., Brandao, D.C., Mourato, I.P. and Britto, M.C.A. (2018) 'Six-minute walk test as a determinant of the functional capacity of children and adolescents with cystic fibrosis: A systematic review', *Respiratory Medicine*, 137, pp. 83–88. doi: 10.1016/j.rmed.2018.02.016.

Armstrong, N. and Welsman, J. (2019) 'Development of peak oxygen uptake from 11–16 years determined using both treadmill and cycle ergometry', *European Journal of Applied Physiology*, 119(3), pp. 801–812. doi: 10.1007/s00421-019-04071-3.

Aurora, P., Gustafsson, P., Bush, A., Lindblad, A., Oliver, C., Wallis, C.E. and Stocks, J. (2004) 'Multiple breath inert gas washout as a measure of ventilation distribution in children with cystic fibrosis', *Thorax*, 59(12), pp. 1068–1073. doi: 10.1136/thx.2004.022590.

Balfour-Lynn, I.M., Prasad, S.A., Laverty, A., Whitehead, B.F. and Dinwiddie, R. (1998) 'A step in the right direction: Assessing exercise tolerance in cystic fibrosis', *Pediatric Pulmonology*, 25(4), pp. 278–284. doi: 10.1002/(sici)1099-0496(199804)25:4<278::Aid-ppul8>3.0.Co;2-g.

Barker, A.R., Williams, C.A., Jones, A.M. and Armstrong, N. (2011) 'Establishing maximal oxygen uptake in young people during a ramp cycle test to exhaustion', *British Journal of Sports Medicine*, 45(6), pp. 498–503. doi: 10.1136/bjsm.2009.063180.

Baxter-Jones, A.G. (2017) 'Growth and maturation', in Armstrong, N. and van Mechelen, W. (eds.), *Children's sport and exercise medicine*. 3rd ed. New York, NY: Oxford University Press.

Beydon, N., Davis, S.D., Lombardi, E., Allen, J.L., Arets, H.G., Aurora, P., Bisgaard, H., Davis, G.M., Ducharme, F.M., Eigen, H. and Gappa, M. (2007). An official American Thoracic Society/European Respiratory Society statement: Pulmonary function testing in preschool children. *American Journal of Respiratory and Critical Care Medicine*, 175(12), 1304–1345. doi: 10.1164/rccm.200605-642ST.

Bilton, D., Canny, G., Conway, S., Dumcius, S., Hjelte, L., Proesmans, M., Tümmler, B., Vavrova, V. and De Boeck, K. (2011) 'Pulmonary exacerbation: Towards a definition for use in clinical trials. Report from the EuroCareCF Working Group on outcome parameters in clinical trials', *Journal of Cystic Fibrosis*, 10, pp. S79–S81. doi: 10.1016/s1569-1993(11)60012-x.

Bland, J.M. and Altman, D.G. (1986) 'Statistical methods for assessing agreement between two methods of clinical measurement', *The Lancet*, 327(8476), pp. 307–310. doi: 10.1016/S0140-6736(86)90837-8.

Bongers, B.C., van Brussel, M., Hulzebos, E.H.J. and Takken, T. (2014) *Pediatric norms for cardiopulmonary exercise testing*. 2nd edn. 's-Herogenbosch, the Netherlands: Uitgeverij BOXPress.

British Thoracic Society (2019) *BTS/SIGN British guideline on the management of asthma*, Edinburgh, UK: Healthcare Improvement Scotland.

Bruce, R.A., Kusumi, F. and Hosmer, D. (1973) 'Maximal oxygen intake and nomographic assessment of functional aerobic impairment in cardiovascular disease', *American Heart Journal*, 85(4), pp. 546–562. doi: 10.1016/0002-8703(73)90502-4.

Burghard, M.M., Berkers, G.G., Ghijsen, S.S., Hollander-Kraaijeveld, F.F., de Winter-de Groot, K.K., van der Ent, C.K., Heijerman, H.H., Takken, T.T. and Hulzebos, H.E. (2020) 'Long-term effects of ivacaftor on nonpulmonary outcomes in individuals with cystic fibrosis, heterozygous for a S1251N mutation', *Pediatric Pulmonology*, 55(6), pp. 1400–1405. doi: 10.1002/ppul.24745.

Choi, I.S., Koh, Y.I. and Lim, H. (2002) 'Peak expiratory flow rate underestimates severity of airflow obstruction in acute asthma', *Korean Journal of Internal Medicine*, 17(3), pp. 174–179. doi: 10.3904/kjim.2002.17.3.174.

Cooper, B.G., Stocks, J., Hall, G.L., Culver, B., Steenbruggen, I., Carter, K.W., Thompson, B.R., Graham, B.L., Miller, M.R., Ruppel, G., Henderson, J., Vaz Fragoso, C.A. and Stanojevic, S. (2017) 'The Global Lung Function Initiative (GLI) Network: Bringing the world's respiratory reference values together', *Breathe*, 13(3), pp. e56–e64. doi: 10.1183/20734735.012717.

Davies, J., Sheridan, H., Bell, N., Cunningham, S., Davis, S.D., Elborn, J.S., Milla, C.E., Starner, T.D., Weiner, D.J., Lee, P.S. and Ratjen, F. (2013) 'Assessment of clinical response to ivacaftor with lung clearance index in cystic fibrosis patients with a G551D-CFTR mutation and preserved spirometry: A randomised controlled trial', *The Lancet Respiratory Medicine*, 1(8), pp. 630–638. doi: 10.1016/s2213-2600(13)70182-6.

de Jong, P.A., Lindblad, A., Rubin, L., Hop, W.C., de Jongste, J.C., Brink, M. and Tiddens, H.A. (2006) 'Progression of lung disease on computed tomography and pulmonary function tests in children and adults with cystic fibrosis', *Thorax*, 61(1), pp. 80–85. doi: 10.1136/thx.2005.045146.

del Corral, T., Gómez Sánchez, Á. and López-de-Uralde-Villanueva, I. (2019) 'Test-retest reliability, minimal detectable change and minimal clinically important differences in modified shuttle walk test in children and adolescents with cystic fibrosis', *Journal of Cystic Fibrosis*, 19(3), pp. 442–448. doi: 10.1016/j.jcf.2019.10.007.

Elkins, M.R., Dentice, R.L. and Bye, P.T. (2009) 'Validation of the MST-25: An extension of the modified shuttle test (MST)', *Journal of Cystic Fibrosis*, 8, pp. S70. doi: 10.1016/s1569-1993(09)60276-9.

Emerson, J., Rosenfeld, M., McNamara, S., Ramsey, B. and Gibson, R.L. (2002) 'Pseudomonas aeruginosa and other predictors of mortality and morbidity in young children with cystic fibrosis', *Pediatric Pulmonology*, 34(2), pp. 91–100. doi: 10.1002/ppul.10127.

Flume, P.A., Mogayzel, P.J., Jr., Robinson, K.A., Goss, C.H., Rosenblatt, R.L., Kuhn, R.J., Marshall, B.C. and Clinical Practice Guidelines (2009) 'Cystic fibrosis pulmonary guidelines treatment of pulmonary exacerbations', *American Journal of Respiratory and Critical Care Medicine*, 180(9), pp. 802–808. doi: 10.1164/rccm.200812-1845PP.

Foster, C., Jackson, A.S., Pollock, M.L., Taylor, M.M., Hare, J., Sennett, S.M., Rod, J.L., Sarwar, M. and Schmidt, D.H. (1984) 'Generalized equations for predicting functional capacity from treadmill performance', *American Heart Journal*, 107(6), pp. 1229–1234. doi: 10.1016/0002-8703(84)90282-5.

Fuchs, S.I., Eder, J., Ellemunter, H. and Gappa, M. (2009) 'Lung clearance index: Normal values, repeatability, and reproducibility in healthy children and adolescents', *Pediatric Pulmonology*, 44(12), pp. 1180–1185. doi: 10.1002/ppul.21093.

Fuchs, S.I., Ellemunter, H., Eder, J., Mellies, U., Grosse-Onnebrink, J., Tummler, B., Staab, D., Jobst, A., Griese, M., Ripper, J., Rietschel, E., Zeidler, S., Ahrens, F. and Gappa, M. (2012) 'Feasibility and variability of measuring the Lung Clearance Index in a multi-center setting', *Pediatric Pulmonology*, 47(7), pp. 649–657. doi: 10.1002/ppul.21610.

Fuchs, S.I., Gappa, M., Eder, J., Unsinn, K.M., Steinkamp, G. and Ellemunter, H. (2014) 'Tracking Lung Clearance Index and chest CT in mild cystic fibrosis lung disease over a period of three years', *Respiratory Medicine*, 108(6), pp. 865–874. doi: 10.1016/j.rmed.2014.03.011.

Gaffin, J.M., Shotola, N.L., Martin, T.R. and Phipatanakul, W. (2010) 'Clinically useful spirometry in preschool-aged children: Evaluation of the 2007 American Thoracic Society Guidelines', *Journal of Asthma*, 47(7), pp. 762–767. doi: 10.3109/02770903.2010.485664.

Godfrey, S., Davies, C.T.M., Wozniak, E. and Barnes, C.A. (1971) 'Cardio-respiratory response to exercise in normal children', *Clinical Science*, 40(5), pp. 419–431. doi: 10.1042/cs0400419.

Graham, B.L., Steenbruggen, I., Miller, M.R., Barjaktarevic, I.Z., Cooper, B.G., Hall, G.L., Hallstrand, T.S., Kaminsky, D.A., McCarthy, K., McCormack, M.C., Oropez, C.E., Rosenfeld, M., Stanojevic, S., Swanney, M.P. and Thompson, B.R. (2019) 'Standardization of Spirometry 2019 Update. An Official American Thoracic Society and European Respiratory Society Technical Statement', *American Journal of Respiratory and Critical Care Medicine*, 200(8), pp. e70–e88. doi: 10.1164/rccm.201908-1590ST.

Gruet, M., Peyre-Tartaruga, L.A., Mely, L. and Vallier, J.M. (2016) 'The 1-minute sit-to-stand test in adults with cystic fibrosis: Correlations with cardiopulmonary exercise test, 6-minute walk test, and quadriceps strength', *Respiratory Care*, 61(12), pp. 1620–1628. doi: 10.4187/respcare.04821.

Gulmans, V.A.M., van Veldhoven, N.H.M.J., de Meer, K. and Helders, P.J.M. (1996) 'The six-minute walking test in children with cystic fibrosis: Reliability and validity', *Pediatric Pulmonology*, 22(2), pp. 85–89. doi: 10.1002/(sici)1099-0496(199608)22:2<85::aid-ppul1>3.0.co;2-i.

Gustafsson, P.M., De Jong, P.A., Tiddens, H.A. and Lindblad, A. (2008) 'Multiple-breath inert gas washout and spirometry versus structural lung disease in cystic fibrosis', *Thorax*, 63(2), pp. 129–134. doi: 10.1136/thx.2007.077784.

Halbeisen, F.S., Jose, A., de Jong, C., Nyilas, S., Latzin, P., Kuehni, C.E. and Goutaki, M. (2019) 'Spirometric indices in primary ciliary dyskinesia: Systematic review and meta-analysis', *ERJ Open Research*, 5(2). doi: 10.1183/23120541.00231-2018.

Hebestreit, H., Arets, H.G., Aurora, P., Boas, S., Cerny, F., Hulzebos, E.H., Karila, C., Lands, L. C., Lowman, J.D., Swisher, A., Urquhart, D.S. and European Cystic Fibrosis Exercise Working Group (2015) 'Statement on exercise testing in cystic fibrosis', *Respiration*, 90(4), pp. 332–351. doi: 10.1159/000439057.

Hebestreit, H., Hulzebos, E.H.J., Schneiderman, J.E., Karila, C., Boas, S.R., Kriemler, S., Dwyer, T., Sahlberg, M., Urquhart, D.S., Lands, L.C., Ratjen, F., Takken, T., Varanistkaya, L., Rucker, V., Hebestreit, A., Usemann, J., Radtke, T. and Prognostic Value of CPET in CF Study Group (2019) 'Cardiopulmonary exercise testing provides additional prognostic information in cystic fibrosis', *American Journal of Respiratory and Critical Care Medicine*, 199(8), pp. 987–995. doi: 10.1164/rccm.201806-1110OC.

Hebestreit, H., Schmid, K., Kieser, S., Junge, S., Ballmann, M., Roth, K., Hebestreit, A., Schenk, T., Schindler, C., Posselt, H.G. and Kriemler, S. (2014) 'Quality of life is associated with physical activity and fitness in cystic fibrosis', *BMC Pulmonary Medicine*, 14, pp. 26. doi: 10.1186/1471-2466-14-26.

Holland, A.E., Spruit, M.A., Troosters, T., Puhan, M.A., Pepin, V., Saey, D., McCormack, M.C., Carlin, B.W., Sciurba, F.C., Pitta, F., Wanger, J., MacIntyre, N., Kaminsky, D.A., Culver, B.H., Revill, S.M., Hernandes, N.A., Andrianopoulos, V., Camillo, C.A., Mitchell, K.E., Lee, A.L., Hill, C.J. and Singh, S.J. (2014) 'An official European Respiratory Society/American Thoracic Society technical standard: Field walking tests in chronic respiratory disease', *European Respiratory Journal*, 44(6), pp. 1428–1446. doi: 10.1183/09031936.00150314.

Hulzebos, E.H., Bomhof-Roordink, H., van de Weert-van Leeuwen, P.B., Twisk, J.W., Arets, H. G., van der Ent, C.K. and Takken, T. (2014) 'Prediction of mortality in adolescents with cystic fibrosis', *Medicine and Science in Sports and Exercise*, 46(11), pp. 2047–2052. doi: 10.1249/MSS.0000000000000344.

Jones, N.L., Makrides, L., Hitchcock, C., Chypchar, T. and McCartney, N. (1985) 'Normal standards for an incremental progressive cycle ergometer test', *American Review of Respiratory Disease*, 131(5), pp. 700–708. doi: 10.1164/arrd.1985.131.5.700.

Kent, L., Reix, P., Innes, J.A., Zielen, S., Le Bourgeois, M., Braggion, C., Lever, S., Arets, H.G., Brownlee, K., Bradley, J.M. and Bayfield, K. (2014) 'Lung clearance index: Evidence for use in clinical trials in cystic fibrosis', *Journal of Cystic Fibrosis*, 13(2), pp. 123–138. doi: 10.1016/j.jcf.2013.09.005.

Kirkby, J., Bountziouka, V., Lum, S., Wade, A. and Stocks, J. (2016) 'Natural variability of lung function in young healthy school children', *European Respiratory Journal*, 48(2), pp. 411–419. doi: 10.1183/13993003.01795-2015.

Kivastik, J. and Kingisepp, P.H. (1997) 'Differences in lung function and chest dimensions in school-age girls and boys', *Clinical Physiology*, 17(2), pp. 149–157. doi: 10.1046/j.1365-2281.1997.02121.x.

Klijn, P.H.C., van der Net, J., Kimpen, J.L., Helders, P.J.M. and van der Ent, C.K. (2003) 'Longitudinal determinants of peak aerobic performance in children with cystic fibrosis', *Chest*, 124(6), pp. 2215–2219. doi: 10.1378/chest.124.6.2215.

Lammers, A.E., Hislop, A.A., Flynn, Y. and Haworth, S.G. (2008) 'The 6-minute walk test: Normal values for children of 4-11 years of age', *Archives of Disease in Childhood*, 93(6), pp. 464–468. doi: 10.1136/adc.2007.123653.

Lang, R.L., Stockton, K., Wilson, C., Russell, T.G. and Johnston, L.M. (2020) 'Exercise testing for children with cystic fibrosis: A systematic review', *Pediatric Pulmonology*, 55(8), pp. 1996–2010. doi: 10.1002/ppul.24794.

Lanza, F.C., Reimberg, M.M., Ritti-Dias, R., Scalco, R.S., Wandalsen, G.F., Sole, D., van Brussel, M., Hulzebos, H.J., Dal Corso, S. and Takken, T. (2018) 'Validation of the modified shuttle test to predict peak oxygen uptake in youth asthma patients under regular treatment', *Frontiers in Physiology*, 9, pp. 919. doi: 10.3389/fphys.2018.00919.

Lanza, F.C., Zagatto, E.P., Silva, J.C., Selman, J.P., Imperatori, T.B., Zanatta, D.J., de Carvalho, L.N., Reimberg, M.M. and Dal Corso, S. (2015) 'Reference equation for the incremental shuttle walk test in children and adolescents', *Journal of Pediatrics*, 167(5), pp. 1057–1061. doi: 10.1016/j.jpeds.2015.07.068.

Li, A.M., Yin, J., Au, J.T., So, H.K., Tsang, T., Wong, E., Fok, T.F. and Ng, P.C. (2007) 'Standard reference for the six-minute-walk test in healthy children aged 7 to 16 years', *American Journal of Respiratory and Critical Care Medicine*, 176(2), pp. 174–180. doi: 10.1164/rccm.200607-883OC.

Linnane, B.M., Hall, G.L., Nolan, G., Brennan, S., Stick, S.M., Sly, P.D., Robertson, C.F., Robinson, P.J., Franklin, P.J., Turner, S.W., Ranganathan, S.C. and Arest, C.F. (2008) 'Lung function in infants with cystic fibrosis diagnosed by newborn screening', *American Journal of Respiratory and Critical Care Medicine*, 178(12), pp. 1238–1244. doi: 10.1164/rccm.200804-551OC.

Logie, K., Welsh, L. and Ranganathan, S.C. (2019) 'Telehealth spirometry for children with cystic fibrosis', *Archives of Disease in Childhood*, 105(12), pp. 1203–1205. doi: 10.1136/archdischild-2019-317147.

Lum, S., Stocks, J., Stanojevic, S., Wade, A., Robinson, P., Gustafsson, P., Brown, M., Aurora, P., Subbarao, P., Hoo, A.F. and Sonnappa, S. (2013) 'Age and height dependence of lung clearance index and functional residual capacity', *European Respiratory Journal*, 41(6), pp. 1371–1377. doi: 10.1183/09031936.00005512.

Marthin, J.K., Petersen, N., Skovgaard, L.T. and Nielsen, K.G. (2010) 'Lung function in patients with primary ciliary dyskinesia: A cross-sectional and 3-decade longitudinal study', *American Journal of Respiratory and Critical Care Medicine*, 181(11), pp. 1262–1268. doi: 10.1164/rccm.200811-1731OC.

Milani, R.V., Lavie, C.J. and Mehra, M.R. (2004) 'Cardiopulmonary exercise testing: How do we differentiate the cause of dyspnea?', *Circulation*, 110(4), pp. e27–31. doi: 10.1161/01.CIR.0000136811.45524.2F.

Miller, M.R., Dickinson, S.A. and Hitchings, D.J. (1992) 'The accuracy of portable peak flow meters', *Thorax*, 47(11), pp. 904–909. doi: 10.1136/thx.47.11.904.

Narang, I., Pike, S., Rosenthal, M., Balfour-Lynn, I.M. and Bush, A. (2003) 'Three-minute step test to assess exercise capacity in children with cystic fibrosis with mild lung disease', *Pediatric Pulmonology*, 35(2), pp. 108–113. doi: 10.1002/ppul.10213.

Neve, V., Girard, F., Flahault, A. and Boule, M. (2002) 'Lung and thorax development during adolescence: Relationship with pubertal status', *European Respiratory Journal*, 20(5), pp. 1292–1298. doi: 10.1183/09031936.02.00208102.

Orenstein, D.M. (1993) 'Assessment of exercise pulmonary function', in Rowland, T. (ed.), *Pediatric laboratory exercise testing*. Champaign IL, USA: Human Kinetics, pp. 141–163.

Pastre, J., Prevotat, A., Tardif, C., Langlois, C., Duhamel, A. and Wallaert, B. (2014) 'Determinants of exercise capacity in cystic fibrosis patients with mild-to-moderate lung disease', *BMC Pulmonary Medicine*, 14, pp. 74. doi: 10.1186/1471-2466-14-74.

Pellegrino, R., Viegi, G., Brusasco, V., Crapo, R.O., Burgos, F., Casaburi, R., Coates, A., van der Grinten, C.P., Gustafsson, P., Hankinson, J., Jensen, R., Johnson, D.C., MacIntyre, N., McKay, R., Miller, M.R., Navajas, D., Pedersen, O.F. and Wanger, J. (2005) 'Interpretative strategies for lung function tests', *European Respiratory Journal*, 26(5), pp. 948–968. doi: 10.1183/09031936.05.00035205.

Pérez, M., Groeneveld, I.F., Santana-Sosa, E., Fiuza-Luces, C., Gonzalez-Saiz, L., Villa-Asensi, J. R., López-Mojares, L.M., Rubio, M. and Lucia, A. (2014) 'Aerobic fitness is associated with lower risk of hospitalization in children with cystic fibrosis', *Pediatric Pulmonology*, 49(7), pp. 641–649. doi: 10.1002/ppul.22878.

Pianosi, P., LeBlanc, J. and Almudevar, A. (2005a) 'Peak oxygen uptake and mortality in children with cystic fibrosis', *Thorax*, 60(1), pp. 50–54. doi: 10.1136/thx.2003.008102.

Pianosi, P., LeBlanc, J. and Almudevar, A. (2005b) 'Relationship between FEV_1 and peak oxygen uptake in children with cystic fibrosis', *Pediatric Pulmonology*, 40(4), pp. 324–329. doi: 10.1002/ppul.20277.

Poole, D.C. and Jones, A.M. (2017) 'Measurement of the maximum oxygen uptake VO_{2max}: VO_{2peak} is no longer acceptable', *Journal of Applied Physiology*, 122(4), pp. 997–1002. doi: 10.1152/japplphysiol.01063.2016.

Quanjer, P.H., Stanojevic, S., Cole, T.J., Baur, X., Hall, G.L., Culver, B.H., Enright, P.L., Hankinson, J.L., Ip, M.S., Zheng, J., Stocks, J. and E.R.S. Global Lung Function Initiative (2012) 'Multi-ethnic reference values for spirometry for the 3-95-yr age range: The global lung function 2012 equations', *European Respiratory Journal*, 40(6), pp. 1324–1343. doi: 10.1183/09031936.00080312.

Radtke, T., Crook, S., Kaltsakas, G., Louvaris, Z., Berton, D., Urquhart, D.S., Kampouras, A., Rabinovich, R.A., Verges, S., Kontopidis, D., Boyd, J., Tonia, T., Langer, D., De Brandt, J., Goertz, Y.M.J., Burtin, C., Spruit, M.A., Braeken, D.C.W., Dacha, S., Franssen, F.M.E., Laveneziana, P., Eber, E., Troosters, T., Neder, J.A., Puhan, M.A., Casaburi, R., Vogiatzis, I. and Hebestreit, H. (2019) 'ERS statement on standardisation of cardiopulmonary exercise testing in chronic lung diseases', *European Respiratory Review*, 28(154). doi: 10.1183/16000617.0101-2018.

Ramos, K.J., Smith, P.J., McKone, E.F., Pilewski, J.M., Lucy, A., Hempstead, S.E., Tallarico, E., Faro, A., Rosenbluth, D.B., Gray, A.L., Dunitz, J.M. and C. F. Lung Transplant Referral Guidelines Committee (2019) 'Lung transplant referral for individuals with cystic fibrosis: Cystic Fibrosis Foundation Consensus guidelines', *Journal of Cystic Fibrosis*, 18(3), pp. 321–333. doi: 10.1016/j.jcf.2019.03.002.

Rand, S., Prasad, S.A. and Main, E. (2015) 'New incremental field step-test (iSTEP) is valid and feasible in measuring near maximal exercise performance in children with cystic fibrosis', *Physiotherapy*, 101, pp. e931–e932. doi: 10.1016/j.physio.2015.03.1777.

Ranganathan, S.C., Stocks, J., Dezateux, C., Bush, A., Wade, A., Carr, S., Castle, R., Dinwiddie, R., Hoo, A.F., Lum, S., Price, J., Stroobant, J. and Wallis, C. (2004) 'The evolution of airway function in early childhood following clinical diagnosis of cystic fibrosis', *American Journal of Respiratory and Critical Care Medicine*, 169(8), pp. 928–933. doi: 10.1164/rccm.200309-1344OC.

Ranu, H., Wilde, M. and Madden, B. (2011) 'Pulmonary function tests', *Ulster Medical Journal*, 80(2), pp. 84–90. PMCID: PMC3229853.

Ruf, K., Winkler, B., Hebestreit, A., Gruber, W. and Hebestreit, H. (2010) 'Risks associated with exercise testing and sports participation in cystic fibrosis', *Journal of Cystic Fibrosis*, 9(5), pp. 339–345. doi: 10.1016/j.jcf.2010.05.006.

Saunders, C., Bayfield, K., Irving, S., Short, C., Bush, A. and Davies, J.C. (2017) 'Developments in multiple breath washout testing in children with cystic fibrosis', *Current Medical Research and Opinion*, 33(4), pp. 613–620. doi: 10.1080/03007995.2016.1268999.

Saynor, Z.L., Barker, A.R., Oades, P.J., Tomlinson, O.W. and Williams, C.A. (2016) 'Validity and reliability concerns associated with cardiopulmonary exercise testing young people with cystic fibrosis', *Respiration*, 92(1), pp. 61–62. doi: 10.1159/000447642.

Saynor, Z.L., Barker, A.R., Oades, P.J. and Williams, C.A. (2013a) 'A protocol to determine valid VO_{2max} in young cystic fibrosis patients', *Journal of Science and Medicine in Sport*, 16(6), pp. 539–544. doi: 10.1016/j.jsams.2013.01.010.

Saynor, Z.L., Barker, A.R., Oades, P.J. and Williams, C.A. (2013b) 'Reproducibility of maximal cardiopulmonary exercise testing for young cystic fibrosis patients', *Journal of Cystic Fibrosis*, 12(6), pp. 644–650. doi: 10.1016/j.jcf.2013.04.012.

Selvadurai, H.C., Blimkie, C.J., Meyers, N., Mellis, C.M., Cooper, P.J. and Van Asperen, P.P. (2002) 'Randomized controlled study of in-hospital exercise training programs in children with cystic fibrosis', *Pediatric Pulmonology*, 33(3), pp. 194–200. doi: 10.1002/ppul.10015.

Selvadurai, H.C., Cooper, P.J., Meyers, N., Blimkie, C.J., Smith, L., Mellis, C.M. and Van Asperen, P.P. (2003) 'Validation of shuttle tests in children with cystic fibrosis', *Pediatric Pulmonology*, 35(2), pp. 133–138. doi: 10.1002/ppul.10197.

Shakkottai, A., Kaciroti, N., Kasmikha, L. and Nasr, S.Z. (2018) 'Impact of home spirometry on medication adherence among adolescents with cystic fibrosis', *Pediatric Pulmonology*, 53(4), pp. 431–436. doi: 10.1002/ppul.23950.

Singh, S.J., Morgan, M.D., Scott, S., Walters, D. and Hardman, A.E. (1992) 'Development of a shuttle walking test of disability in patients with chronic airways obstruction', *Thorax*, 47(12), pp. 1019–1024. doi: 10.1136/thx.47.12.1019.

Sly, P.D., Cahill, P., Willet, K. and Burton, P. (1994) 'Accuracy of mini peak flow meters in indicating changes in lung function in children with asthma', *BMJ*, 308(6928), pp. 572–574. doi: 10.1136/bmj.308.6928.572.

Stahl, M., Joachim, C., Blessing, K., Hammerling, S., Sommerburg, O., Latzin, P. and Mall, M.A. (2014) 'Multiple breath washout is feasible in the clinical setting and detects abnormal lung function in infants and young children with cystic fibrosis', *Respiration*, 87(5), pp. 357–363. doi: 10.1159/000357075.

Stanojevic, S., Filipow, N. and Ratjen, F. (2020) 'Paediatric reproducibility limits for the forced expiratory volume in 1 s', *Thorax*, 75(10), pp. 891–896. doi: 10.1136/thoraxjnl-2020-214817.

Stanojevic, S., Wade, A., Cole, T.J., Lum, S., Custovic, A., Silverman, M., Hall, G.L., Welsh, L., Kirkby, J., Nystad, W., Badier, M., Davis, S., Turner, S., Piccioni, P., Vilozni, D., Eigen, H., Vlachos-Mayer, H., Zheng, J., Tomalak, W., Jones, M., Hankinson, J.L., Stocks, J. and Asthma, U. K.S.C.G. (2009) 'Spirometry centile charts for young Caucasian children: The Asthma UK Collaborative Initiative', *American Journal of Respiratory and Critical Care Medicine*, 180(6), pp. 547–552. doi: 10.1164/rccm.200903-0323OC.

Stanojevic, S., Wade, A., Stocks, J., Hankinson, J., Coates, A.L., Pan, H., Rosenthal, M., Corey, M., Lebecque, P. and Cole, T.J. (2008) 'Reference ranges for spirometry across all ages: A new approach', *American Journal of Respiratory and Critical Care Medicine*, 177(3), pp. 253–260. doi: 10.1164/rccm.200708-1248OC.

Stevens, D., Oades, P.J., Armstrong, N. and Williams, C.A. (2010) 'A survey of exercise testing and training in UK cystic fibrosis clinics', *Journal of Cystic Fibrosis*, 9(5), pp. 302–306. doi: 10.1016/j.jcf.2010.03.004.

Sylvester, K.P., Clayton, N., Cliff, I., Hepple, M., Kendrick, A., Kirkby, J., Miller, M., Moore, A., Rafferty, G.F., O'Reilly, L., Shakespeare, J., Smith, L., Watts, T., Bucknall, M. and Butterfield, K. (2020) 'ARTP statement on pulmonary function testing 2020', *BMJ Open Respiratory Research*, 7(1). doi: 10.1136/bmjresp-2020-000575.

Szczesniak, R., Heltshe, S.L., Stanojevic, S. and Mayer-Hamblett, N. (2017) 'Use of FEV_1 in cystic fibrosis epidemiologic studies and clinical trials: A statistical perspective for the clinical researcher', *Journal of Cystic Fibrosis*, 16(3), pp. 318–326. doi: 10.1016/j.jcf.2017.01.002.

Teoh, O.H., Trachsel, D., Mei-Zahav, M. and Selvadurai, H. (2009) 'Exercise testing in children with lung diseases', *Paediatric Respiratory Reviews*, 10(3), pp. 99–104. doi: 10.1016/j.prrv.2009.06.004.

Tomlinson, O.W., Barker, A.R., Trott, J., Withers, N.J., Oades, P.J. and Williams, C.A. (2019) 'WS02-3-1 Validity of prediction equations for evaluating aerobic fitness in cystic fibrosis', *Journal of Cystic Fibrosis*, 18. doi: 10.1016/s1569-1993(19)30125-0.

Tomlinson, O.W., Trott, J., Williams, C.A., Withers, N.J. and Oades, P.J. (2020) 'Challenges in implementing routine cardiopulmonary exercise testing in cystic fibrosis clinical practice: A single-centre review', *SN Comprehensive Clinical Medicine*, 2(3), pp. 327–331. doi: 10.1007/s42399-020-00239-7.

Urquhart, D.S. and Saynor, Z.L. (2018) 'Exercise testing in cystic fibrosis: Who and why?', *Paediatric Respiratory Reviews*, 27, pp. 28–32. doi: 10.1016/j.prrv.2018.01.004

Vandekerckhove, K., Keyzer, M., Cornette, J., Coomans, I., Pyl, F., De Baets, F., Schelstraete, P., Haerynck, F., De Wolf, D., Van Daele, S. and Boone, J. (2017) 'Exercise performance and quality of life in children with cystic fibrosis and mildly impaired lung function: Relation with antibiotic treatments and hospitalization', *European Journal of Pediatrics*, 176(12), pp. 1689–1696. doi: 10.1007/s00431-017-3024-7.

Vandenbroucke, N.J., Zampoli, M. and Morrow, B. (2020) 'Lung function determinants and mortality of children and adolescents with cystic fibrosis in South Africa 2007-2016', *Pediatric Pulmonology*, 55(6), pp. 1381–1387. doi: 10.1002/ppul.24726.

Vermeulen, F., Proesmans, M., Boon, M., Havermans, T. and De Boeck, K. (2014) 'Lung clearance index predicts pulmonary exacerbations in young patients with cystic fibrosis', *Thorax*, 69(1), pp. 39–45. doi: 10.1136/thoraxjnl-2013-203807.

Weir, E., Burns, P.D., Devenny, A., Young, D. and Paton, J.Y. (2017) 'Cardiopulmonary exercise testing in children with cystic fibrosis: One centre's experience', *Archives of Disease in Childhood*, 102(5), pp. 440–444. doi: 10.1136/archdischild-2016-310651.

Werkman, M.S., Hulzebos, E.H., Helders, P.J., Arets, B.G. and Takken, T. (2014) 'Estimating peak oxygen uptake in adolescents with cystic fibrosis', *Archives of Disease in Childhood*, 99(1), pp. 21–25. doi: 10.1136/archdischild-2012-303439.

Zolin, A., Bossi, A., Cirilli, N., Kashirskaya, N. and Padoan, R. (2018) 'Cystic fibrosis mortality in childhood. Data from European Cystic Fibrosis Society Patient Registry', *International Journal of Environmental Research and Public Health*, 15(9). doi: 10.3390/ijerph15092020.

3 The Physiology and Psychological Consequence of Breathlessness in Children

Jayne Trott, Holly Jones, and Patrick J. Oades

Introduction

Breathing is essential to life and is usually under subconscious control. It can be modified voluntarily, (e.g., breath-holding), involuntarily (e.g., coughing or sneezing), or by emotional responses (e.g., crying, laughing, gasping, and hyperventilating). An awareness of breathing occurs when our consciousness takes over; when it is disordered, uncomfortable, or in anticipation of physical exertion. The threshold of awareness varies between persons and within individuals over time, which can be helpful or problematic depending on individual circumstances.

Breathlessness has been defined as a subjective experience of breathing discomfort that consists of qualitatively distinct sensations that vary in intensity (Parshall *et al.*, 2012). Breathlessness and dyspnoea are often used interchangeably within the literature, and there is clear overlap between these definitions. Some define breathlessness as an unpleasant symptom that an individual senses and reports to others, which may initially be invisible to an observer. Dyspnoea is the noticeable increase in the rate and work of breathing that appears laboured and uncomfortable. Symptoms of breathlessness and physical signs of respiratory distress need to be distinguished in paediatric practice (Schweitzer and Marchal, 2009). Generally, dyspnoea is used to describe the physical signs of respiratory distress in young children while breathlessness describes the reported symptom in older children.

In health, breathlessness is a mark of normal physiological limitation related to individual fitness levels and can be associated with a positive sense of challenge. In poor health, breathlessness can be a chronic symptom that individuals live alongside, compromising activities, or marking decline. Numerous medical disorders can present with breathlessness (Bhatia *et al.*, 2019), and unrecognised illnesses need differentiating from normal physiological limitation (Weinberger and Abu-Hasan, 2007).

Accurate assessment and management of breathlessness in individuals requires a breadth of competencies including knowledge of the mechanics and control of normal breathing and utilisation of subjective and objective measures of breathlessness to assess exercise performance or monitor

DOI: 10.4324/9781003020462-3

illness progression. The perception and impact of breathlessness varies both between individuals, and within their own lifespan. This explains discordance between objective physiology and self-reported severity of symptoms. Interventions to manage breathlessness and maintain physical activity levels are important to reduce the personal and financial costs of repeated healthcare attendances, morbidity, and under-achievement.

Much of the understanding of breathlessness in children is derived from research involving children with asthma or the extrapolation of work with adults. Studies in wider paediatric populations are needed to improve our understanding of the specific needs of this age group.

Mechanisms

Neurology of Breathing

The breathing rhythm is generated by respiratory centres located in the medulla and pons of the brainstem. Motor neurone efferent pathways communicate via the spinal cord then peripheral nerves to action responses from the muscles of respiration (Ikeda *et al.*, 2017). Breathing patterns change through the integration of sensory feedback about the chemical and mechanical status of breathing, and input from higher mental functions (Lumb, 2017).

Mechanoreceptors in the lungs and chest wall communicate information about their physical state to the respiratory centres. Stretch receptors in airway smooth muscle detect over-inflation, while irritant receptors throughout the respiratory tract can trigger defensive reflexes such as coughing, sneezing, and bronchoconstriction. As physical activity and metabolism increase, more oxygen is needed, and more carbon dioxide is produced. Carotid and aortic arterial chemoreceptors detect changes in the partial pressures of carbon dioxide ($PaCO_2$) and oxygen (PaO_2), while hydrogen ion receptors on the surface of the medulla detect a fall in the pH of cerebrospinal fluid when $PaCO_2$ rises or if lactate rises with anaerobic metabolism. Ventilation is adjusted to maintain homeostasis and to provide adequate arterial oxygenation to fuel and maintain the function of working tissues. Breathing can be consciously controlled by the motor cortex, while the hypothalamus and limbic system formulate the perception of discomfort and emotions leading to responses such as gasping or hyperventilation.

Mechanics of Breathing

Ventilation is the cycle of inspiration and expiration in order to achieve gas exchange. Airflow occurs via the upper airways and trachea when there is a pressure gradient between the inside and outside of the lungs. The lungs are enclosed within the thoracic cage and remain inflated by negative pressure around them, generated by the elastic properties of lung tissue. The volume of the thoracic cavity changes rhythmically due to the actions of the respiratory muscles and the diaphragm. During inspiration, intercostal muscles contract and lift the ribs, which hinge on the spine, upwards and outwards. Simultaneously, the diaphragm contracts, causing its dome shape to flatten. Consequently, thoracic volume increases, generating a greater negative pressure causing the lungs to expand and air flows inwards. Expiration at rest is a passive process where the respiratory muscles and diaphragm relax allowing the elastic recoil of the lungs to reduce thoracic volume. With exercise, there is coordinated and sequential recruitment of muscle action to increase ventilation. Initially abdominal and subsequently ribcage muscles are brought into action to force expiration, increasing pressure and flow. Tidal volume increases by reducing end expiratory and increasing end inspiratory lung volumes. Subsequently the respiratory rate rises to further increase ventilation. The expiratory muscles guard against inefficient ribcage distortions and unload the diaphragm, which has a key role in generating flow (Macklem, 2014). Accessory muscles of respiration anchored around the neck and shoulders contribute to postural stability and pressure generation.

The precise mechanism of breathlessness is still debated (Parshall *et al.*, 2012). Key components of ventilation help clinicians understand factors that contribute to the symptoms of breathlessness (Jones, 1995). Breath volume, respiratory rate, and airflow relate to the magnitude, frequency, and velocity of respiratory muscle contraction respectively, while the inspiratory time relates to the duration of inspiratory muscle contraction per breath. Expiration is passive at rest, but becomes active, with expiratory muscle contraction during exercise or when airway obstruction requires more work. Thus, when the work of breathing is greater, opposing inspiratory and expiratory muscles synchronise alternate concentric and eccentric contraction. Overall, these constitute the respiratory muscle performance characteristics and are limited by an individual's respiratory muscle capacity. As with any working muscle, the maximum force generated falls as the velocity of contraction increases or when the muscle is lengthened. Less force is generated by respiratory muscles at higher respiratory rates and by expiratory muscles when tidal volumes are high, or when there is hyperinflation, such as in an asthma attack. The respiratory muscle performance characteristics also determine that resting maximal spirometry measurements are not attained during exercise. During high-intensity exercise, tidal volumes are only 55–60% of vital capacity, inspiratory flows rarely exceed 75% of the resting maximum and expiratory flows only approach maximal levels at low lung volumes. In health, respiratory muscle capacity limits exercise performance more than ventilatory capacity (Takken *et al.*, 2020).

Breathlessness in Children

Promoting the health benefits of exercise is a valuable public health message, and it is important to recognise if breathlessness becomes a barrier to physical activity. Breathlessness during physical activity is a common human experience, but there are multiple factors that influence how it is perceived, interpreted, and reported. These include physical health and fitness status, the environment and context in which the activity is undertaken, previous experiences and psychological co-morbidities such as panic-induced hyperventilation.

Exercise Limitation

Awareness of increased respiratory effort occurs at about 40% of maximum ventilation in children (Pianosi *et al.*, 2015). Further increments in physical exercise depend on effort, motivation (reward or performance target), and the subjective tolerance of incremental discomfort. Breathlessness relates to the perceived effort of breathing as the respiratory muscle capacity is approached highlighted by negative sensory feedback about the state of lung mechanics and airway irritation related to cooling and drying at high breathing rates. Feelings of 'chest tightness,' 'air hunger,' or inadequate 'breath satisfaction' can become the focus of attention. Poor air quality can contribute to discomfort, especially at higher breathing rates. Muscle weakness develops when the force expected cannot be generated and fatigue when contraction cannot be sustained. Although different symptoms may predominate in individuals, symptoms eventually combine with faltering performance and concentration and the individual must stop.

When the level of breathlessness is under personal control, tolerance in individuals will be variable, some rationalising symptoms as evidence that they are exercising hard, aligning with their goals. For others, breathlessness will be considered unpleasant and best avoided. The discomfort of breathlessness may act as a warning that physical performance is at risk, analogous to pain signalling possible injury. In evolutionary terms, faltering performance increases vulnerability and breathlessness may signal the need to slow down and seek safety. Healthy children are most likely to experience breathlessness during competitive sporting activities, but as school physical education lessons involve relatively low-intensity activities and time spent playing outside has declined, children in modern society may experience less breathlessness through activity than previous generations.

Paediatric Respiratory Illness and Breathlessness

Globally, respiratory diseases in children are a major cause of morbidity and mortality. Conditions are diverse and range from acute infections to chronic non-communicable diseases. Pneumonia is the most common acute infection, responsible for more than 1 million childhood deaths per year (Zar and Ferkol, 2014). Asthma is the most common non-communicable chronic condition affecting 8% of 0–17 year-olds in the U.S.A. (Zahran *et al.*, 2018).

Respiratory diseases may compromise lung function acutely, recurrently, and/or progressively, and often with a degree of overlap. Symptoms including breathlessness will therefore worsen, remit, or progress depending on the nature and course of the disease. Different types of lung damage and examples of the diseases responsible are outlined in Table 3.1.

Table 3.1 Paediatric Respiratory Diseases Associated with Breathlessness

Paediatric Respiratory Diseases Associated with Breathlessness			
Impairment	*Examples*	*Mechanism*	*Additional Notes*
Reduced lung volume	Pneumonia[a] Pleural effusion[a] Pneumothorax[a] Thoracic cage[b] deformity	Consolidation Fluid compresses lung Lung collapse Restriction and external compression	Common Can form around pneumonia Puncture of lung or thoracic wall
Reduced airway calibre (Increased airflow resistance leads to air trapping and hyperinflation)	Asthma[b] Bronchiolitis[a] Bronchiectasis[b] Croup[a]	Bronchospasm, inflammatory swelling and mucus plugging Inflammatory swelling and mucus plugging Thin floppy saccular airways damaged by inflammation Upper airway and laryngeal swelling	Episodic and/or chronic. Very common Acute illness in infants E.g., cystic fibrosis Acute illness usually due to viral infection
Impaired gas exchange	Pulmonary fibrosis[b] Interstitial lung disease[b] Oedema[a] Collapse/ consolidation[a]	Thickened alveolar membrane as barrier to diffusion or loss of alveolar surface area. Reduced lung volume	Very rare Very rare
Reduced lung compliance and elasticity	Pulmonary fibrosis[b] Interstitial lung disease[b]	Restricted lung function and greater work needed to achieve ventilation	
Impaired mechanics of breathing	Neuromuscular disease[b] Thoracic cage deformity, especially spinal scoliosis[b]	Respiratory muscle weakness. Poor cough. Retention of secretions Reduced or limited chest expansion	Often associated with scoliosis. Frequent co-morbidities e.g., gastro-oesophageal reflux and aspiration
Non-respiratory conditions that can cause breathlessness	Cardiovascular disease Anaemia Metabolic acidosis	Reduced oxygen delivery Reduced oxygen delivery Respiration stimulated to buffer acidosis by lowering $PaCO_2$	Compensatory increase in ventilation may masquerade as respiratory illness, e.g., diabetic ketoacidosis

[a]Acute conditions, often presenting with respiratory distress and breathlessness at rest.
[b]Chronic conditions but which can be complicated by episodic exacerbations of disease activity leading to variations in exercise tolerance and symptoms.

Breathlessness in poor health is qualitatively different from that in exercise; it is often accompanied by other symptoms, arises at lower levels of activity and may be linked with frightening healthcare episodes. '*Pathological breathlessness*' cannot be rationalised in relation to physical activity or controlled in the same way as physiological breathlessness; it can cause frustration, fear, and panic. It can arise at rest in acute severe illness or may develop following a progressive decline in exercise tolerance in chronic disease, thus compromising an individual's daily living and peer group activities to impair quality of life. The fear of breathlessness can lead to early cessation or avoidance of activities with an increased perception of disability relative to pulmonary function and true exercise capacity. This may drive a spiral of decline where poor fitness becomes a confounding factor (Parshall *et al*, 2012).

While health professionals understand breathlessness as a physiological symptom or sensation residing in the respiratory system, they often lack personal experience of it. Breathlessness in disease states can dominate thoughts, restrict behaviours, and remind individuals of their mortality. Experts by experience have questioned whether it is possible to understand the extent of fear and debilitation that arise with pathological breathlessness without ever experiencing it (Carel, 2018).

Dysfunctional Breathing

Dysfunctional breathing is a term that encompasses episodic abnormalities in the pattern or mechanics of breathing that lead to inefficiencies or physiologically inappropriate hyperventilation, causing a variety of uncomfortable respiratory or non-respiratory symptoms in the absence of an underlying condition. It affects 10% of the general adult population (Freitas *et al.*, 2013), but information about the prevalence, treatment, or prognosis in children is lacking (Barker *et al.*, 2020). It rarely presents in early childhood, but is more common in adolescence, affecting girls more than boys. There are significant associations with psychological co-morbidities such as anxiety and emotional stress.

Dysfunctional breathing can be categorised into thoracic or laryngeal types (Depiazzi and Everard, 2016). '*Breathing pattern disorders*' describes the thoracic form, including hyperventilation, periodic deep sighing, thoracic-abdominal asynchrony, and over or underuse of different respiratory muscle groups (Boulding *et al.*, 2016). Symptoms include breathlessness, chest discomfort or tightness, fatigue, anxiety, abdominal bloating, panting, and periodic maximal inspirations, linked to a sensation of not being able to take a deep breath (Morgan, 2002). Wheezing can be heard if there is forced expiration at low lung volumes, easily confused with asthma. Hyperventilation results in a lower $PaCO_2$ and metabolic alkalosis causing dizziness, paraesthesia and, if severe, involuntary muscle spasm (Bott *et al.*, 2009).

Laryngeal disorders can co-exist with breathing pattern disorders, and symptoms can overlap, but additional features include prolonged inspiration with stridor and throat tightness. The term inducible laryngeal obstruction (ILO) is preferred to laryngeal dysfunction or paradoxical vocal cord motion. Two forms are described, one with severe episodes at rest affecting young adults and sometimes adolescents, often with psychological difficulties. Exercise-associated ILO (EILO) typically affects high achieving, athletically competitive individuals but without obvious psychological disturbance, although competitive activities may trigger anxiety and anticipation of underperformance. The diagnosis of EILO is discussed in Chapter 7.

Dysfunctional breathing disorders frequently co-exist as comorbidities in young people with respiratory disease, such as asthma and poor treatment responses should prompt suspicion of the diagnosis (Connett and Thomas, 2018). The overlap of symptoms may cause confusion and accurate diagnosis depends on careful clinical assessment which can be supported by observation of episodes by a physiotherapist ideally using field-testing protocols to classify the problem. Individuals with dysfunctional breathing disorders may struggle to accept that their symptoms may be a conditioned response to psychological problems.

Assessment of Breathlessness

The clinical management of illness-related breathlessness requires a range of assessment methods. When a child is more breathless than expected, the initial assessment should include a thorough medical history, identifying associated symptoms such as cough, illness duration, provoking factors, the social and environmental settings in which breathlessness has arisen and the response to any treatments (Haddad *et al.*, 2015). The use of reliable and valid assessments to capture both subjective and objective measures of breathlessness is important. As children's symptom reporting may be influenced by tests or interaction with technicians, subjective reports should be taken first (Rietveld *et al.*, 1996).

Subjective Measures

An individual's description of their breathlessness can be helpful for understanding the underlying cause (Scano *et al.*, 2005), for example, reported chest tightness is often indicative of asthma. School age children use age-related language to convey breathlessness, such as 'bad breathing' or 'feeling puffed-out' (Carrieri *et al.*, 1991).

Numerous scales and questionnaires have been designed to standardise breathlessness and effort reporting in adults. The Borg Rating of Perceived Exertion (RPE), Borg scale (6–20), and Borg CR-10 have been widely used in adults, but their use with children is less well understood. Simplification of perception scales in the Borg CR-10 improved its use with children, but some authors have noted that children younger than 11 years may struggle correlating words or sentences to describe exercise. A review by Martins *et al.* (2014) concluded that there was no gold standard to date, but that each scale had its own descriptors or images to enhance understanding. Children under 10 years have demonstrated ability to use Visual Analogue Scales (VAS) to report asthma symptoms, although the relationships between VAS scores and objective measures were weaker in older children (Horak *et al.*, 2003). The VAS consists of a 100 mm vertical or horizontal line with anchors indicating the extremes of perception, from 'not breathless at all' to 'extremely breathless.' Scoring is performed according to the distance from the beginning of the scale to the point indicated by the subject. Vertical lines and linear scales appear to be more easily understood by younger children and the addition of pictures and symbols can help in their interpretation of numerical perception scales, such as the children's OMNI scale, validated in 8- to 12-year-olds (Robertson *et al.*, 2000).

The Dalhousie Dyspnoea and Perceived Exertion scales are pictorial sequences depicting three dyspnoea constructs; chest tightness, throat closure, and breathing effort. A further series depicts leg exertion and fatigue (McGrath *et al.*, 2005). Used with children aged 7 years and above, they have been shown to track breathlessness in objectively induced bronchospasm and have been validated in formal cardiopulmonary exercise testing of both healthy children and those with respiratory disease (Pianosi *et al.*, 2015). A non-linear increase in perceived dyspnoea and exertion was observed during incremental exercise and perception did not appear to be influenced by gender or health status. Good short-term intra-individual reproducibility was observed, although there was marked inter-individual variability in ratings at similar relative levels of exertion, emphasising how perception can be discordant with the level of relative work and health status. The Nijmegen Questionnaire (NQ) is a symptom scoring tool that can identify dysfunctional breathing in both asthmatic and non-asthmatic adults (Thomas *et al.*, 2005). In a cross-sectional study of 203 asthmatic children, the NQ identified hyperventilation in 5.3%, was more prevalent in girls and was associated with poorer asthma control (de Groot *et al.*, 2013).

When using rating scales, children frequently score perceptions beneath the scale maximum despite reaching their maximum exercise capacity. This concurs with the variability in children's ability to detect asthma symptoms (van Gent *et al.*, 2007) and the poor prediction of exercise-induced asthma by self-reported breathlessness in school age children (De Baets *et al.*, 2005). The inter-individual variability in rating trajectory significantly undermines comparisons in breathlessness between different disease groups (Pianosi *et al.*, 2015). Although children over 10 years can usually comprehend adult terms used to describe breathlessness, it would be better to have validated terms, scores, and tests designed specifically for children and adolescents. Valid and reliable child-friendly tools are needed to explore the quality and magnitude of breathlessness in children and to understand how symptoms relate to measures of disease status (Lands, 2017).

Objective Measures

Clinical signs of respiratory distress in children are influenced by anatomical factors, but do not fully convey what a child is feeling (Figure 3.1).

The reliance on clinical signs to assess breathlessness in younger children has led to the development of a number of composite '*dyspnoea severity scores*' to monitor children with acute breathing difficulty. In a prospective study in children aged 0–8 years, five scoring tools were evaluated: Asthma Score (AS), Asthma Severity Score (ASS), Clinical Asthma Evaluation Score 2 (CAES-2), Paediatric Respiratory Assessment Measure (PRAM), and the Respiratory rate, Accessory muscle use, Decreased breath sounds (RAD) (Eggink *et al.*, 2016). When tested in clinical practice, all had insufficient validity or reliability and they lacked sufficient discriminative and evaluative power to be used a sole outcome measures in acute care. Thus, more valid and reliable tools are needed to support clinicians managing children with acute respiratory illness.

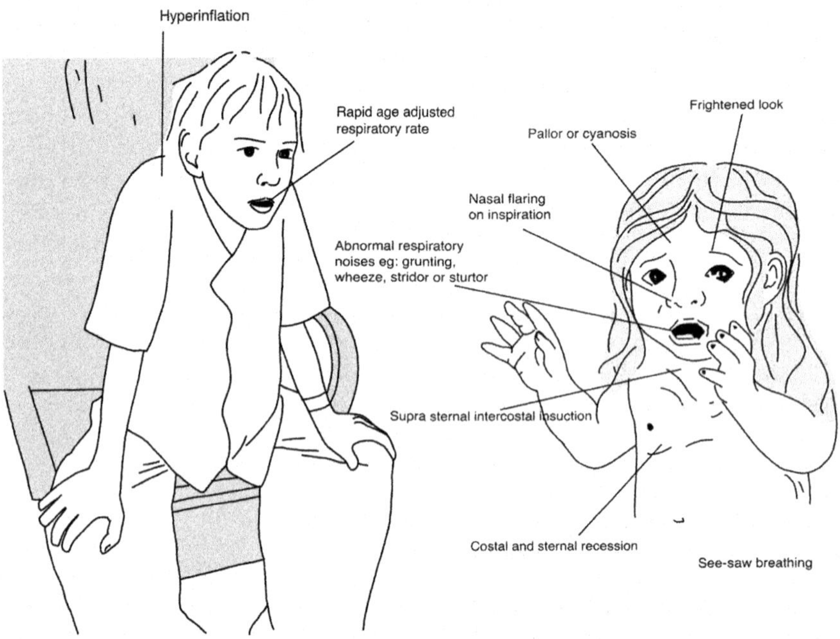

Figure 3.1 Clinical signs of respiratory distress in children. The flexible cartilage ribcage in children increases chest wall compliance allowing paradoxical costal and sternal recession during inspiration when the diaphragm contracts, pushing the abdomen out, causing characteristic '*see-sawing*' of the abdomen and thorax. Such deformations undermine the efficiency of breathing as effort increases. Respiratory muscles in young children are relatively underdeveloped and prone to fatigue and the accessory muscles are less well anchored, '*head bobbing*' is a feature of this. Obstruction of smaller airways in children causes air trapping and chest hyperinflation. '*Nasal flaring*', on inspiration is a sign of increased effort and audible expiratory '*grunting*' in infants generates positive airway pressure, splinting them and helping prevent alveolar collapse.

Paediatric Early Warning Systems (PEWS) continue to be refined in order to score age-appropriate physiological parameters and so generically identify children at risk of clinical deterioration, prompting timely escalation in care (Zachariasse *et al.*, 2020).

The 15-count breathlessness score (Prasad *et al.*, 2000) is an objective evaluation of breathlessness validated in children as young as 7 years who can confidently count to 15. The number of breaths taken is recorded and has been shown to increase with exercise. It is also higher in children with respiratory disease than in healthy controls after defined exercise bouts, although the test does not convey how the children feel.

Perception of Breathlessness

Accurate symptom perception is important for the management of paediatric respiratory conditions (Horak *et al.*, 2003), but there is variability in children's ability to detect symptoms (van Gent *et al.*, 2007). Low-perception thresholds may result in overmedication, frequent hospital attendances, and school absences. High thresholds may delay treatment and result in serious health consequences including life-threatening asthma attacks and death in young people (McQuaid *et al.*, 2007). However, the ability to distinguish between breathlessness caused by bronchoconstriction, anxiety, or other factors is a complex process that involves sensory input, affect, life experience, and beliefs (von Leupoldt *et al.*, 2006). Consequently, an awareness of cognitive, social, emotional, and developmental factors is important.

Cognitive

The brain holds a mental model of the world that is updated following discrepancies between what the brain expects (predictions) and what the brain receives (sensory signals) (Rao and Ballard, 1999). Individuals use a representation of levels of breathlessness associated with certain activities to recognise exacerbations, change activity levels, alert caregivers, and access treatment (Wilson and Jones, 1990). Perceptions that are closely related to the real world predict accurate outcomes, and perceptions that are distorted in comparison predict inaccurate outcomes; this mismatch between predictions and sensory signals is referred to as 'prediction error.' When predictions about breathlessness are based on negative experiences, such as hospitalisation, breathlessness may be perceived as severe, even in the absence of objective markers (Boulay and Boulet, 2013).

Functional neuroimaging has identified brain areas that are active during, but not specific to breathlessness. These include the anterior cingulate cortex, insula, amygdala, and sensory processing areas (Stoeckel *et al.*, 2016). Drawing on pain research, common networks underpinning the perception of aversive physical sensations have been identified (von Leupoldt *et al.*, 2009). The anterior insula is activated during the processing of both pain and breathlessness, and the hypothalamus and limbic system in the perception of pain and emotions that trigger gasping or hyperventilation. However, there are inter- and intra-individual variations in the activation of brain regions associated with adverse sensations (Hayen *et al.*, 2013) and searching for localised activity in a specific '*breathlessness brain region*' is unlikely to be successful. Instead, investigating the brain networks that generate breathlessness may inform understanding beyond where breathlessness is processed, to how it is processed.

Social

The way that parents model their own health beliefs and manage physical complaints influences how children deal with physical sensations (McQuaid *et al.*, 2007). Parents who are symptom-focused and ignore or minimise symptoms may model unhelpful behaviour that does not to equip their child with the skills to perceive and manage their symptoms effectively. Ambiguous physical sensations such as dizziness and tiredness can be misinterpreted as warning signs of an asthma attack. Children may also monitor and report symptoms more frequently if parental attention and school absence is a secondary gain (Bouton *et al.*, 2001). This emphasises the importance of exploring how the child and family manage symptoms to encourage accurate symptom perception and timely treatment to reduce morbidity.

Emotional

An individual's emotional disposition, mood, anxiety, and stress can intensify and distort the perception of respiratory symptoms (Peiffer, 2008). Breathlessness, feelings of choking, chest pain, and discomfort are all part of the definition of panic attacks in the Diagnostic and Statistical Manual of Mental Disorders (DSM-5: American Psychiatric Association, Edition F., 2013). Panic and fear as comorbidities in asthmatic adults increase healthcare visits, activity restriction, and rescue medication usage despite no increase in asthma severity (Feldman *et al.*, 2009). Intense breathlessness can be induced in teenage asthmatics after exposure to negative emotions and stress, independent of respiratory function (Rietveld and Prins, 1998). von Leupoldt *et al.* (2006) found that the perception of respiratory load was decreased in children age 6–12 years when watching an amusing film clip (the 'Jungle Book') compared to when sad or neutral clips were viewed during exercise. Children with asthma who were told that pre-recorded wheezy breathing sounds were their own, reported significantly more breathlessness than those listening to normal breathing sounds, or than children without asthma (Rietveld *et al.*, 1997). Children's memory of severe asthma attacks can have a long-term negative impact on their physical and emotional wellbeing (Lands, 2017; Woodgate, 2009).

Anticipatory anxiety is felt in anticipation of events to which negative experiences are attached. Perceived breathlessness increases in situations in which individuals have previously been breathless, even in the absence of the original stimulus (Herzog *et al.*, 2018). An initially neutral stimulus (e.g., the playground) attracts negative breathlessness associations, and a conditioned response develops. On exposure to the negatively cued stimuli, the anticipation of breathlessness can increase the perception of respiratory symptoms; children anticipate that playtime is approaching, and they expect to feel out of breath. Individuals with asthma can feel breathless on mislaying their inhaler. Lansing *et al.* (2009) proposes a model where primary sensory (intensity) and affective (unpleasantness) components are followed by a secondary, cognitive-affective component; this leads to a long-term emotional response (suffering) that shapes future breathlessness-related behaviour. However, replicating the emotional component of breathlessness in laboratory settings is difficult as the fears encountered in real life are hard to simulate.

Developmental

Symptom perception is not a static trait and fluctuates across developmental stages. As life experiences accrue during the different developmental stages (preschool, school age, adolescence, and adulthood), the potential for the perception of breathlessness to become less aligned to objective physiological measures increases. This may account for the increased incidence of dysfunctional breathing patterns in the second decade of life. The perception of breathlessness may be reduced in early developmental stages compared with adults, making children with respiratory conditions vulnerable to underreporting of symptoms. In children awareness of breathing begins at around 40% of maximum exercise capacity, compared to 20–40% in adults (Pianosi *et al.*, 2015), and adolescents are more likely to under-perceive their symptoms (Rhee *et al.*, 2011). Furthermore, the transition in perception from comfortable to extreme discomfort is more abrupt in youth compared to a steadier exponential rise in adults. Children who have more acute onset of symptoms may be more attuned to respiratory changes, warning them of exacerbations than those who have a more insidious changes in disease activity. In chronic disease, sedentary individuals may not complain of breathlessness unless compelled to do something strenuous (climbing stairs when the elevator is broken); whereas active children will notice their performance faltering at an early disease stage.

In a study of 7–17 year-old asthmatics, spirometer devices provided objective feedback about pulmonary function to help children interpret their symptoms (Feldman *et al.*, 2007), morbidity was less in those with the ability to perceive asthma symptoms accurately. While overperception of symptoms was common, ~20% of those using feedback spirometry underestimated their symptoms, suggesting that monitoring may reduce their risk of delay in identifying an asthma attack. Further work is required to determine whether symptom perception can be improved by the provision of tools to provide feedback on pulmonary function as this would have the potential to improve adherence and clinical outcomes.

Therapeutic Approaches

Despite disease-specific treatments, breathlessness is often inadequately treated and can undermine an individual's quality of life. Treatment outcomes depend on treatment adherence, which can be influenced by many factors including miscommunications, misunderstandings, patient capacity, and capability (Kaplan and Price, 2020). Treatment approaches may target different stages of the symptom's development and include interventions to reduce an individual's metabolic demand, improve the efficiency of the cardiorespiratory gas exchange, dampen central respiratory drive, or modify the perception of discomfort and anxiety. This work is often undertaken in collaboration with clinicians from different disciplines.

Physiotherapists play a central role in this, advising on exercise training, activity modifications, positioning, and breathing techniques. Even adjustment of a person's environment, modifying sensory input, such as the provision of an electric fan (Barnes-Harris *et al.*, 2019), playing music, and the promotion of relaxation techniques like meditation or yoga can alleviate breathlessness (Norweg and Collins, 2013).

Physical Training

Hallstrand *et al.* (2000) reported a decrease in dyspnoea, better resting lung function and less exercise-induced bronchospasm in children with mild asthma following aerobic training. Exercise training and education in adults with COPD can improve reported breathlessness without measurable effects on lung function (Janssens *et al.*, 2011).

One systemic review found only limited evidence that aerobic and/or anaerobic exercise training is beneficial to exercise capacity and health-related quality of life in people with cystic fibrosis (CF), (Radtke *et al.*, 2017). A further meta-analysis of the benefits of a variety of exercise training programs in children with chronic lung disease, primarily asthma, and CF, found significant improvement in aerobic capacity; (standard mean difference (SMD) 1.16; $p < 0.0001$), disease-related quality of life scores (SMD 1.27) and some evidence for improved muscle strength and reduced inflammation (Joschtel *et al.*, 2018). Although breathlessness was not specifically measured, benefit is implied in relation to exercise tolerance and physical functioning. However, there was no stratification of benefit in relation to the mode, frequency, intensity, or duration of training employed. An eight-week intervention of high-intensity interval training in young adults with CF accelerated $\dot{V}O_2$ kinetics at lower intensity exercise and increased time to exhaustion at higher intensity exercise, implying an improvement in the tolerance of activity bursts during daily living (Reuveny *et al.*, 2020). However, dyspnoea scores did not improve in participants. Further standardisation of training programs and high-quality randomised controlled trials are needed to comprehensively assess the benefits of exercise training in children with chronic lung disease and more evidence is needed to determine whether measures to relieve breathlessness and related anxiety can help adherence to exercise training programmes (Norweg and Collins, 2013).

Breathing Techniques, Exercises, and Positioning

Breathing techniques such as breathing control, paced breathing, 'pursed-lip' breathing, and 'blow as you go' are all techniques that aim to reduce the work of breathing and improve alveolar ventilation (Garrod *et al.*, 2005). Pursed-lip breathing generates positive expiratory pressure, lengthening expiratory time, increasing functional residual capacity, and reduces air trapping. It encourages a slower breathing frequency, increases the efficiency of inspiratory muscle work, and decreases breathlessness. Although these techniques are firmly embedded in practice and endorsed by patients, usage is based on physiological theory and there remains little evidence of their benefit in relieving breathlessness in children.

Breathing retraining exercises focus on diaphragmatic and nose breathing while reducing respiratory rate and minute ventilation. They form part of wider behavioural intervention programmes and can improve outcomes and reduce health-care costs in adults but evidence in children is limited (Barker *et al.,* 2013). Rapid shallow breathing (RSB) is a feature of anxiety-related hyperventilation but may be observed in respiratory illness and obesity in children (Fitzgerald, 2017). Although RSB has a lower energy cost than deep breathing, in ventilatory terms, it is much less efficient. When recognised, RSB may be amenable to breathing retraining.

Breathing exercises can improve breathlessness but, appropriate application requires understanding of why someone is breathless. Exercises that aim to slow the rate and depth of breathing can be beneficial in dysfunctional breathing but will increase breathlessness in someone with respiratory disease who is working hard to maintain adequate ventilation. There is a body of evidence advocating the use of breathing exercises in adult respiratory disease, including, The Papworth Method (Holloway and West, 2007) and Breathing Freely (Bruton *et al.*, 2018). In a systematic review, breathing exercises, including Buteyko and Yoga had some positive effects on quality of life, hyperventilation symptoms, and lung function in adults with asthma (Santino *et al.*, 2020).

Breathing exercises are viewed to have a positive effect on asthma symptoms, quality of life, and bronchodilator use in adults but evidence of benefit in children is limited (British Thoracic Society, 2019). In a literature review of breathing exercises in children with asthma, only three studies were included due to methodological problems, and no reliable conclusions could be determined (Macêdo *et al.*, 2016). A three-week Buteyko programme in asthmatic children aged 7–12 years improved lung function, reduced school absences, and reliever medication use compared to controls (Mendonca *et al.*, 2017).

A systematic review of targeted inspiratory muscle training (IMT) in children and adolescents with neuromuscular disease suggested that inspiratory muscle strength and endurance improved and that early, dose-dependent IMT may slow vital capacity decline, but the authors concluded that evidence was insufficient to guide clinical IMT practice (Human *et al.*, 2017). In a systematic review of IMT usage in adults and children with CF, no clinical benefit was identified (Reid *et al.*, 2008).

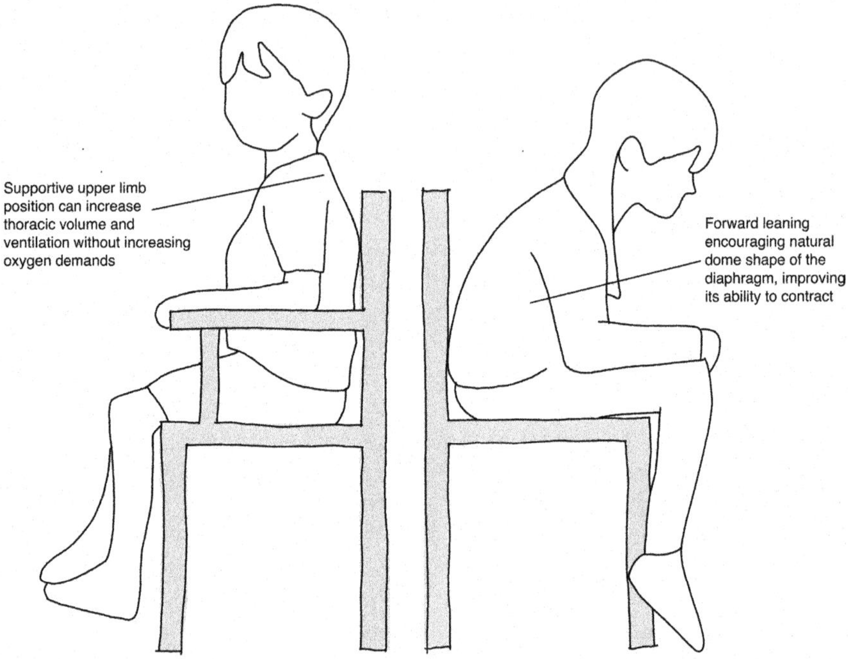

Figure 3.2 Positioning to reduce work of breathing and relieve breathlessness in respiratory distress. A child will naturally fix their upper limbs to anchor the accessory muscles, reversing the origin and insertion of muscles such as latissimus dorsi to assist in lifting the rib cage during inspiration. Additional muscle work to fix the shoulder girdle can increase thoracic volume and ventilation, but positioning a child's upper limbs as illustrated, achieves the same effect without increasing oxygen demands (Bott et al., 2009).

Positioning can alleviate the sensation of breathlessness by optimising the efficiency of the respiratory muscles. Children will often assume a posture that optimises the mechanics of their breathing, reducing work, and guarding against fatigue. Sitting up relieves abdominal pressure on the diaphragm and holding onto something firm with the upper limbs helps maintain posture and anchor the accessory muscles. In obstructive diseases, gas trapping causing hyperinflation can compromise diaphragmatic and respiratory muscle efficiency. Some muscle adaptation can occur but often the accessory muscles are recruited during inspiration. By leaning forward the natural dome shape of the diaphragm is encouraged, improving its ability to contract (Figure 3.2).

Psychological Interventions

Psychological interventions for individuals with physical illness can support symptom management, illness-related anxiety, low mood, and treatment adherence. A comprehensive assessment informs a Bio-Psycho-Social formulation; a working hypothesis that identifies which biological, psychological, and social factors determine vulnerability to problems, triggers, or perpetuates them or prevents them getting worse (Engel, 1981). Mapping problems in this way emphasises the relationship between psychological and physical health, and the value of a multidisciplinary approach in respiratory health and exercise.

Mind-body links are often explored using evidence-based approaches including Cognitive Behaviour Therapy (CBT) (Figure 3.3), (Christie and Wilson, 2005); Acceptance and Commitment Therapy (ACT), (Hayes *et al.*, 2009), and Motivational Interviewing (MI) (Rollnick *et al.*, 2008). Psychoeducation about breathlessness, anxiety, and panic can help children and families understand the underlying physiological and psychological processes to improve awareness. Techniques including guided imagery and relaxation can help individuals tolerate unpleasant symptoms during exacerbations, exercise, or physiotherapy treatments. Anxious thoughts that cause early cessation of exercise can be managed through cognitive restructuring, defusion, or acceptance techniques. Behavioural interventions can target the vicious cycle of anxiety and avoidance, encourage planned and paced physical exertion, and invite individuals to commit their actions towards value-based, as opposed to goal-based living. Traditionally, psychological interventions have been provided in person to facilitate the therapeutic relationship. More recently, the value of telehealth and video sessions is being recognised to minimise cross infection in hospital settings, and reduce the financial, social, and educational impact of travelling to face-to-face appointments (Lang *et al.*, 2019).

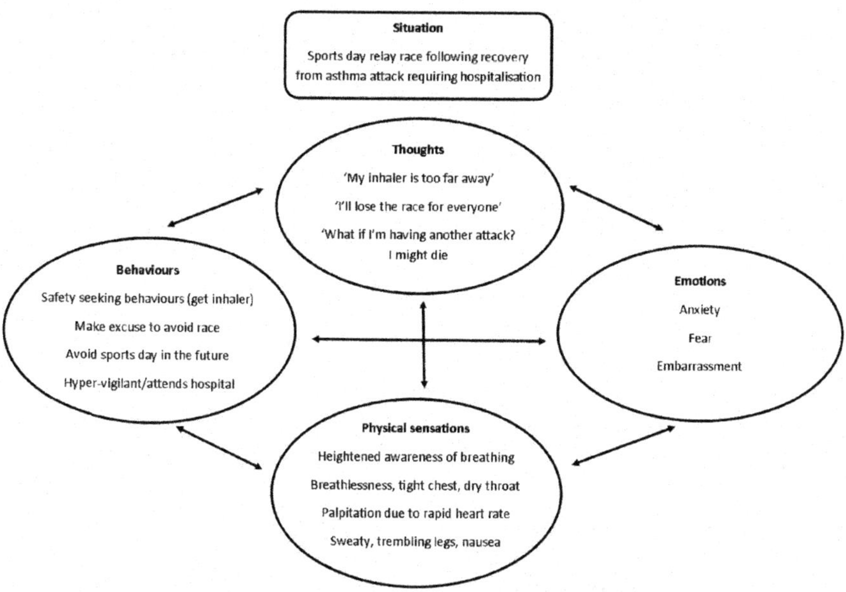
Situation
Sports day relay race following recovery from asthma attack requiring hospitalisation
Thoughts
'My inhaler is too far away'
'I'll lose the race for everyone'
'What if I'm having another attack? I might die
Behaviours
Safety seeking behaviours (get inhaler)
Make excuse to avoid race
Avoid sports day in the future
Hyper-vigilant/attends hospital
Emotions
Anxiety
Fear
Embarrassment
Physical sensations
Heightened awareness of breathing
Breathlessness, tight chest, dry throat
Palpitation due to rapid heart rate
Sweaty, trembling legs, nausea

Figure 3.3 A Cognitive Behaviour Therapy construct of psychological considerations in managing breathlessness in a child with asthma.

Symptom overlap can make it difficult to determine whether a child who presents with breathlessness and anxiety is overperceiving symptoms, suffering an exacerbation, or having a panic attack. Failing to distinguish the independent contribution of panic from a respiratory condition can have adverse consequences. The patient with asthma whose breathlessness is triggered by a panic attack may benefit from anxiolytics or talking therapy and may worsen if asthma treatments are escalated. Conversely, erroneously attributing breathlessness to panic could lead to potentially life-threatening illness. Psychologists in physical health and exercise settings are well placed to manage the anxiety of healthcare staff working with these challenges, to encourage reflection, peer supervision, and self-care. Knowing how to respond to breathlessness with either encouragement or caution can be confusing and may cause anxiety and moral uncertainty amongst carers.

Pharmacological Intervention and Respiratory Support Measures

Neuronal pathways involved in the perception of breathlessness may be modified by medications. Drugs to alter the perception of discomfort and anxiety can be considered and are primarily used in palliative care. The therapeutic usefulness of agents needs to be balanced against the risk of harm.

Low doses of opioids, such as morphine, can modify the perception of both pain and breathlessness whist simultaneously suppressing the cough reflex. Higher doses result in a progressive reduction in respiratory drive paralleling a reduction in conscious level. Thus, these actions are valuable in treating breathlessness in severe disease but tailoring the dose for different clinical scenarios can be challenging (Pieper *et al.*, 2018). Benzodiazepines, such as midazolam, have sedative and anxiolytic properties which can help to reduce breathlessness and distress, although high doses cause respiratory depression (Prommer, 2020). Bronchodilators such as salbutamol and theophylline are stimulants and can worsen anxiety especially if taken inappropriately for dysfunctional breathing or hyperventilation complicating respiratory illness.

In palliative care for advanced disease, supplemental oxygen via mask or nasal cannula does not relieve breathlessness in non-hypoxic patients (Davey and Pursell, 2015). Caregivers can overestimate benefit and underestimate risk associated with oxygen administration for breathlessness (Collier *et al.*, 2017). Non-invasive respiratory support such as continuous positive airway pressure (CPAP) can reduce the work of breathing and help reduce breathlessness although the benefits need to be balanced against the discomfort and physical restrictions associated with their application (Ringuier *et al.*, 2017).

Future Research

Despite the prevalence and impact of breathlessness in children, there is a poor evidence base to inform its management. While adult research has been helpful in some areas, child-specific research is needed, including diseases other than CF and asthma such as neuromuscular disorders. Further work is needed to improve the validity and reliability of subjective breathlessness rating scales and to determine their clinical significance. These need to be designed with a developmental perspective to be sensitive to the ways in which perception is modified through childhood and adolescence. Standardisation of exercise training is needed with research to determine what is effective, acceptable, and time efficient for children with respiratory disease and whether interventions that alter the perception or tolerance of breathlessness can improve adherence to such programs.

Conclusion

Breathlessness is a distressing symptom that can significantly impair the quality of life of children with respiratory conditions and limit their physical activity. The physiological, psychological, and social factors relevant to the assessment, diagnosis, and management of breathlessness in paediatric respiratory health and exercise settings are complex. Discordance between the objective assessment of breathlessness and the subjective experience of it can leave patients feeling misunderstood and lead to avoidance of physical activity, greater morbidity, overuse of medical services, and inappropriate interventions. A multi-disciplinary approach to assessment and management of breathlessness is advocated and must involve physiologists, clinicians, physiotherapists, and psychologists.

Key Points

- The experience of breathlessness is complex and multi-dimensional.
- Evidence supporting the assessment and treatment of breathlessness in children is sparse, with a lack of randomised controlled trials and systematic reviews. Most evidence has been drawn from adult studies or from a limited number of conditions.
- More valid and reliable tools to measure breathlessness in children are needed.
- The comprehensive assessment and management of breathlessness demands a multi-disciplinary approach, and this should be reflected in future research.

References

Barnes-Harris, M., Allgar, V., Booth, S., Currow, D., Hart, S., Phillips, J., Swan, F. and Johnson, M.J. (2019). Battery operated fan and chronic breathlessness: Does it help? *BMJ Supportive and Palliative Care* 9(4), 478–481. Doi: 10.1136/bmjspcare-2018-001749.

Barker, N.J., Jones, M., O'Connell, N.E. and Everard, M.L. (2013). Breathing exercises for dysfunctional breathing/hyperventilation syndrome in children. *Cochrane Database of Systematic Reviews* 12. Doi: 10.1002/14651858.CD010376.pub2.

Barker, N., Thevasagayam, R., Ugonna, K. and Kirkby, J. (2020). Pediatric dysfunctional breathing: Proposed components, mechanisms, diagnosis, and management. *Frontiers in Pediatrics* 8: 379. Doi: 10.3389/fped.2020.00379.

Bhatia, R., Abu-Hasan, M. and Weinberger, M. (2019). Exercise-induced dyspnea in children and adolescents: Differential diagnosis. *Pediatric Annals* 48(3), e121–e127. Doi: 10.3928/19382359-20190219-02.

Bott, J., Blumenthal, S., Buxton, M., Ellum, S., Falconer, C., Garrod, R., Harvey, A., Hughes, T., Lincoln, M., Mikelsons, C. and Potter, C. (2009). Guidelines for the physiotherapy management of the adult, medical, spontaneously breathing patient. *Thorax* 64(Suppl 1), i1–i52. Doi: 10.1136/thx.2008.110726.

Boulay, M.E. and Boulet, L.P. (2013). Discordance between asthma control clinical, physiological and inflammatory parameters in mild asthma. *Respiratory Medicine 107*(4), 511–518. Doi: 10.1016/j.rmed.2012.12.015.

Boulding, R., Stacey, R., Niven, R. and Fowler, S.J. (2016). Dysfunctional breathing: A review of the literature and proposal for classification. *European Respiratory Review* 25(141), 287–294. Doi: 10.1183/16000617.0088-2015.

Bouton, M.E., Mineka, S. and Barlow, D.H. (2001). A modern learning theory perspective on the etiology of panic disorder. *Psychological Review 108*(1), 4–32. Doi: 10.1037/0033-295X.108.1.4.

British Thoracic Society, Scottish Intercollegiate Guidelines Network (2019). British guideline on the management of asthma. SIGN 158. Available at: www.sign.ac.uk/assets/sign158.pdf.

Bruton, A., Lee, A., Yardley, L., Raftery, J., Arden-Close, E., Kirby, S., Zhu, S., Thiruvothiyur, M., Webley, F., Taylor, L. and Gibson, D. (2018). Physiotherapy breathing retraining for asthma: A randomised controlled trial. *The Lancet Respiratory Medicine* 6(1), 19–28. Doi: 10.1016/S2213-2600(17)30474-5.

Carel, H. (2018). Breathlessness: The rift between objective measurement and subjective experience. *The Lancet Respiratory Medicine* 6(5), 332–333. Doi: 10.1016/S2213-2600(18)30106-1.

Carrieri, V.K., Kieckhefer, G., Janson-Bjerklie, S. and Souza, J. (1991). The sensation of pulmonary dyspnea in school-age children. *Nursing Research* 40, 81–85. Doi: 10.1177/1479972308096710.

Christie, D. and Wilson, C. (2005). CBT in paediatric and adolescent health settings: A review of practice-based evidence. *Pediatric Rehabilitation* 8(4), 241–247. Doi: 10.1080/13638490500066622.

Collier, A., Breaden, K., Phillips, J.L., Agar, M., Litster, C. and Currow, D.C. (2017). Caregivers' perspectives on the use of long-term oxygen therapy for the treatment of refractory breathlessness: A qualitative study. *Journal of Pain and Symptom Management* 53(1), 33–39. Doi: 10.1016/j.jpainsymman.2016.06.007.

Connett, G.J. and Thomas, M. (2018). Dysfunctional breathing in children and adults with asthma. *Frontiers in Pediatrics* 6, 406. Doi:10.3389/fped.2018.00406.

Davey, C. and Pursell, J. (2015). Oxygen therapy: emergency use and long-term treatment. *Clinical Pharmacist* 7(5). Doi: 10.1211/CP.2015.20068717.

De Baets, F., Bodart, E., Dramaix-Wilmet, M., Van Daele, S., De Bilderling, G., Masset, S., Vermeire, P. and Michel, O. (2005). Exercise-induced respiratory symptoms are poor predictors of bronchoconstriction. *Pediatric Pulmonology* 39(4), 301–305. Doi: 10.1002/ppul.20185.

De Groot, E.P., Duiverman, E.J. and Brand, P.L., (2013). Dysfunctional breathing in children with asthma: A rare but relevant comorbidity. *European Respiratory Journal* 41(5), 1068–1073. Doi: 10.1183/09031936.00130212.

Depiazzi J. and Everard ML. (2016). Dysfunctional breathing and reaching one's physiological limit as causes of exercise-induced dyspnoea. *Breathe*, 12, 120–129. Doi: 10.1183/20734735.007216.

DSM-5, American Psychiatric Association. Edition, F. (2013). Diagnostic and statistical manual of mental disorders. *American Psychiatric Association*, 21. ISBN 978-0-89042-555-8.

Eggink, H., Brand, P., Reimink, R. and Bekhof, J. (2016). Clinical scores for dyspnoea severity in children: A prospective validation study. *PloS ONE*, 11(7). Doi: 10.1371/journal.pone.0157724.

Engel, G.L. (1981). The clinical application of the biopsychosocial model. *Journal of Medicine and Philosophy: A Forum for Bioethics and Philosophy of Medicine* 6(2), 101–124. Oxford University Press.

Feldman, J.M., McQuaid, E.L., Klein, R.B., Kopel, S.J., Nassau, J.H., Mitchell, D.K., Wamboldt, M.Z. and Fritz, G.K. (2007). Symptom perception and functional morbidity across a 1-year follow-up in pediatric asthma. *Pediatric Pulmonology* 42(4), 339–347. Doi: 10.1002/ppul.20584.

Feldman, J.M., Siddique, M.I, Thompson, N.S, Lehrer, P.M. (2009). The role of panic-fear in comorbid asthma and panic disorder. *Journal of Anxiety Disorders* 23(2), 178–184. Doi: 10.1016/j.janxdis.2008.06.005.

Fitzgerald, D.A. (2017). The weighty issue of obesity in paediatric respiratory medicine. *Paediatric Respiratory Reviews* 24, 4–7. Doi: 10.1016/j.prrv.2017.06.008.

Freitas, D.A., Holloway, E.A., Bruno, S.S., Chaves, G.S., Fregonezi, G.A. and Mendonca, K.M. (2013). Breathing exercises for adults with asthma. *Cochrane Database of Systematic Reviews* (10). Doi: 10.1002/14651858.CD001277.pub3.

Garrod R, Dallimore K, Cook J, Davis, V. Quade, K. (2005). An evaluation of the acute impact of pursed lips breathing on walking distance in nonspontaneous pursed lips breathing chronic obstructive pulmonary disease patients. *Chronic Respiratory Disease* 2, 67–72. Doi: 10.1191/1479972305cd068oa.

Haddad, F., Finocchiaro, G. and Myers, J. (2015). 3A. Personal history: Have you ever had excessive shortness of breath or fatigue with exercise beyond what is expected for your level of fitness? *Current Sports Medicine Reports* 14(3), 257–259. Doi: 10.1097/01.CSMR.0000465138.47875.3d.

Hallstrand, T.S., Bates, P.W. and Schoene, R.B. (2000). Aerobic conditioning in mild asthma decreases the hyperpnea of exercise and improves exercise and ventilatory capacity. *Chest* 118(5), 1460–1469. Doi:10.1378/chest.118.5.1460.

Hayen, A., Herigstad, M. and Pattinson, K.T. (2013). Understanding dyspnea as a complex individual experience. *Maturitas* 76(1), 45–50. Doi: 10.1016/j.maturitas.2013.06.005.

Hayes, S.C., Strosahl, K.D. and Wilson, K.G. (2009). *Acceptance and Commitment Therapy*. Washington, DC: American Psychological Association.

Herzog, M., Sucec, J., Van Diest, I., Van den Bergh, O., Chenivesse, C., Davenport, P., Similowski, T. and von Leupoldt, A. (2018). Observing dyspnoea in others elicits dyspnoea, negative affect and brain responses. *European Respiratory Journal* 51(4). Doi: 10.1183/13993003.02682-2017.

Holloway, E.A. and West, R.J. (2007). Integrated breathing and relaxation training (The Papworth Method) for adults with asthma in primary care: A randomised controlled trial. *Thorax* 62(12), 1039–1042. Doi: 10.1136/thx.2006.076430.

Horak, E., Grässl, G., Skladal, D. and Ulmer, H. (2003). Lung function and symptom perception in children with asthma and their parents. *Pediatric Pulmonology* 35(1), 23–28. Doi: 10.1002/ppul.10218.

Human, A., Corten, L., Jelsma, J. and Morrow, B. (2017). Inspiratory muscle training for children and adolescents with neuromuscular diseases: A systematic review. *Neuromuscular Disorders* 27(6), 503–517. Doi: 10.1016/j.nmd.2017.03.009.

Ikeda, K., Kawakami, K., Onimaru, H., Okada, Y., Yokota, S., Koshiya, N., Oku, Y., Iizuka, M. and Koizumi, H. (2017). The respiratory control mechanisms in the brainstem and spinal cord: Integrative views of the neuroanatomy and neurophysiology. *The Journal of Physiological Sciences* 67(1), 45–62. Doi: 10.1007/s12576-016-0475-y.

Janssens, T., De Peuter, S., Stans, L., Verleden, G., Troosters, T., Decramer, M. and Van den Bergh, O. (2011). Dyspnea perception in COPD: Association between anxiety, dyspnea-related fear, and dyspnea in a pulmonary rehabilitation program. *Chest* 140(3), 618–625. Doi: 10.1378/chest.10-3257.

Jones, N.L. (1995). Respiratory function during exercise. (1995). In: Brewis R.A.L., Corrin B., Geddes D.M., Gibson G.J. (eds), *Respiratory Medicine.* 2nd edn. London: WB Saunders, pp. 163–170.

Joschtel, B., Gomersall, S.R., Tweedy, S., Petsky, H., Chang, A.B. and Trost, S.G. (2018). Effects of exercise training on physical and psychosocial health in children with chronic respiratory disease: A systematic review and meta-analysis. *BMJ Open Sport and Exercise Medicine* 4(1). Doi: 10.1136/bmjsem-2018-000409.

Kaplan, A. and Price, D. (2020). Treatment adherence in adolescents with asthma. *Journal of Asthma and Allergy* 13, 39–49. Doi: 10.2147/JAA.S233268.

Lands, L.C. (2017). Dyspnea in children: What is driving it and how to approach it? *Paediatric respiratory reviews* 24, 29–31. Doi: 10.1016/j.prrv.2017.03.013.

Lang, R.L., Wilson, C., Stockton, K., Russell, T. and Johnston, L.M. (2019). CyFiT telehealth: Protocol for a randomised controlled trial of an online outpatient physiotherapy service for children with cystic fibrosis. *BMC Pulmonary Medicine* 19(1), 21. Doi: 10.1186/s12890-019-0784-z.

Lansing, R.W., Gracely, R.H. and Banzett, R.B. (2009). The multiple dimensions of dyspnea: Review and hypotheses. *Respiratory Physiology and Neurobiology* 167(1), 53–60. Doi: 10.1016/j.resp.2008.07.012.

Lumb, A.B. (2017). *Control of Breathing. Nunn's Applied Respiratory Physiology.* 8th edn. London, United Kingdom: Elsevier, pp. 51–72.

Macêdo, T.M., Freitas, D.A., Chaves, G.S., Holloway, E.A. and Mendonça, K.M. (2016). Breathing exercises for children with asthma. *Cochrane Database of Systematic Reviews* (4). Doi: 10.1002/14651858.

Macklem (2014). Mechanics of breathing: New insights from new technologies. In Aliverti, A. and Pedotti, A. (eds), *The Act of Breathing.* Verlag, Italia: Springer, pp. 3–9.

Martins, R., Assumpção, M.S., and Schivinski, C.I. (2014). Perceived exertion and dyspnea in pediatrics: a review of rating scales. *Medicina* (Ribeirão Preto) 47(1), 25–35. Doi: 10.11606/issn.2176-7262.v47i1p25-35.

McGrath, P.J., Pianosi, P.T., Unruh, A.M. and Buckley, C.P. (2005). Dalhousie dyspnea scales: Construct and content validity of pictorial scales for measuring dyspnea. *BMC Pediatrics*, 5(1), 33. Doi: 10.1186/1471-2431-5-33.

McQuaid, E.L., Koinis Mitchell, D., Walders, N., Nassau, J.H., Kopel, S.J., Klein, R.B., Wamboldt, M.Z. and Fritz, G.K. (2007). Pediatric asthma morbidity: The importance of symptom perception and family response to symptoms. *Journal of Pediatric Psychology* 32(2), 167–177. Doi: 10.1093/jpepsy/jsj112.

Mendonca, K.M., Freitas, D.A., Macedo, T.M., Silva, A.C., Amaral, C.T., Santino, T.A. and McKeown, P. (2017). Buteyko method for children with asthma: A randomized controlled trial. *American Thoracic Society.* https://www.atsjournals.org/doi/abs/10.1164/ajrccm-conference.2017.195.1_MeetingAbstracts.A2203.

Morgan, M. (2002). Dysfunctional breathing in asthma: Is it common, identifiable and correctable? *Thorax* 57(Suppl 2): ii31–ii35. PMID: 12364708.

Norweg, A. and Collins, E.G. (2013). Evidence for cognitive–behavioral strategies improving dyspnea and related distress in COPD. *International Journal of Chronic Obstructive Pulmonary Disease* 8, 439–451. Doi: 10.2147/COPD.S30145.

Parshall, M.B., Schwartzstein, R.M., Adams, L., Banzett, R.B., Manning, H.L., Bourbeau, J., Calverley, P.M., Gift, A.G., Harver, A., Lareau, S.C. and Mahler, D.A. (2012). An official American Thoracic Society statement: Update on the mechanisms, assessment, and management of dyspnea. *American Journal of Respiratory and Critical Care Medicine* 185(4), 435–452. Doi:10.1164/rccm.201111-2042ST.

Peiffer, C. (2008). Dyspnea and emotion: What can we learn from functional brain imaging? *American Journal of Respiratory and Critical Care Medicine* 177(9), 937–939. Doi: 10.1164/rccm.200802-298ED.

Pianosi, P.T., Huebner, M., Zhang, Z., Turchetta, A. and McGrath, P.J. (2015). Dalhousie pictorial scales measuring dyspnea and perceived exertion during exercise for children and adolescents. *Annals of the American Thoracic Society* 12(5), 718–726. Doi: 10.1513/annalsats.201410-477oc.

Pieper, L., Zernikow, B., Drake, R., Frosch, M., Printz, M. and Wager, J. (2018). Dyspnea in children with life-threatening and life-limiting complex chronic conditions. *Journal of Palliative Medicine* 21(4), 552–564. Doi: 10.1089/jpm.2017.0240.

Prasad, S.A., Randall, S.D. and Balfour-Lynn, I.M. (2000). Fifteen-count breathlessness score: An objective measure for children. *Pediatric Pulmonology* 30(1), 56–62. Doi: 10.1002/1099-0496.

Prommer, E. (2020). Midazolam: An essential palliative care drug. *Palliative Care and Social Practice* 14, Doi: 10.1177/2632352419895527.

Radtke, T., Nevitt, S.J., Hebestreit, H. and Kriemler, S. (2017). Physical exercise training for cystic fibrosis. *Cochrane Database of Systematic Reviews* (11). Doi: 10.1002/14651858.CD002768.pub4.

Rao, R.P. and Ballard, D.H. (1999). Predictive coding in the visual cortex: A functional interpretation of some extra-classical receptive-field effects. *Nature Neuroscience* 2(1), 79–87. Doi: 10.1038/4580.

Reid, W.D., Geddes, E.L., O'Brien, K., Brooks, D. and Crowe, J. (2008). Effects of inspiratory muscle training in cystic fibrosis: A systematic review. *Clinical Rehabilitation* 22(10–11), 1003–1013. Doi: 10.1177/0269215508090619.

Reuveny, R., DiMenna, F.J., Gunaratnam, C., Arad, A.D., McElvaney, G.N., Susta, D., Peled, M. and Moyna, N.M. (2020). High-intensity interval training accelerates oxygen uptake kinetics and improves exercise tolerance for individuals with cystic fibrosis. *BMC Sports Science, Medicine and Rehabilitation* 12, 1–13. Doi: 10.1186/s13102-020-0159-z.

Rhee, H., Belyea, M.J. and Halterman, J.S. (2011). Adolescents' perception of asthma symptoms and health care utilization. *Journal of Pediatric Health Care* 25(2), 105–113. Doi: 10.1016/j.pedhc.2009.10.003.

Rietveld, S., Kolk, A.M. and Prins, P.J. (1996). The influence of lung function information on self-reports of dyspnea by children with asthma. *Journal of Pediatric Psychology* 21(3), 367–377. Doi: 10.1093/jpepsy/21.3.367.

Rietveld, S., Kolk, A.M., Prins, P.J. and Colland, V.T. (1997). The influence of respiratory sounds on breathlessness in children with asthma: a symptom-perception approach. *Health Psychology* 16(6), 547. Doi 10.1037/0278-6133.16.6.547.

Rietveld, S. and Prins, P.J. (1998). The relationship between negative emotions and acute subjective and objective symptoms of childhood asthma. *Psychological Medicine* 28(2), 407–415. Doi: 10.1017/s0033291797006387.

Ringuier, B., Troussier, F., Boussicault, G., Chapotte, C. and Rachieru, P. (2017). Non-invasive ventilation and pediatric palliative care. A French survey. *Archives de Pediatrie: Organe Officiel de la Societe Francaise de Pediatrie* 24(8), 712–719. Doi: 10.1016/j.arcped.2017.05.007.

Robertson, R.J., Goss, F.L., Boer, N.F., Peoples, J.A., Foreman, A.J., Dabayebeh, I.M., Millich, N.B., Balasekaran, G., Riechman, S.E., Gallagher, J.D. And Thompkins, T. (2000). Children's OMNI scale of perceived exertion: Mixed gender and race validation. *Medicine and Science in Sports and Exercise* 32(2), 452–458. Doi: 10.1097/00005768-200002000-00029.

Rollnick, S., Miller, W.R. and Butler, C. (2008). *Motivational Interviewing in Health Care: Helping Patients Change Behaviour.* New York: Guilford Press.

Santino, T.A., Chaves, G.S., Freitas, D.A., Fregonezi, G.A. and Mendonça, K.M. (2020). Breathing exercises for adults with asthma. *Cochrane Database of Systematic Reviews* (3). Doi: 10.1002/14651858.CD001277.pub4.

Scano, G., Stendardi, L. and Grazzini, M. (2005). Understanding dyspnoea by its language. *European Respiratory Journal* 25(2), 380–385. Doi: 10.1183/09031936.05.00059404.

Schweitzer, C. and Marchal, F. (2009). Dyspnoea in children. Does development alter the perception of breathlessness? *Respiratory Physiology and Neurobiology* 167(1), 144–153. Doi: 10.1016/j.resp.2008.12.001.

Stoeckel, M.C., Esser, R.W., Gamer, M., Büchel, C. and von Leupoldt, A. (2016). Brain responses during the anticipation of dyspnea. *Neural Plasticity.* Doi: 10.1155/2016/6434987.

Takken, T., Sonbahar Ulu, H. and Hulzebos, E.H. (2020). Clinical recommendations for cardiopulmonary exercise testing in children with respiratory diseases. *Expert Review of Respiratory Medicine*, 1–11. Doi: 10.1080/17476348.2020.1752195.

Thomas, M., McKinley, R.K., Freeman, E., Foy, C. and Price, D. (2005). The prevalence of dysfunctional breathing in adults in the community with and without asthma. *Primary Care Respiratory Journal* 14(2), 78–82. Doi: 10.1016/j.pcrj.2004.10.007.

van Gent, R., van Essen-Zandvliet, L.E.M., Rovers, M.M., Kimpen, J.L., deMeer, G., van der Ent, C.K. (2007). Poor perception of dyspnoea in children with undiagnosed asthma. *European Respiratory Journal* 30, 887–891. Doi: 10.1183/09031936.00031407.

von Leupoldt, A., Riedel, F. and Dahme, B. (2006). The impact of emotions on the perception of dyspnea in pediatric asthma. *Psychophysiology* 43(6), 641–644. Doi: 10.1111/j.1469-8986.2006.00453.

von Leupoldt, A., Sommer, T., Kegat, S., Baumann, H.J., Klose, H., Dahme, B. and Büchel, C. (2009). Dyspnea and pain share emotion-related brain network. *Neuroimage* 48(1), 200–206. Doi: 10.1016/j.neuroimage.2009.06.015.

Weinberger, M. and Abu-Hasan, M. (2007). Pseudo-asthma: when cough, wheezing, and dyspnea are not asthma. *Pediatrics* 120(4), 855–864. Doi: 10.1542/peds.2007-0078.

Welsh, L., Kemp, J.G. and Roberts, R.G. (2005). Effects of physical conditioning on children and adolescents with asthma. *Sports Medicine* 35(2), 127–141. Doi: 10.2165/00007256-200535020-00003.

Wilson, R.C. and Jones, P.W. (1990). Influence of prior ventilatory experience on the estimation of breathlessness during exercise. *Clinical Science* 78(2), 149–153. Doi: 10.1042/cs0780149.

Woodgate, R. (2009). The experience of dyspnea in school-age children with asthma. *MCN: The American Journal of Maternal/Child Nursing* 34(3), 154–161. Doi: 10.1097/01.NMC.0000351702.58632.9e.

Zachariasse, J.M., Nieboer, D., Maconochie, I.K., Smit, F.J., Alves, C.F., Greber-Platzer, S., Tsolia, M.N., Steyerberg, E.W., Avillach, P., van der Lei, J. and Moll, H.A. (2020). Development and validation of a Paediatric Early Warning Score for use in the emergency department: A multicentre study. *The Lancet Child & Adolescent Health* 4(8), 583–591. Doi: 10.1016/S2352-4642(20)30139-5.

Zahran, H.S., Bailey, C.M., Damon, S.A., Garbe, P.L. and Breysse, P.N. (2018). Vital signs: Asthma in children—United States, 2001–2016. *Morbidity and Mortality Weekly Report* 67(5), 149. Doi: 10.15585/mmwr.mm6705e1.

Zar, H.J. and Ferkol, T.W. (2014). The global burden of respiratory disease—impact on child health. *Pediatric Pulmonology* 49(5), 430–434. Doi: 10.1002/ppul.23030.

4 Towards a Comprehensive Assessment of Physical Function in Young People with Cystic Fibrosis and Non-cystic Fibrosis Bronchiectasis

Zoe Saynor, Donald Urquhart, Thomas Radtke, Melitta McNarry, and Mathieu Gruet

Introduction

Bronchiectasis is associated with considerable morbidity, exercise intolerance, and may negatively impact quality of life. Typically, a distinction is made between bronchiectasis caused by cystic fibrosis (CF) and non-CF bronchiectasis. CF is the most common cause of childhood bronchiectasis and the most well studied with regards to exercise. The clinical utility of evaluating the physical function of people with CF is well-recognised, with certain tests demonstrating functional and prognostic value. However, despite clinical similarities between these diseases, the study, and utility of exercise evaluations in people with non-CF bronchiectasis are less established. Following insight into how the pathophysiology of childhood bronchiectasis may affect a child's ability to exercise, this chapter provides a contemporary review of best practice recommendations to comprehensively evaluate the physical function of children with bronchiectasis.

Paediatric Bronchiectasis

Originally described in 1819, bronchiectasis is a chronic lung disease caused by chronic airway infection and inflammation. Mucus accumulation in the airways and persistent inflammation cause structural damage to the bronchial walls, leading to permanent dilation and scarring (O'Donnell, 2018). The extent and severity of these anatomical changes are confirmed using high-resolution computed tomography thoracic imaging. Bronchiectasis is heterogeneous, with variable aetiologies and wide-ranging disease severities. It is impacted by the degree of lung involvement, microbiological changes, and co-morbidities (O'Donnell, 2018). Distinction is typically made between the bronchiectasis caused by CF and all other presentations, which include genetic abnormalities, immunologic conditions, autoimmune diseases, obstructing airway lesions, or chronic aspiration. Indeed, the aetiology in the majority of children with non-CF bronchiectasis is thought to be prior

DOI: 10.4324/9781003020462-4

infection although many are considered idiopathic. CF remains, however, the most common cause of bronchiectasis in childhood.

There are reportedly 70,000 people with CF worldwide, of which ~40% are ≤16 years of age. CF is an inherited disorder caused by mutations in a single gene on the long arm of chromosome 7 that encodes for a complex protein; cystic fibrosis transmembrane conductance regulator (CFTR), important for trans-epithelial chloride transport. CF mutations render the epithelial membrane relatively impermeable to the chloride ion, adversely, but variably affecting many organ systems, including the lungs, upper airway, pancreas, liver, intestine, and reproductive organs.

The story of CF over the past 75 years is truly remarkable and inspiring. From the original description of the disease, causing death in early life (Andersen, 1938), to the elucidation of the basic physiological defect and identification of the CF gene. Improved understanding of the pathophysiology of this disease with innovation and improvement in medical care have contributed to median survival rising to 40 years today. In the UK, mortality rates decreased annually by 2% between 2006 and 2015, with median survival from birth in Phe508-del homozygotes currently 46 years for men and 41 years for women (Keogh *et al.*, 2018). Similar decline in mortality rates has been reported in the United States (MacKenzie *et al.*, 2014). If mortality continues to drop at the same rate, reports suggest that men and women with CF will soon have median life expectancies of 65 and 56 years, respectively (Keogh *et al.*, 2018).

CFTR modulator therapy looks set to dramatically change the clinical course of those fortunate enough to receive it, however, people with CF will continue to need close, lifelong follow-up and careful monitoring. Whilst the improvement in life expectancy associated with CF represents a major medical achievement, an ageing CF population brings new challenges, including CF-related diabetes (CFRD), bone disease, and CF-associated arthritis. Obesity is another key consideration for the future; successful comprehensive multidisciplinary care addressing CF-related nutritional complications has been accompanied by a significant rise in overweight and obese children and adults with CF.

High-quality paediatric care is the foundation for a long and healthy life with CF, within which exercise is considered an essential component. It is vital that CF healthcare providers adapt to meet both the existing and emerging needs of this population, as well as young people with non-CF bronchiectasis, for whom few clear standards for clinical exercise testing exist.

Exercise Testing in Paediatric Bronchiectasis

Why?

As noted in Chapter 2, exercise stress testing provides unique insights into physiological changes that are not detectable from more static measures.

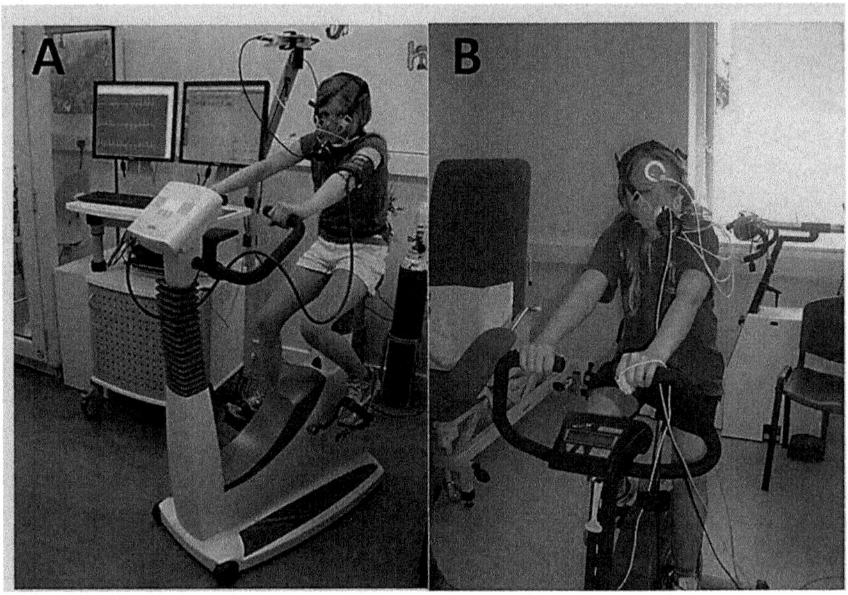

Figure 4.1 An illustration of children with cystic fibrosis performing cycle-based cardiopulmonary exercise testing using electrocardiography (A) or thoracic impedance cardiography (B) to assess cardiac function during exercise.

Note: The child in panel B is exercising on the pediatric specific Baby Lode ergometer and has pediatric specific electrode placement.

Comprehensive cardiopulmonary exercise testing (CPET) offers an integrated, objective assessment of the efficiency and performance of the cardiovascular, respiratory, and musculoskeletal systems, see Figure 4.1. Exercise testing is also needed to identify exercise-related adverse events, such as hypoxaemia or arrhythmias. Appropriate exercise testing can also assess interval changes in clinical status (Urquhart and Saynor, 2018), with several CPET outcome measures demonstrating prognostic value in CF (Nixon *et al.*, 1992, Pianosi *et al.*, 2005, Hebestreit *et al.*, 2019) – such that tests identifying poor exercise capacity relative to lung function act as an early warning of decline prompting further assessment and intervention. Despite comparably less literature concerning exercise testing in non-CF childhood bronchiectasis, the British Thoracic Society guidelines suggest that exercise tests have a key role in investigating children in whom symptoms are incongruent with lung function or high-resolution computed tomography measurements, which unlike exercise testing involves ionising radiation.

It is important to highlight the wealth of information that comprehensive exercise testing can provide. Specifically, not only can it provide information regarding an individual's functional ability but also the underpinning mechanism(s) responsible, see Figure 4.2. It is therefore unsurprising that it is being increasingly used as an endpoint for clinical trials. Exercise testing can also

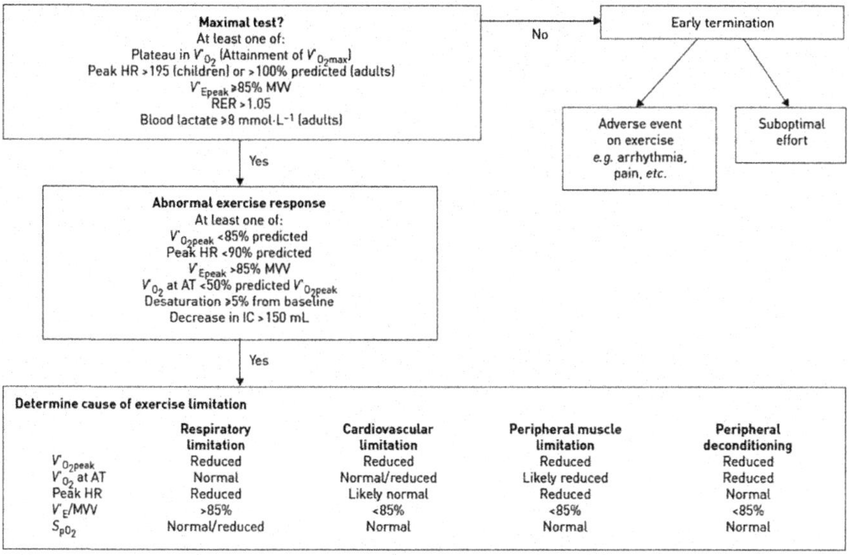

Figure 4.2 Schematic overview of how to determine whether a maximal effort has been given during a cardiopulmonary exercise testing and the cause(s) of any exercise limitation.

Source: Radtke *et al.*, (2019); with permission.

be empowering, demonstrating that a child can exercise at a higher intensity than expected, freeing them from personal uncertainty and/or parental fears (Urquhart and Saynor, 2018). High-intensity exercise can, however, also trigger negative emotions in some individuals, particularly those who fear breathlessness. Effort should therefore be made to promote enjoyment. Finally, comprehensive, appropriate evaluation of physical function facilitates the development of individualised exercise programmes.

Who?

The most recent European statement, endorsed by the European Respiratory Society (ERS), recommends exercise testing for all people with CF ≥10 years of age (Hebestreit *et al.*, 2015), although the age at which regular routine testing begins should also consider the type of test being undertaken and the physical and cognitive capabilities of the child. This age is primarily a guide for those undertaking CPET on a cycle ergometer, since participants must be able to reach the pedals (minimum height 128 cm for many ergometers) and maintain a set pedalling speed, which some children find difficult. However, valid CPET has been performed in children from six years of age and paediatric cycle ergometers (see Figure 4.1), and treadmill safety harnesses make it possible to test smaller children. While technically acceptable tests can be achieved in younger children, the introduction to ergometer testing helps familiarise them with procedures, providing motivation and guidance for exercise participation. For younger children (6–9 years) who are not able to use ergometry, validated field-based tests are suitable, several of which are discussed in Chapter 2. Although guidance has to date focused on chronological age for testing, in the future considering biological age will be valuable.

When?

At least annual exercise testing is internationally recommended for all people with CF (Hebestreit *et al.*, 2015) ideally undertaken at a similar time to the clinical annual review. Additionally, appropriate and relevant exercise testing should be undertaken before and after any significant intervention(s), e.g., a new treatment or exercise programme. In people with more severe lung disease, exercise testing plays a valuable role in pre-transplant assessment.

Potential Contributors to Impaired Physical Function

The disordered physiological processes that are associated with both CF and non-CF bronchiectasis have the potential to profoundly alter a young person's exercise physiology, even if they are physically active. The knowledge concerning the contribution of pulmonary, muscular, and cardiovascular impairments to this are outlined below.

Pulmonary Contributors

In an era of increased life expectancy and new treatments, children and adolescents with CF may have similar, or even sometimes greater, exercise capacity than their healthy peers. However, several pathophysiological and lifestyle factors may still contribute to reduced fitness in young people with CF (Figure 4.2). In mild disease, ventilatory limitation is often not observed during exercise; even at exhaustion. However, as lung disease progresses, ventilatory limitation during exercise is common, with multifaceted causes. Specifically, dead space increases as lung disease progresses and is exacerbated during exercise, requiring a higher minute ventilation (Urquhart and Saynor, 2018). Additionally, airway obstruction due to mucus within the airways (+/− airway hyper-reactivity) may be present, requiring greater inspiratory airflows generated by greater respiratory muscle effort to achieve the required ventilation rate. However, as strategies to treat the pulmonary manifestations of CF improve, children and adolescents are likely to be limited by non-pulmonary factors.

Muscular Contributors

Reduced muscle mass and muscle strength, particularly in the lower limbs, is common in people with CF. Muscle weakness can have a significant impact on exercise tolerance and the capacity to undertake the activities of daily living (Troosters *et al.*, 2009). Although physical inactivity may play a key role in this, it cannot solely explain these changes. Additional factors known to contribute to skeletal muscle dysfunction in chronic respiratory disease include inflammation, metabolic abnormalities, and/or oxidative stress.

Specific to CF, other structural and functional changes are evident. CFTR is expressed in skeletal muscle cells (Lamhonwah *et al.*, 2010) and lack of CFTR has been shown to predispose mice with CF to muscle wasting and diaphragm muscle pump failure (Divangahi *et al.*, 2009). Furthermore, reduced antioxidant capacity, due to increased systemic inflammation and/or oxidative damage, which has been shown to characterise individuals with CF even when clinically stable (Causer *et al.*, 2020), may also lower mitochondrial efficiency (Valdivieso and Santa-Coloma, 2013) and contribute to peripheral muscle dysfunction. A pro-inflammatory state in CF may also promote muscle catabolism. However, evidence supporting reduced respiratory muscle strength remains equivocal and so the debate regarding the contribution of CF-specific factors to muscle dysfunction remains open.

Cardiovascular Contributors

Bronchiectasis is associated with an increased risk of cardiovascular disease, which may link to specific markers of severity, including pulmonary exacerbation frequency and the degree of lung function impairment. Whilst this excess risk is likely causally linked to increased systemic inflammation, bronchiectasis caused by CF may present additional risk factors. CFTR is involved in the regulation of cardiomyocyte contraction (Sellers *et al.*, 2010), suggesting that there may be a direct effect of CF on cardiac function itself (Labombarda *et al.*, 2016). Adding to previously scattered reports of cardiac abnormalities in people with CF, recent evidence suggests early indications of potential myocardial impairment in children/adolescents with mild CF lung disease (Giacchi *et al.*, 2015), although exercise-induced cardiac arrhythmias are very rare in children and adolescents with CF (Ruf *et al.*, 2010).

Micro- and macrovascular endothelial perturbations have also been reported in young people with CF (Poore *et al.*, 2013, Rodriguez-Miguelez *et al.*, 2016), and show weak to moderately strong associations with aerobic fitness. Although questions remain regarding the mechanisms underlying these changes, CFTR has been implicated. CFTR is expressed in human endothelial cells in the lung microvascular circulation (Tousson *et al.*, 1998), umbilical vein (Tousson *et al.*, 1998), and pulmonary arteries (Plebani *et al.*, 2017, Totani *et al.*, 2017) with a functional role reported in pulmonary endothelial cells (Khalaf *et al.*, 2020). Despite recent pharmacological advances in the medical management of CF, it is still likely that as individuals with CF and non-CF bronchiectasis live longer, more will enter the age range where cardiovascular abnormalities become apparent and may suffer cardiovascular complications, making assessment of cardiac activity and the haemodynamic response to exercise important.

Additional Mediators

A recent report published by the American Heart Association (AHA), (Raghuveer *et al.*, 2020), suggested that the time spent sedentary makes up as much as 75% of a 15-year old's waking hours, which between 2003 and 2016 increased from a mean of 7–8.2 hours per day in adolescents in England and the United States. Children with a chronic condition may further restrict their physical activity (PA) as a consequence of real or perceived limitations imposed by their condition. Indeed, the environmental and social factors contributing to inactivity (e.g., increased *'screen time'*) and the increased prevalence of obesity in otherwise healthy children are similarly at work in children with chronic disease and disability, contributing to the significant rise in overweight and obesity in children (Hanna and Weiner, 2015) and adults (Harindhanavudhi *et al.*, 2020, Stephenson *et al.*, 2013) with CF.

Risks of Exercise Testing

Although exercise testing in CF is generally safe, it is pertinent to be aware of potential risks. In people with CF, adverse events such as cardiac arrhythmias, pneumothorax, and hypoglycaemia associated with exercise are possible, but reportedly occur in less than 1% of ~1,000 from a survey of 37 CF centres across Germany (Ruf *et al.*, 2010). However, contraindications to exercise do exist and may be absolute or relative, and can depend on the individual's clinical status, i.e., be more common in people with more advanced disease and/or additional complications such as CF-related diabetes (CFRD). Infection control is also an important consideration when undertaking exercise testing in people with CF.

Motivation and Volition during Exercise Testing

Verbal encouragement is commonly used to motivate individuals to enhance effort investment during maximal exercise testing. In children, however, motivation and volition are more challenging, as intrinsic motivation and time awareness are still developing. Most children can be motivated to exercise to exhaustion, but it requires skill and experience from the practitioner. Time should be taken to gain this experience, since verbal encouragement can improve performance during exercise testing. Personality differences between individuals should be considered, since these influence the effects of verbal encouragement on motivation. Appropriate familiarisation with the testing environment, equipment, and requirements can help, as well as using age-appropriate language and contextualising the testing in relation to personal functional goals. For individuals who are particularly breathless during exercise, additional support may be needed to facilitate testing.

What Test?

Physical fitness is a multidimensional construct and there is no single, standardised approach to clinical exercise testing in children and adolescents. It is important to consider that some assessments are most suitable for laboratory-based research and others for clinical practice. Tests employed may differ or be adapted depending on the indication for testing, the individual's age, fitness level, and exercise interests. CPET alone does not reflect the entire exercise testing toolkit and single exercise tests may not fully reflect day-to-day activities. Considering both time and cost constraints, we cannot test everything in everybody. However, given that people with CF are living longer and children in particular are fitter than ever, it is important to consider the needs and sporting interests of the individual as well as providing an appropriate level of challenge.

Most physiological assessments performed on athletes can also be performed on children with disease (Wells and Norris, 2009). For the assessment of physical function to inform an individualised physical training programme for a young person with bronchiectasis, particularly those who do not have ventilatory limitation, multi-modal, and perhaps safe and appropriate sport-specific, modalities of exercise testing should be considered. Multimodal assessments of aerobic fitness, muscle function, and other components of physical fitness using reproducible tests represent an important next step in our exercise testing practices for children and adolescents with bronchiectasis.

Aerobic Fitness

Aerobic fitness refers to the capacity of the circulatory and respiratory systems to supply oxygen to skeletal muscle mitochondria for energy production needed during PA. Low aerobic fitness is a strong, independent predictor of poor cardio-metabolic health and premature cardiovascular disease (Högström *et al.*, 2014), greater total adiposity (Lee and Arslanian, 2007), lower academic achievement (Santana *et al.*, 2017), and mental health problems (Lubans *et al.*, 2016). To date, much of the focus of exercise testing in youth with bronchiectasis has been on the evaluation of aerobic fitness, given its association with survival (Nixon *et al.*, 1992, Pianosi *et al.*, 2005, Hebestreit *et al.*, 2019) and hospitalisation risk in CF (Pérez *et al.*, 2014). The highest oxygen uptake attained during a graded maximal exercise test to volitional exhaustion ($\dot{V}O_{2peak}$) is considered the single best indicator of aerobic fitness.

As noted in Chapter 2, tests of aerobic fitness range from comprehensive laboratory CPETs to '*field*' tests.

Cardiopulmonary Exercise Testing (CPET)

Incremental CPET is a maximal progressive exercise test that can be performed with or without gas analysis. The best practice recommendations for people with CF involves standardised cycle or treadmill protocols to exhaustion, while measuring oxygen consumption, pulse oximetry, and electrocardiography (ECG) throughout exercise and into recovery (Hebestreit *et al.*, 2015). When testing children, equipment should be appropriately sized (Takken *et al.*, 2020) if necessary, with a paediatric cycle ergometer. Treadmills do not have a height limit, but a harness may be used, however this must not restrict chest expansion.

As shown in Chapter 2, there are significant logistical considerations to be made with regards to exercise modality (e.g., cycle vs. treadmill) and protocol (e.g., 'step' vs. 'ramp'). Irrespective of the protocol chosen, CPET should involve progressive increases in work rate with the endpoints of either volitional exhaustion, the appearance of clinical signs and symptoms (e.g., hypoxaemia, dizziness, chest pain), or a predetermined submaximal endpoint (e.g., 85% of age-predicted heart rate). It is generally recommended that the test should last 8–12 minutes, a duration needed to examine responses to exercise but short enough to avoid undue fatigue, or perhaps boredom. For younger children though, 6–10 minutes may be more realistic. When a low $\dot{V}O_{2peak}$ is anticipated due to clinical concerns, it is important that smaller work rate increments are utilised to avoid premature termination of the test with failure to achieve a true maximal effort.

Irrespective of exercise modality, a brief resting period before initiation of exercise should be included to allow the participant to familiarise themselves with the testing apparatus and resting measurements to be taken. Resting measures, especially the respiratory exchange ratio, can be particularly useful for identifying individuals who may be demonstrating an anticipatory hyperventilatory response prior to exercise and is common when a mouthpiece/face mask is fitted. Data can be compared with that obtained during maximal effort in order to assist interpretation.

Outside of the clinical annual review, other modalities of CPET may be considered for children and adolescents who regularly participate in and enjoy different sports. Physiological assessment equipment continues to become smaller and more portable, meaning that clinicians and exercise physiologists can now evaluate physiological function in more realistic *'field'* situations with laboratory quality measurements. Testing children outdoors using a mobile cardiopulmonary exercise unit worn in a backpack represents an alternative to standard treadmill testing and an example of a water-based CPET in an adolescent swimmer with CF who did not enjoy or feel motivated by her cycle test is presented in Figure 4.3. New technologies are now available to augment physiological measurements during CPET; including non-invasive measurements of cardiac output (e.g., PhysioFlow) and muscle oxygenation (near-infrared spectroscopy), see Figure 4.1B.

It is acknowledged that CPET can be time-consuming and costly, due to the requirement of trained exercise scientists and specialised equipment. CPET may be performed without gas analysis in lieu of the gold standard (Hebestreit *et al.*, 2015). Additionally, the Steep Ramp Test (SRT) provides

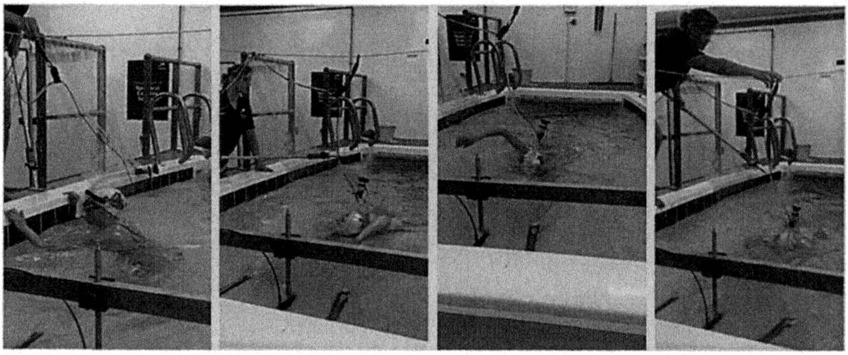

Figure 4.3 An illustration of a child with cystic fibrosis performing swimming-based cardiopulmonary exercise testing.

as a less sophisticated and time-intensive incremental exercise test without respiratory gas analysis (Bongers and Takken, 2014). The SRT is completed to maximal exertion on a cycle ergometer, with the attained W_{peak} being its primary outcome measure. In children and adolescents with CF, comparable $\dot{V}O_{2peak}$ values have been reported when compared to CPET (Werkman *et al.*, 2011). However, if access to a cycle ergometer and trained examiner remains limited, a field test may be chosen (Hebestreit *et al.*, 2015, Lang *et al.*, 2020).

Field Tests

Non-laboratory or field tests of aerobic fitness include shuttle and step tests. These are logistically easier to perform as they are usually portable and require less formalised equipment, as highlighted in Chapter 2. Simple field tests of aerobic fitness cannot replace a full CPET, but they are often used as an alternative to assess both functional capacity and treatment effects. Traditional shuttle and step tests are outlined in Chapter 2, however several new step tests for children with bronchiectasis are in development.

The iStep test is an incremental step test developed for children with CF, and early evidence suggests it is valid and feasible (Rand *et al.*, 2015), demonstrating a near-maximal physiological response in 66% of participants. However, a ceiling effect may exist for fitter patients. The Chester Step Test (CST) is a 10-minute submaximal standardised multistage test that was originally designed for workplace screening and is now widely used for exercise prescription in the UK cardiac population, albeit commonly in adults. The CST is reproducible in chronic obstructive pulmonary disease and reliable in people with bronchiectasis and, since it is often too strenuous for people with more severe lung disease (de Camargo *et al.*, 2011, Camargo *et al.*, 2013), it may be useful for the fitter children. Finally, as part of a small feasibility study, Button and Wilson developed The Alfred or *'A-Step'* test. Although there are no published reviews, the proposed test will allow for early detection of declines in physical function in the day-to-day clinical setting. This test is an incremental, maximal, externally paced step test with a protocol suitable for adults with CF, which is applicable to all levels of fitness and disease states and is in line with current exercise testing recommendations.

Anaerobic Fitness

The anaerobic glycolytic system is the primary energy system involved in shorter activities of high intensity and is critically important for events lasting more than a few seconds through to several minutes (e.g., sprint running, many swimming events, and track cycling sprint events), as well as for most team sports that require bursts of high-intensity activity (e.g., basketball, volleyball, soccer, hockey). Typically, children demonstrate greater resistance to the muscular fatigue often associated with high-intensity exercise than adults; however, children with chronic disease may have a reduced anaerobic fitness compared to their healthy peers.

In the laboratory setting, anaerobic fitness is usually measured using the Wingate test. This involves a 30-second all-out test on a cycle ergometer and is feasible in children with CF (Boas *et al.*, 1996). Performance on Wingate testing is reportedly reduced in youth with CF, with most of the variance explained by reduced fat-free mass. One of the drawbacks of this test is that it requires a specialised ergometer and software. Anaerobic fitness can also be tested more functionally using various indoor and outdoor field tests. Such tests may better reflect day-to-day activities and include the 30-second and 1-minute sit-to-stand test (STS1'), the vertical jump, triple hop distance, and stair climbing power tests, all of which have been used in young adults with CF (Gruet *et al.*, 2016b, Radtke *et al.*, 2016, Sheppard *et al.*, 2019).

STS1' testing is increasingly being used in respiratory disease as a simple functional test which predominantly measures anaerobic capacity. The primary outcome of this test is the number of repetitions that can be performed within the time limit (1 minute) and has demonstrated strong associations with W_{peak} derived from a CPET in CF adults (Radtke *et al.*, 2016). However, in most people with CF, particularly younger adults, STS1' performance is often near that of healthy controls (Gruet *et al.*, 2016b, Radtke *et al.*, 2016), highlighting the lack of sensitivity of the STS1' to detect functional alterations in the fitter CF individuals. This ceiling effect may be problematic in the paediatric CF population and it can be reasonably expected that this test may not provide a sufficient challenge. It is also important to consider that while jumping, cycling, sprinting, and STS test performance may represent interesting markers of anaerobic capacity in people with CF, they are also dependent on subject abilities (e.g., balance, coordination) and may be liable to a significant learning effect (Radtke *et al.*, 2016). It thus seems premature to use these tests as a valid surrogate of limb muscle function, and important measurements such as muscle strength and endurance should be measured directly.

Localised Muscle Function Testing

Muscle function is a broad term that encompasses different variables such as strength, endurance, and fatigability. From a scientific perspective, strength is a specific construct that refers to the ability of a muscle (single or group) to produce measurable force, torque, or moment, about a single joint or multiple joints, under a defined set of controlled conditions. Muscle strength is a multifaceted, performance-related, fitness component, which is underpinned by muscular, neural, and mechanical factors, as well as motivation. Although, as outlined earlier in this chapter, many aspects of childhood bronchiectasis may contribute to impaired muscle function, influencing measures of respiratory and peripheral muscle strength or endurance. To date, such consequences have been somewhat overlooked in the clinical assessment of people with bronchiectasis. Whilst practical issues such as the availability of size-appropriate equipment may influence testing method selection, a variety of options to assess both peripheral and respiratory muscles are available.

Peripheral Muscle

Methods to assess localised peripheral muscle function in children include isokinetic dynamometry, custom-built chairs with strain gauges, and hand-held dynamometry. Computerised dynamometry is generally considered the gold standard method to assess isometric limb muscle strength. It is also useful in evaluating local muscle endurance and fatigability from isokinetic protocols (e.g., repetition of maximal voluntary contractions at a given angular velocity; usually ranging from 60 to $300°\cdot s^{-1}$) (Evans *et al.*, 2015), although the clinimetric properties of these tests are yet to be assessed in people with CF. If computerised dynamometry is unavailable due to technical or cost limitations, strain gauge measurements are an alternative (Gruet and Saynor, 2019). Chairs with a fixed strain gauge, see Figure 4.4A, offer an attractive, although often underutilised alternative for measuring limb muscle strength in people with chronic respiratory disorders and are easily transportable. Strain gauge measures are valid for quadriceps strength (one of the most affected muscle groups in chronic respiratory disorders) when compared to computerised dynamometry (Machado Rodrigues *et al.*, 2017) and are reliable for use in young adults with CF (Gruet *et al.*, 2010). Strain gauge can also be used to measure limb muscle endurance and fatigability in CF (Gruet *et al.*, 2010, 2016a). Until now, these tests have been mostly used for research purposes (e.g., investigating the peripheral factors associated with muscle fatigability in CF using volitional and magnetically-evoked contractions (Gruet *et al.*, 2016a), see Figure 4.4B. Investigating the clinimetric properties of these evaluations in children with CF is an important next step to determine utility in clinical practice. Hand-held dynamometry (especially with belt-stabilisation) may represent an even cheaper alternative to measure limb muscle strength, even though measurements are slightly less reliable compared to strain

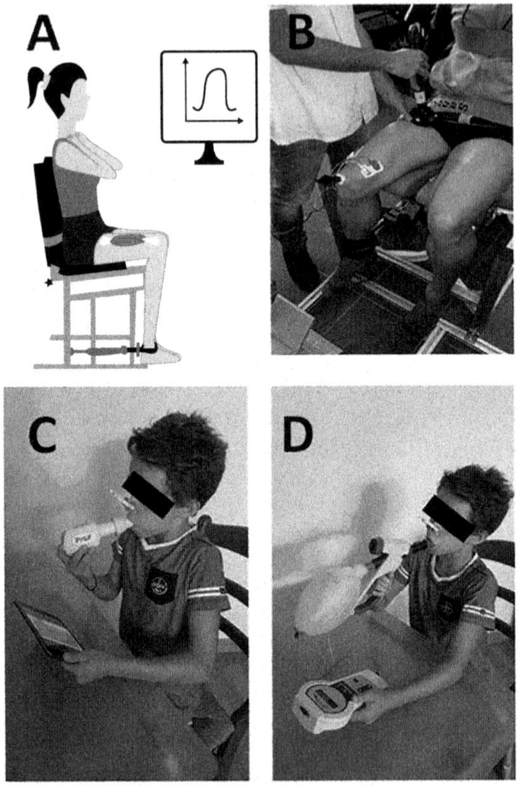

Figure 4.4 Schematic illustration of peripheral and respiratory muscle testing. (A) Isometric knee extensors strength testing using a chair with a fixed strain gauge; adapted and modified from Gruet (2020). (B) Standard evaluation of neuromuscular function using volitional and magnetically-evoked contractions. Strength is recorded using a fixed strain gauge and electrical activity of the muscles is recorded using surface electromyography. This set-up can be used to assess the peripheral and central factors associated with muscle fatigability during endurance testing, see Gruet *et al.*, (2016a) for the use of such methodology in people with CF; adapted from Gruet (2018). (C) Inspiratory resistive breathing endurance test using the PrO2® device. Such device permits the realisation of intermittent incremental inspiratory tests (e.g. Larribaut *et al.*, 2020) with participants inspiring through a mouthpiece attached to the device and expiring outside the device. The device can be connected to a smartphone or a digital tablet, allowing continuous visual feedback of the inspiratory pressures produced during the test. (D) Isocapnic hyperpnea endurance test using the Spirotiger® device. Such device permits partial CO_2 rebreathing, ensuring to maintain normocapnic ventilation throughout the test. Participants are asked to breathe at a given frequency through a mouthpiece attached to a tube connected by a bi-directional valve to a rebreathing bag and ambient air. Such set-up allows the realization of incremental endurance test, using progressive increments of breathing frequency (e.g. Larribaut *et al.*, 2020). The device provides continuous audio and visual feedbacks to control for breathing frequency and tidal volume throughout the test.

gauges. New portable devices have recently been developed and validated to measure quadriceps strength in clinical settings. Such devices, allowing rapid and valid measurement of limb muscle strength, should facilitate the understanding of peripheral muscle function in CF by enabling the quantitative measurement of strength to be included as an outcome in clinical trials.

Beyond quadriceps force assessment, it is also possible to measure the strength of the upper-limb muscles, even though they are generally less affected in CF (Gruet, 2018). Handgrip strength may offer a simple indicator of '*global*' muscle strength and has been studied in people with CF (Gibson *et al.*, 2018, Martínez-García *et al.*, 2020). Future work needs to evaluate the clinical usefulness of this very simple and inexpensive functional assessment in youth with CF and non-CF bronchiectasis, notably by investigating its associations with important clinical markers of disease severity.

Respiratory Muscle

Similar to skeletal muscles, the respiratory muscles are subject to fatigue and assessment of respiratory muscle function should be considered for people with bronchiectasis. Assessment is important to monitor functional changes, since impairment of (inspiratory and expiratory) respiratory muscles is a common clinical finding in people with primary lung disease, contributed to by a variety of factors, including hyperinflation, nutritional status (Dekerlegand *et al.*, 2017), systemic corticosteroid use, chronic *Pseudomonal* infection, and inactivity (Dassios, 2015). Postural abnormalities, including thoracic kyphosis, may also contribute to a restrictive lung function defect that increases demand on the respiratory pump (Denton *et al.*, 1981, Aris *et al.*, 1998). People with more advanced CF lung disease may therefore exhibit an imbalance between ventilatory load and respiratory muscle capacity, which can predispose inefficient breathing patterns. Devices exist to train the respiratory muscles, however, as for peripheral muscle training, an evaluation is required to calibrate training intensities for individuals.

Of the tests available, maximal inspiratory pressure (MIP) and expiratory pressure (MEP) are the most common assessments of global respiratory muscle function. While the MIP manoeuvre is reliable in CF, information concerning the clinimetric properties of expiratory muscle function assessments is lacking (Combret *et al.*, 2020). Assessment of MEP may be of particular interest in CF as this indicator was a powerful predictor of W_{peak} during a CPET in children and young adults with CF (Sovtic *et al.*, 2018). However, one should have in mind that maximal respiratory pressures are rarely required in daily life situations and such measurements may not detect early impairments in respiratory muscle function. This assumption is supported by the fact that many people with CF present normal or sometimes above normal respiratory muscle strength values (Heinzmann Filho *et al.*, 2012). Respiratory muscle endurance (RME) may be more representative of daily respiratory muscle effort and plays an important role in ensuring adapted ventilation and gas exchange over extended periods of PA. RME has been scarcely investigated in youth with CF. However, decreased RME has been reported in youth with CF despite preserved inspiratory muscle strength (Vendrusculo *et al.*, 2016). Future studies in youth with CF should evaluate the clinimetric properties of RME assessments, including isocapnic hyperpnea and/or inspiratory resistive breathing tests, see Figures 4.4(C and D), which have recently shown satisfactory test-retest reliability in young healthy adults (Larribaut *et al.*, 2020).

Reporting the Exercise Test

Applying a standardised approach to conducting, analysing, and interpreting exercise test data will enhance its value as a clinical tool for diagnostic, prognostic, and evaluative purposes in paediatrics. Not only does detailed analysis of an exercise test provide data-driven support for physiological reasoning and clinical decision-making, but it also enables comparisons between clinical centres, which are useful in both clinical audit and research applications. There has been an international effort to standardise the reporting of exercise tests in people with chronic respiratory disease, particularly CPET (Radtke *et al.*, 2019, Takken *et al.*, 2020).

CPET provides a wealth of information and generates a large dataset usually displayed in a series of graphs, known as the 9-panel plot. This is one of its key advantages over other testing methods, but presents a significant challenge in terms of selection, display, management, and interpretation of the data obtained. A systematic approach should be followed for the interpretation of CPET data (Radtke *et al.*, 2019). A correct interpretation of the CPET parameters requires knowledge about the normal response to exercise of these parameters and several key articles are recommended to the reader to assist with this (Urquhart and Saynor, 2018, Takken *et al.*, 2020). Briefly, after checking data quality, it should be established whether $\dot{V}O_{2peak}$ and maximum workload are normal relative to appropriate normative reference data (age, sex, and ethnicity). It is also important to consider whether maximum effort has been reached with respect to HR_{peak}, respiratory exchange ratio at peak exercise and whether $\dot{V}O_{2peak}$ has plateaued at the end of exercise. If maximal exercise endpoints are unclear, supramaximal exercise testing to verify $\dot{V}O_{2peak}$ can be considered (Saynor *et al.*, 2013, Causer *et al.*, 2018). An abnormally low exercise capacity is defined as $\dot{V}O_{2peak}$ <80% predicted. It is important to note that it is not only $\dot{V}O_{2peak}$ that has prognostic value in CF, W_{peak} as well as other submaximal measures have utility in this context (Hulzebos *et al.*, 2014, Hebestreit *et al.*, 2019), so correct determination is important.

The next challenge is to identify whether reduced $\dot{V}O_{2peak}$ may be due to ventilatory limitation, cardiovascular impairment, peripheral muscle abnormality, and/or poor fitness and deconditioning. A schematic overview of how to determine exercise function and/or cause of any dysfunction in individuals with CF is presented in Figure 4.2. The normal mechanism for exercise termination in a healthy individual is cardiac limitation, with HR_{peak} being attained (no cardiac reserve) and minute ventilation ($\dot{V}_E$) falling short of estimated maximal voluntary ventilation (MVV) – exercise $\dot{V}_E$ < 85% MVV (Hebestreit *et al.*, 2015). The physiology in children differs from adults, and expected HR_{peak} falls with age, whilst children with CF often achieve a HR_{max} > 200 beats·min^{-1} during CPET. The point at which anaerobic metabolism begins to predominate, known as the ventilatory threshold or gas exchange threshold (GET), provides a submaximal indicator of an individual's aerobic fitness. Deconditioning results in an early-onset anaerobic threshold (AT), indicative of reduced efficiency to transfer and utilise O_2 at the muscular level. An AT occurring <50% predicted $\dot{V}O_{2peak}$ (in the absence of cardiac disease or muscle abnormalities) is likely to be associated with deconditioning and can be improved with training.

As the physiological responses to exercise change during growth and development, the use of appropriate paediatric reference values is essential for proper interpretation of exercise testing data and can significantly distort interpretation. Growth, sex, ethnicity, and geographical region are all important and efforts should be made to source the most appropriate set of reference values that best reflect the characteristics of the participant tested, and equipment and methodology used. It is advised that after performing any exercise test, the results be documented in a clear report. To assist with this, a guidance document was recently published for chronic respiratory disease (Radtke *et al.*, 2019), which provides a standardised template for the interpretation (Figure 4.2) and reporting of CPET results. This may need to be modified, but the general template can be applied across testing modalities. Ideally, the person responsible for the test should write the report, as they will have observational information about participant effort and symptomatology. To summarise, as a minimum, an exercise test report should include:

- Basic information on the participant
- Technical report
- Responses to exercise (aerobic/anaerobic performance, cardiovascular, ventilatory, gas exchange, and metabolic)
- Report summary

Several key measures should be obtained across testing modalities and protocols. Objective measurement of HR and SpO_2 should be measured before, during, and following exercise, through a defined recovery period. Monitoring should be continuous and recorded where possible, to facilitate a more thorough assessment. Dependent on the exercise test chosen and the equipment available, specific outcome measures should be reported, e.g., W_{peak} and $\dot{V}O_{2peak}$ for CPET and distance covered or steps completed in field tests. If an individual experiences hypoxaemia during exercise, the corresponding intensity of exercise (e.g., HR, work rate, effort rating) should be recorded, as this can then be used to guide 'safe zones' for exercise prescription. Subjective measures of perceived exertion, breathlessness, or fatigue should also be used to assess symptoms during exercise. Providing participants with age-appropriate lay reports can be valuable in promoting their interest and cooperation with testing.

Assessment of Habitual Physical (in) Activity – the Missing Piece of the Puzzle?

Regular exercise testing allows for early detection of physical deconditioning, however, additional assessment of habitual PA in children with bronchiectasis is an important consideration. Such evaluations take into account the amount and intensity of activity, as well as sedentary behaviours, which is important since many children with a chronic condition or disability are less active. New research into PA suggests that it is no longer sufficient just to meet minimum levels recommended by health guidelines in order to reduce cardiovascular risk. Physical fitness, physical inactivity, and sedentary behaviour all bring their own health hazards and need individual consideration in order to be addressed. A recent survey exploring perceptions of PA monitoring among young people with CF and their health care providers (HCPs) reported that HCPs recognised the potential benefits of the devices in clinical practice (Shelley *et al.*, 2018). However, PA assessment is not commonplace or consistent in clinical practice, despite its association with quality of life in people with CF (Hebestreit *et al.*, 2014). To aid in the uptake in clinical practice, several key articles have recently been published (Hulzebos *et al.*, 2013, Shelley *et al.*, 2019) including an expert consensus statement from the European CF Society (Bradley *et al.*, 2015).

Motion sensors, activity questionnaires, and diaries are all useful to gauge an individual's general PA behaviours and as with exercise testing, the purpose of data collection will guide the choice of tool, along with cost and ease of use. The most recent ECFS position statement recommended that activity monitors (e.g., ActiGraph) offer informed choices to facilitate a comprehensive assessment of physical (in)activity, and should, as a minimum, report on dimensions of PA including energy expenditure, step count, and cumulative time spent in different activity intensities and being sedentary (Bradley *et al.*, 2015). The guidelines are perhaps out of date with a surfeit of available wearables being used by the population at large, including those with CF to monitor PA. Importantly, data from the UK suggest that people with CF enjoy wearing monitoring devices and demonstrate good compliance, particularly with wrist-worn devices and those providing feedback (Shelley *et al.*, 2018). Sophisticated activity monitoring, although more technical and costly, can eliminate the subjective evaluation of activity and can provide useful input for PA counselling.

Simple pedometers offer an inexpensive alternative and there is some evidence supporting their use in CF (Hulzebos *et al.*, 2013), although they are limited in the information recorded. The current European recommendation, to increase pedometer standardisation across clinics, is to use the DigiWalker pedometer (Bradley *et al.*, 2015). Questionnaires can also provide an appreciation of an individual's perception of their PA. They may be useful as a screening tool to guide further discussion about exercise patterns, goal setting, and subsequent exercise prescription. However they do depend on subject recall and should be used with caution, particularly in children and adolescents. Although there is insufficient data to recommend the use of one diary over another, the Habitual Activity Estimation Scale (HAES) is currently promoted as a reliable and valid instrument (Bradley *et al.*, 2015).

Conclusion

There is clear evidence that exercise testing in children and adolescents with CF and non-CF bronchiectasis is of real benefit, not only for monitoring disease progression and response to intervention, but perhaps more importantly in tailoring appropriate and individualised exercise prescriptions. We suggest that a combined approach, using multimodal assessments of aerobic fitness and skeletal muscle function, represents an important next step in advancing our understanding of how the pathophysiology of CF and non-CF bronchiectasis and how new treatments *truly* impact on physical function. This will help achieve the goal of individualised exercise prescription and personalised medicine.

Key Points

- Exercise testing children and adolescents with CF and non-CF bronchiectasis is important to monitor disease progression and response to intervention, and to inform prescription of individualised exercise programmes.
- The test chosen will depend on the indications for testing, participant age, and resources available.
- We suggest that a combined approach, using multimodal assessments of aerobic fitness and skeletal muscle function, represents an important next step in the evaluation of children with bronchiectasis and which may be applicable to other respiratory diseases.
- Details of individual habitual PA and sedentary time should constitute part of the comprehensive assessment of children with respiratory disease.

References

Andersen, D. H. 1938. Cystic fibrosis of the pancreas and its relation to celiac disease: a clinical and pathologic study. *American Journal of Diseases of Children*, 56, 344–399. doi:10.1001/archpedi.1938.01980140114013.

Aris, R. M., Renner, J. B., Winders, A. D., Buell, H. E., Riggs, D. B., Lester, G. E. & Ontjes, D. A. 1998. Increased rate of fractures and severe kyphosis: sequelae of living into adulthood with cystic fibrosis. *Annals of Internal Medicine*, 128, 186–193. doi:10.7326/0003-4819-128-3-199802010-00004.

Boas, S. R., Joswiak, M. L., Nixon, P. A., Fulton, J. A. & Orenstein, D. M. 1996. Factors limiting anaerobic performance in adolescent males with cystic fibrosis. *Medicine and Science in Sports and Exercise*, 28, 291–298. doi: 10.1097/00005768-199603000-00004.

Bongers, B. C. & Takken, T. 2014. The paediatric version of the steep ramp test. *Journal of Physiotherapy*, 60, 113. doi: 10.1016/j.jphys.2014.03.002.

Bradley, J., O'neill, B., Kent, L., Hulzebos, E. H., Arets, B., Hebestreit, H., Alison, J., Arets, B., Boas, S. & Bradley, J. 2015. Physical activity assessment in cystic fibrosis: a position statement. *Journal of Cystic Fibrosis*, 14, e25–e32. doi: 10.1016/j.jcf.2015.05.011.

Camargo, A. A., Lanza, F. C., Tupinambá, T. & Corso, S. D. 2013. Reproducibility of step tests in patients with bronchiectasis. *Brazilian Journal of Physical Therapy*, 17, 255–262. doi: 10.1590/s1413-35552012005000089.

Causer, A. J., Shute, J. K., Cummings, M. H., Shepherd, A. I., Bright, V., Connett, G., Allenby, M. I., Carroll, M. P., Daniels, T. & Saynor, Z. L. 2018. Cardiopulmonary exercise testing with supramaximal verification produces a safe and valid assessment of VO^{2max} in people with cystic fibrosis: a retrospective analysis. *Journal of Applied Physiology*, 125, 1277–1283. doi: 10.1152/japplphysiol.00454.2018.

Causer, A. J., Shute, J. K., Cummings, M. H., Shepherd, A. I., Gruet, M., Costello, J. T., Bailey, S., Lindley, M., Pearson, C. & Connett, G. 2020. Circulating biomarkers of antioxidant status and oxidative stress in people with cystic fibrosis: a systematic review and meta-analysis. *Redox Biology*, 32, 101436. doi: 10.1016/j.redox.2020.101436.

Combret, Y., Medrinal, C., Bonnevie, T., Gravier, F. E., Le Roux, P., Lamia, B., Prieur, G. & Reychler, G. 2020. Clinimetric evaluation of muscle function tests for individuals with cystic fibrosis. *Journal of Cystic Fibrosis*, S1569-1993, 30164–30168. doi: 10.1016/j.jcf.2020.05.014.

Dassios, T. 2015. Determinants of respiratory pump function in patients with cystic fibrosis. *Paediatric Respiratory Reviews*, 16, 75–79. doi: 10.1016/j.prrv.2014.01.001.

de Camargo, A. A., Justino, T., De Andrade, C. H. S., Malaguti, C. & Dal Corso, S. 2011. Chester step test in patients with COPD: reliability and correlation with pulmonary function test results. *Respiratory Care*, 56, 995–1001. doi: 10.4187/respcare.01047.

Dekerlegand, R. L., Hadjiliadis, D., Swisher, A. K., Parrott, J. S., Heuer, A. J. & Myslinski, M. J. 2017. Clinical predictors of inspiratory muscle strength in adults with stable cystic fibrosis: a pilot study. *Cardiopulmonary Physical Therapy Journal*, 28, 136–146. doi: 10.1097/CPT.0000000000000064.

Denton, J. R., Tietjen, R. & Gaerlan, P. F. 1981. Thoracic kyphosis in cystic fibrosis. *Clinical Orthopaedics and Related Research (1976–2007)*, 155, 71–74.

Divangahi, M., Balghi, H., Danialou, G., Comtois, A. S., Demoule, A., Ernest, S., Haston, C., Robert, R., Hanrahan, J. W. & Radzioch, D. 2009. Lack of CFTR in skeletal muscle predisposes to muscle wasting and diaphragm muscle pump failure in cystic fibrosis mice. *PLoS Genetics*, 5, e1000586. doi: 10.1371/journal.pgen.1000586.

Evans, R. A., Kaplovitch, E., Beauchamp, M. K., Dolmage, T. E., Goldstein, R. S., Gillies, C. L., Brooks, D. & Mathur, S. 2015. Is quadriceps endurance reduced in COPD?: a systematic review. *Chest*, 147, 673–684. doi: 10.1378/chest.14-1079.

Giacchi, V., Rotolo, N., Amato, B., Di Dio, G., Betta, P., La Rosa, M., Leonardi, S. & Sciacca, P. 2015. Heart involvement in children and adults with cystic fibrosis: correlation with pulmonary indexes and inflammation markers. *Heart, Lung and Circulation*, 24, 1002–1010. doi: 10.1016/j.hlc.2015.03.006.

Gibson, H. T., Mcdonald, C. M., Derrick, J. W., Eggett, D. L. & Bellini, S. G. 2018. Evaluating changes in handgrip strength in children with cystic fibrosis: a pilot study. *Nutrition in Clinical Practice*, 33, 261–267. doi: 10.1002/ncp.10067.

Gruet, M. 2018. Fatigue in chronic respiratory diseases: theoretical framework and implications for real-life performance and rehabilitation. *Frontiers in Physiology*, 9, 1285. doi: 10.3389/fphys.2018.01285.

Gruet, M. 2020. Tolérance à l'effort global et fatigabilité musculaire dans les maladies respiratoires chroniques: Méthodes d'évaluation et identification des mécanismes neuromusculaires sous-jacents. Habilitation à diriger des recherches. Université de Toulon.

Gruet, M., Decorte, N., Mely, L., Vallier, J.-M., Camara, B., Quetant, S., Wuyam, B. & Verges, S. 2016a. Skeletal muscle contractility and fatigability in adults with cystic fibrosis. *Journal of Cystic Fibrosis*, 15, e1–e8. doi: 10.1016/j.jcf.2015.05.004.

Gruet, M., Peyré-Tartaruga, L. A., Mely, L. & Vallier, J.-M. 2016b. The 1-minute sit-to-stand test in adults with cystic fibrosis: correlations with cardiopulmonary exercise test, 6-minute walk test, and quadriceps strength. *Respiratory Care*, 61, 1620–1628. doi: 10.4187/respcare.04821.

Gruet, M. & Saynor, Z. 2019. Assessment of peripheral muscle function in cystic fibrosis: why and how? *Respiratory Care*, 64, 238–240. doi: 10.4187/respcare.06692.

Gruet, M., Vallier, J., Mely, L. & Brisswalter, J. 2010. Long term reliability of EMG measurements in adults with cystic fibrosis. *Journal of Electromyography and Kinesiology*, 20, 305–312. doi: 10.1016/j.jelekin.2009.05.001.

Hanna, R. M. & Weiner, D. J. 2015. Overweight and obesity in patients with cystic fibrosis: a center-based analysis. *Pediatric Pulmonology*, 50, 35–41. doi: 10.1002/ppul.23033.

Harindhanavudhi, T., Wang, Q., Dunitz, J., Moran, A. & Moheet, A 2020. Prevalence and factors associated with overweight and obesity in adults with cystic fibrosis: a single-center analysis. Prevalence and factors associated with overweight and obesity in adults with cystic fibrosis: a single-center analysis, *Journal of Cystic Fibrosis*, 19, 139–145. doi: 10.1016/j.jcf.2019.10.004.

Hebestreit, H., Arets, H. G., Aurora, P., Boas, S., Cerny, F., Hulzebos, E. H., Karila, C., Lands, L. C., Lowman, J. D. & Swisher, A. 2015. Statement on exercise testing in cystic fibrosis. *Respiration*, 90, 332–351. doi: 10.1159/000439057.

Hebestreit, H., Hulzebos, E. H., Schneiderman, J. E., Karila, C., Boas, S. R., Kriemler, S., Dwyer, T., Sahlberg, M., Urquhart, D. S. & Lands, L. C. 2019. Cardiopulmonary exercise testing provides additional prognostic information in cystic fibrosis. *American Journal of Respiratory and Critical Care Medicine*, 199, 987–995. doi: 10.1164/rccm.201806-1110OC.

Hebestreit, H., Schmid, K., Kieser, S., Junge, S., Ballmann, M., Roth, K., Hebestreit, A., Schenk, T., Schindler, C. & Posselt, H.G. 2014. Quality of life is associated with physical activity and fitness in cystic fibrosis. *BMC Pulmonary Medicine*, 14, 26. doi: 10.1186/1471-2466-14-26.

Heinzmann Filho, J. P., Marostica, P. J. C. & Donadio, M. V. F. 2012. Ventilatory muscle strength in cystic fibrosis patients: a literature review. *Monaldi Archives for Chest Disease*, 77, 134–138. doi: 10.4081/monaldi.2012.147.

Högström, G., Nordström, A. & Nordström, P. 2014. High aerobic fitness in late adolescence is associated with a reduced risk of myocardial infarction later in life: a nationwide cohort study in men. *European Heart Journal*, 35, 3133–3140. doi: 10.1093/eurheartj/eht527.

Hulzebos, E., Dadema, T. & Takken, T. 2013. Measurement of physical activity in patients with cystic fibrosis: a systematic review. *Expert Review of Respiratory Medicine*, 7, 647–653. doi: 10.1586/17476348.2013.839248.

Hulzebos, E. H., Bomhof-Roordink, H., Van De Weert-Van Leeuwen, P., Twisk, J. W., Arets, H., Van Der Ent, C. K. & Takken, T. 2014. Prediction of mortality in adolescents with cystic fibrosis. *Medicine and Science in Sports and Exercise*, 46, 2047. doi: 10.1249/MSS.0000000000000344.

Keogh, R. H., Szczesniak, R., Taylor-Robinson, D. & Bilton, D. 2018. Up-to-date and projected estimates of survival for people with cystic fibrosis using baseline characteristics: a longitudinal study using UK patient registry data. *Journal of Cystic Fibrosis*, 17, 218–227. doi: 10.1016/j.jcf.2017.11.019.

Khalaf, M. M., Scott-Ward, T. S., Causer, A. J., Saynor, Z. L., Shepherd, A. I., Gorecki, D., Lewis, A., Laight, D. & Shute, J. K. 2020. Cystic fibrosis transmembrane conductance regulator (CFTR) in human lung microvascular endothelial cells controls oxidative stress, reactive oxygen-mediated cell signalling and inflammation. *Frontiers in Physiology*, 11, 879. doi: 10.3389/fphys.2020.00879.

Labombarda, F., Saloux, E., Brouard, J., Bergot, E. & Milliez, P. 2016. Heart involvement in cystic fibrosis: a specific cystic fibrosis-related myocardial changes? *Respiratory Medicine and Research*, 118, 31–38. doi: 10.1016/j.rmed.2016.07.011.

Lamhonwah, A. M., Bear, C. E., Huan, L. J., Chiaw, P. K., Ackerley, C. A. & Tein, I. 2010. Cystic fibrosis transmembrane conductance regulator in human muscle: dysfunction causes abnormal metabolic recovery in exercise. *Annals of Neurology*, 67, 802–808. doi: 10.1002/ana.21982.

Lang, R. L., Stockton, K., Wilson, C., Russell, T. G. & Johnston, L. M. 2020. Exercise testing for children with cystic fibrosis: a systematic review. *Pediatric Pulmonology*, 55, 1996–2010. doi: 10.1002/ppul.24794.

Larribaut, J., Gruet, M., Mcnarry, M., Mackintosh, K. & Verges, S. 2020. Methodology and reliability of respiratory muscle assessment. *Respiratory Physiology and Neurobiology*, 273, 103321. doi: 10.1016/j.resp.2019.103321.

Lee, S. J. & Arslanian, S. A. 2007. Cardiorespiratory fitness and abdominal adiposity in youth. *European Journal of Clinical Nutrition*, 61, 561–565. doi: 10.1038/sj.ejcn.1602541.

Lubans, D., Richards, J., Hillman, C., Faulkner, G., Beauchamp, M., Nilsson, M., Kelly, P., Smith, J., Raine, L. & Biddle, S. 2016. Physical activity for cognitive and mental health in youth: a systematic review of mechanisms. *Pediatrics*, 138, e20161642. doi: 10.1542/peds.2016-1642.

Machado Rodrigues, F., Demeyer, H., Hornikx, M., Camillo, C. A., Calik-Kutukcu, E., Burtin, C., Janssens, W., Troosters, T. & Osadnik, C. 2017. Validity and reliability of strain gauge measurement of volitional quadriceps force in patients with COPD. *Chronic Respiratory Disease*, 14, 289–297. doi: 10.1177/1479972316687210.

Mackenzie, T., Gifford, A. H., Sabadosa, K. A., Quinton, H. B., Knapp, E. A., Goss, C. H. & Marshall, B. C. 2014. Longevity of patients with cystic fibrosis in 2000 to 2010 and beyond: survival analysis of the Cystic Fibrosis Foundation patient registry. *Annals of Internal Medicine*, 161, 233–241. doi: 10.7326/M13-0636.

Martínez-García, M. D. M., Rodríguez-Juan, J. J. & Ruiz-Cárdenas, J. D. 2020. Influence of sex gap on muscle strength and functional mobility in patients with cystic fibrosis. *Physiology, Nutrition, and Metabolism*, 45, 387–392. doi: 10.1139/apnm-2019-0484.

Nixon, P. A., Orenstein, D. M., Kelsey, S. F. & Doershuk, C. F. 1992. The prognostic value of exercise testing in patients with cystic fibrosis. *New England Journal of Medicine*, 327, 1785–1788. doi: 10.1056/NEJM199212173272504.

O'donnell, A. E. 2018. Medical management of bronchiectasis. *Journal of Thoracic Disease*, 10, S3428–S3435. doi: 10.21037/jtd.2018.09.39.

Pérez, M., Groeneveld, I. F., Santana-Sosa, E., Fiuza-Luces, C., Gonzalez-Saiz, L., Villa-Asensi, J. R., López-Mojares, L. M., Rubio, M. & Lucia, A. 2014. Aerobic fitness is associated with lower risk of hospitalization in children with cystic fibrosis. *Pediatric Pulmonology*, 49, 641–649. doi: 10.1002/ppul.22878.

Pianosi, P., Leblanc, J. & Almudevar, A. 2005. Peak oxygen uptake and mortality in children with cystic fibrosis. *Thorax*, 60, 50–54. doi: 10.1136/thx.2003.008102.

Plebani, R., Tripaldi, R., Lanuti, P., Recchiuti, A., Patruno, S., Di Silvestre, S., Simeone, P., Anile, M., Venuta, F. & Prioletta, M. 2017. Establishment and long-term culture of human cystic fibrosis endothelial cells. *Laboratory Investigation*, 97, 1375–1385. doi: 10.1038/labinvest.2017.74.

Poore, S., Berry, B., Eidson, D., Mckie, K. T. & Harris, R. A. 2013. Evidence of vascular endothelial dysfunction in young patients with cystic fibrosis. *Chest*, 143, 939–945. doi: 10.1378/chest.12-1934.

Radtke, T., Crook, S., Kaltsakas, G., Louvaris, Z., Berton, D., Urquhart, D. S., Kampouras, A., Rabinovich, R. A., Verges, S., Kontopidis, D., Boyd, J., Tonia, T., Langer, D., Dr Brandt, J., Goërtz, Y. M. J., Burtin, C., Spruit, M. A., Braeken, D. C. W., Dacha, S., Franssen, F. M. E., Lavaneziana, P., Eber, E., Troosters., T., Neder, J. A., Puhan, M. A., Casaburi, R., Vogiatzis, I. & Hebestreit, H. 2019. ERS statement on standardisation of cardiopulmonary exercise testing in chronic lung diseases. *European Respiratory Review*, 28, 180101. doi: 10.1183/16000617.0101-2018.

Radtke, T., Puhan, M. A., Hebestreit, H. & Kriemler, S. 2016. The 1-min sit-to-stand test—a simple functional capacity test in cystic fibrosis? *Journal of Cystic Fibrosis*, 15, 223–226. doi: 10.1016/j.jcf.2015.08.006.

Raghuveer, G., Hartz, J., Lubans, D. R., Takken, T., Wiltz, J. L., Mietus-Snyder, M., Perak, A. M., Baker-Smith, C., Pietris, N., Edwards, N. M., on behalf of the American Heart Association Young Hearts Athero, Hypertension and Obesity in the Young Committee of the Council on Lifelong Congenital Heart Disease and Heart Health in the Young. 2020. Cardiorespiratory fitness in youth: an important marker of health: a scientific statement from the American Heart Association. *Circulation*, 142, e101–e118. doi: 10.1161/CIR.0000000000000866.

Rand, S., Prasad, S. & Main, E. 2015. New incremental field step-test (iSTEP) is valid and feasible in measuring near maximal exercise performance in children with cystic fibrosis. *Physiotherapy*, 101, e931–e932. doi: 10.1016/j.physio.2015.03.1777.

Rodriguez-Miguelez, P., Thomas, J., Seigler, N., Crandall, R., Mckie, K. T., Forseen, C. & Harris, R. A. 2016. Evidence of microvascular dysfunction in patients with cystic fibrosis. *American Journal of Physiology-Heart and Circulatory Physiology*, 310, H1479–H1485. doi: 10.1152/ajpheart.00136.2016.

Ruf, K., Winkler, B., Hebestreit, A., Gruber, W. & Hebestreit, H. 2010. Risks associated with exercise testing and sports participation in cystic fibrosis. *Journal of Cystic Fibrosis*, 9, 339–345. doi: 10.1016/j.jcf.2010.05.006.

Santana, C. C. A., Hill, J. O., Azevedo, L. B., Gunnarsdottir, T. & Prado, W. L. 2017. The association between obesity and academic performance in youth: a systematic review. *Obesity Reviews*, 18, 1191–1199. doi: 10.1111/obr.12582.

Saynor, Z. L., Barker, A. R., Oades, P. J. & Williams, C. A. 2013. A protocol to determine valid VO^{2max} in young cystic fibrosis patients. *Journal of Science and Medicine in Sport*, 16, 539–544. doi: 10.1016/j.jsams.2013.01.010.

Sellers, Z. M., De Arcangelis, V., Xiang, Y. & Best, P. M. 2010. Cardiomyocytes with disrupted CFTR function require CaMKII and $Ca2^+$-activated Cl^- channel activity to maintain contraction rate. *The Journal of Physiology*, 588, 2417–2429. doi: 10.1113/jphysiol.2010.188334.

Shelley, J., Boddy, L. M., Knowles, Z. R., Stewart, C. E. & Dawson, E. A. 2019. Physical activity and associations with clinical outcome measures in adults with cystic fibrosis; a systematic review. *Journal of Cystic Fibrosis*, 18, 590–601. doi: 10.1016/j.jcf.2019.03.003.

Shelley, J., Fairclough, S. J., Knowles, Z. R., Southern, K. W., Mccormack, P., Dawson, E. A., Graves, L. E. & Hanlon, C. 2018. A formative study exploring perceptions of physical activity and physical activity monitoring among children and young people with cystic fibrosis and health care professionals. *BMC Pediatrics,* 18, 335. doi: 10.1186/s12887-018-1301-x.

Sheppard, E., Chang, K., Cotton, J., Gashgarian, S., Slack, D., Wu, K., Michalski, A., Fox, P., Stephenson, A. L. & Mathur, S. 2019. Functional tests of leg muscle strength and power in adults with cystic fibrosis. *Respiratory Care*, 64, 40–47. doi: 10.4187/respcare.06224.

Sovtic, A., Minic, P., Markovic-Sovtic, G. & Trajkovic, G. Z. 2018. Respiratory muscle strength and exercise performance in cystic fibrosis–a cross sectional study. *Frontiers in Pediatrics*, 6, 244. doi: 10.3389/fped.2018.00244.

Stephenson, A. L., Mannik, L. A., Walsh, S., Brotherwood, M., Robert, R., Darling, P. B., Nisenbaum, R., Moerman, J. & Stanojevic, S. 2013. Longitudinal trends in nutritional status and the relation between lung function and BMI in cystic fibrosis: a population-based cohort study. *The American Journal of Clinical Nutrition*, 97, 872–877. doi: 10.3945/ajcn.112.051409.

Takken, T., Sonbahar Ulu, H. & Hulzebos, E. H. 2020. Clinical recommendations for cardiopulmonary exercise testing in children with respiratory diseases. *Expert Review of Respiratory Medicine*, 14, 1–11. doi: 10.1080/17476348.2020.1752195.

Totani, L., Plebani, R., Piccoli, A., Di Silvestre, S., Lanuti, P., Recchiuti, A., Cianci, E., Dell'elba, G., Sacchetti, S. & Patruno, S. 2017. Mechanisms of endothelial cell dysfunction in cystic fibrosis. *Biochimica et Biophysica Acta (BBA)-Molecular Basis of Disease*, 1863, 3243–3253. doi: 10.1016/j.bbadis.2017.08.011.

Tousson, A., Van Tine, B. A., Naren, A. P., Shaw, G. M. & Schwiebert, L. M. 1998. Characterization of CFTR expression and chloride channel activity in human endothelia. *American Journal of Physiology-Cell Physiology*, 275, C1555–C1564. doi: 10.1152/ajpcell.1998.275.6.C1555.

Troosters, T., Langer, D., Vrijsen, B., Segers, J., Wouters, K., Janssens, W., Gosselink, R., Decramer, M. & Dupont, L. 2009. Skeletal muscle weakness, exercise tolerance and physical activity in adults with cystic fibrosis. *European Respiratory Journal*, 33, 99–106. doi: 10.1183/09031936.00091607.

Urquhart, D. & Saynor, Z. 2018. Exercise testing in cystic fibrosis: who and why? *Paediatric Respiratory Reviews*, 27, 28–32. doi: 10.1016/j.prrv.2018.01.004.

Valdivieso, A. G. & Santa-Coloma, T. A. 2013. CFTR activity and mitochondrial function. *Redox Biology*, 1, 190–202. doi: 10.1016/j.redox.2012.11.007.

Vendrusculo, F. M., Heinzmann-Filho, J. P., Piva, T. C., Marostica, P. J. & Donadio, M. V. 2016. Inspiratory muscle strength and endurance in children and adolescents with cystic fibrosis. *Respiratory Care*, 61, 184–191. doi: 10.4187/respcare.04231.

Wells, G. D. & Norris, S. R. 2009. Assessment of physiological capacities of elite athletes & respiratory limitations to exercise performance. *Paediatric Respiratory Reviews*, 10, 91–98. doi: 10.1016/j.prrv.2009.04.002.

Werkman, M. S., Hulzebos, H. J., Van De Weert-Van, P. B., Arets, H. G., Helders, P. J. & Takken, T. 2011. Supramaximal verification of peak oxygen uptake in adolescents with cystic fibrosis. *Pediatric Physical Therapy*, 23, 15–21. doi: 10.1097/PEP.0b013e318208ca9e.

5 Using Behaviour Change Theory and Evidence to Understand and Support Physical Activity among People with Cystic Fibrosis

Sarah Denford and Paul O'Halloran

Introduction to Behaviour Change

Our behaviour can have a profound impact on our health and wellbeing. Supporting individuals to change their behaviour in order to maximise their health is not easy. Influences on health behaviours are numerous and operate at different levels. Socioeconomic models highlight the range of individual and environmental factors that influence the health and behaviour of an individual. Whilst choices are influenced by beliefs, attitudes, and motivations, these in turn are influenced by social networks and the communities and organisations within which we live, work, and socialise. The physical environment, including the provision of and access to services, will also play a key role in shaping actions. Interventions to promote health behaviours may occur at any one of these levels. For example, to promote physical activity, an intervention could operate at the level of the individual, targeting the regulatory processes or 'determinants' of physical activity within an individual. At a community level, urban planning, the provision of community health and fitness centres, and access to green spaces can also increase (or decrease) participation in physical activity. Changes to organisational policies and/or legislation, such as alterations to physical education classes in schools, will also have an impact on behaviour. Whilst the focus of this chapter will be on the individual level behaviour change, evidence indicates that targeting multiple levels of influence is likely to optimise behaviour change. Throughout this chapter we will introduce the reader to theoretical perspectives on behaviour change, before outlining key determinants of physical activity among young people with cystic fibrosis (CF). The chapter will end with consideration of potentially promising interventions for supporting and promoting physical activity among the CF population and its behaviour change in the context of a chronic condition.

'From handfuls of pills to hours of physiotherapy and making sure you get enough exercise, the burden of treatment for people with CF can be immense. Many people tell us that sticking to their treatment regime can be difficult, with the guilt that comes from not "adhering" to treatment leading to shame and isolation' (Cystic Fibrosis Trust UK, 2020). A recent quote

DOI: 10.4324/9781003020462-5

from a young person with CF eloquently highlighting the realities of living with CF.

When thinking about behaviour change in the context of a chronic condition, we need to consider the influences on behaviour that living with the condition entails. On the one hand, individuals with a chronic condition may be considered to have an additional reason, or motive, to perform health promoting behaviours. It may be assumed that an individual for whom engaging in a particular behaviour (e.g., physical activity, medication adherence, etc.) could be life-extending, should be highly motivated to engage in the behaviour. However, there are a range of psychological (e.g., emotions, acceptance, understanding), social (e.g., treatment by others, self-consciousness), and physical (e.g., illness fluctuations) reasons why people do not engage in health-promoting behaviours. Attempts to change the behaviour of individuals with a chronic condition will likely fail unless efforts are individualised to the needs and circumstances of the individual in question (Brawley, Rejeski and King, 2003; Montori, Gafni and Charles, 2006).

Theoretical Perspectives

The information, motivation, behavioural skills model is a useful framework for thinking about behaviour (Fisher and Fisher, 1992). The model suggests that, in order for behaviour change to occur, an individual would need to be well informed, have all the skills to perform the behaviour, and be highly motivated. It will not always be necessary to focus on all three of the aforementioned regulatory processes, and it is important to identify which of the three need to be targeted. For example, in some situations, simple information campaigns is sufficient to change behaviour, and considerable information exists regarding how to make information persuasive and attractive (Abraham and Kools, 2011). However, it is very common for an individual to be very well informed, yet not act on that knowledge. Indeed, much research has identified that individuals are very well informed about the need to take part in physical activity; however, many people fail to put this into practice (Currie et al., 2004). This may be due to a lack of motivation.

Self-Determination Theory (Deci and Ryan, 1985), whilst not specifically about motivation for physical activity, is often used to explain motivation for physical activity. The theory posits that, rather than viewing motivation in terms of volume (I am more or less motivated toward a particular behaviour), we should think about types of motivation. The theory states that motivation may be intrinsic or extrinsic, autonomous or controlled. There are two main reasons that people are not motivated (or amotivated). The first reason is that they are simply not interested in the behaviour or any of the outcomes associated with the behaviour (Hagberg et al., 2009). For example, they do not enjoy physical activity, or they do not value the benefits associated with physical activity, such as improved health or fitness (Hagberg et al., 2009). The second reason for amotivation is that individuals do not feel sufficiently competent (e.g., as a result of a lack of skill or as a result of health limitations; Oakley, Booth and Patterson, 2001). In either case, amotivated individuals have no intentions to partake in the behaviour in question. In addition to those who are amotivated, there are individuals who may intend to behave in a particular way (e.g., be active), and may even begin the behaviour. However, such efforts are short-term and not sustained (Amireault, Godin and Vézina-Im, 2013). This is because this motivation is controlled as opposed to autonomous. Controlled motivation includes behaviours that are performed as a means to an end. They are performed because there is a belief that they must be physically active – either to avoid a punishment or for short-term reward. This may explain why young people who are prescribed physical activity as 'medicine' may fail to maintain this behaviour in the long-term. In contrast, individuals who are intrinsically motivated are motivated to take part in physical activity for the pleasure of being physically active. This is the most autonomous form of motivation, and self-determined behaviours are most likely to be sustained in the long-term (Deci and Ryan, 1985).

For individuals presenting as amotivated, it may be necessary to check their understanding of the range of benefits associated with physical activity (i.e., enjoyment, improved mental, and social wellbeing – and not just improvements in lung function), as previous research has found that patients and clinicians often have different views regarding what is important. Whilst clinicians may prioritise improvements in clinical markers (e.g., lung function), patients may not value this outcome in the same way. Research suggests that adherence can be improved if clinical teams can identify and focus on outcomes that are important to patients (Britten, 1994), rather than focusing exclusively on clinical outcomes. Whilst some people with CF may be motivated by improvements in lung function, others may consider psycho-social benefits to be more important. The latter group may not be motivated by information relating to the role of physical activity in improving lung function, particularly if improvements in lung function provide no immediate visible patient benefits. Such patients may respond better to information about the psychological benefits. Identifying the outcomes that are important to patients may be more beneficial.

Unsurprisingly, people are unlikely to invest much effort in behaviours that they do not believe they are capable of performing. Self-efficacy refers to an individuals' self-belief in their ability to take control of challenging situations and adapt to overcome such demands. The role of self-efficacy in performance of physical activity behaviour has long been established; with levels of self-efficacy having an influence on the choice of activities, persistence, and effort expended. There is also evidence to suggest that interventions can increase physical activity behaviour as a result of increased self-efficacy (Darker et al., 2010). Bandura identifies four main approaches to self-efficacy enhancement; including past accomplishments, social persuasion, social modelling, and the interpretation of emotional arousal (Bandura, 1997). Indeed, many interventions targeting physical activity behaviour integrate these four approaches to enhance self-efficacy for the behaviour.

Habits and Physical Activity

In some instances, patients can be highly motivated, have the necessary skills and information, but still fail to act. This may be a result of automatic processes. Research indicates that behaviour is controlled by networks of neural activation that may be viewed as two interactive systems; the reflective system and the impulsive system (Strack and Deusch, 2004; Kahneman, 2011). Planning to partake in physical activity using the reflective system is based on values, conscious reasoning, and intentions. For example, highly valuing the behaviour (or outcome of the behaviour), goal setting, and consciously planning how to achieve the goal are all actions performed by the reflective system. In contrast, actions regulated by the impulsive system have low levels of conscious monitoring and are enacted largely in response to behavioural cues with little conscious awareness (Kahneman, 2011). These behaviours are said to be habitual (Verplanken and Aarts, 1999). With repeated performance overtime reinforces the context-behaviour associations; thus strengthening the habit. As a result, the behaviour is performed automatically, and with little thought, in response to the cue or context. There is much evidence that physical activity habits are frequently performed, and that habits dominate over intentions (Gardener, de Bruijn and Lally, 2011). Habitual behavioural patterns are very difficult to change; however, once 'healthy' habits, that is, ones that help you achieve a goal, are established, the likelihood of success increases (Gardener, de Bruijn and Lally, 2011).

Determinants of Physical Activity among People with CF

A large body of work, including a systematic review of seven studies, has explored potential determinants of and barriers and facilitators to physical activity among young people with CF (Denford et al., 2020). These studies included: (i) individual level determinants; age and gender, health status, beliefs and attitudes relating to CF and physical activity, and motivation for physical activity, (ii) social networks; families and peer groups, and (iii) environmental factors; availability of facilities, weather, and pollution.

Age and Gender

Participation in physical activity is very much influenced by demographic factors, such as age (Jago et al., 2019; Farooq et al., 2020), gender (Selvadurai et al., 2004), and socioeconomic status (Gidlow et al., 2006; Ferreira et al., 2007). It is widely accepted that participation in physical activity is lower among women and girls in almost every country in the world (Guthold et al., 2018).

Participation in physical activity also declines with age; with the decline becoming apparent in children as young as six years (Jago et al., 2019). However, declines in physical activity are steeper among girls (Selvadurai et al., 2004) with girls reporting less enjoyment of physical activity, and lower confidence in their ability to be active (Sport England, 2019). This has led to campaigns such as 'This Girl Can' and 'We Are Undefeatable' which have had considerable success in encouraging women and people with long-term health conditions to be more active. However, it is still a challenge to increase participation among those from lower income households (Elhakeem et al., 2017). Furthermore, socioeconomic status and sex and gender remain important determinants of survival from CF; with this effect failing to reduce over time (Barr et al., 2011).

Health

Whilst ill health will have a direct impact on participation in physical activity behaviour, i.e., through exacerbations of illness, being overweight (Jago et al., 2020) or symptoms (Fereday et al., 2009; Moola, Faulkner and Schneiderman, 2012; Moola et al., 2011; Shelley et al., 2018; Swisher and Erickson, 2008), or serious or disruptive events such as hospitalisation and infections (Fereday et al., 2009; Moola, Faulkner and Schneiderman, 2012), it may also accentuate the extent to which physical activity is viewed as unpleasant. Symptoms, such as breathlessness, fatigue, and coughing may exacerbate the perceived unpleasantness associated with physical activity; leading to avoidance of activity whenever possible (Moola et al., 2011; Shelley et al., 2018; Swisher and Erickson, 2008). Furthermore, any decline in ability to partake in physical activity may be interpreted as a decline in health (Denford et al., 2019). In contrast, relative 'wellness' could be inspirational; with individuals being motivated by the fact that they are able to take part in physical activity when others with CF cannot (Shelley et al., 2018).

Beliefs, Attitudes, and Motivations

Physical activity behaviour is strongly influenced by the beliefs and attitudes head by individuals relating to physical activity (Happ et al., 2013; Moola, Faulkner and Schneiderman, 2012; Shelley et al., 2018; Swisher and Erickson, 2008). Attitudes towards physical activity are influenced by previous experience of physical activity, the health of the individual, and the social environment in which physical activity is performed. Positive attitudes, such as enjoyment of physical activity, feelings associated with competency, mastery, achievement, and a sense of autonomy have all been linked to sustained participation in physical activity behaviour (Moola and Faulkner, 2014; Swisher and Erikson, 2008). In contrast, negative perceptions of physical activity include the belief that physical activity is unpleasant, difficult, boring, painful or uncomfortable, and tiring (Happ et al., 2013; Shelley et al.,

2018). For some, feelings of self-consciousness result in young people feeling exposed and vulnerable, despondent, and anxious to avoid physical activity (Street et al., 2016).

Beliefs relating to the importance of physical activity for CF, for example, for improving the general health of people with CF and their families (Happ et al., 2013; Moola et al., 2011; Shelley et al., 2018; Swisher and Erickson, 2008), and in the management of CF (Happ et al., 2013; Moola et al., 2011; Swisher and Erickson, 2008), are likely to increase motivation to take part in physical activity. However, literature consistently shows that beliefs relating to the importance of physical activity are not as important as the positive or negative attitudes held by individuals. Despite being aware of the benefits of physical activity, it is rarely valued if it is perceived to be unpleasant (Moola, Faulkner and Schneiderman, 2012). Indeed, health improvement and CF management do not appear to be sufficiently motivational for those who are not already active.

Motivation for participation in physical activity is also influenced by the range of competing activities one must partake in. Indeed, a lack of time for physical activity is often cited as a key barrier (Happ et al., 2013; Moola, Faulkner and Schneiderman, 2012; Moola et al., 2011). This is particularly the case for people with CF who report spending more than 4 hours per day on their treatment (Happ et al., 2013b). This may interfere with the opportunity to do physical activity (Moola, Faulkner and Schneiderman, 2012). However, for some, having only limited time for physical activity prohibited participation because they would rather spend the time doing something meaningful and enjoyable for them (such as seeing friends) (Moola, Faulkner and Schneiderman, 2012). Furthermore, some individuals have alluded to a lack of time in a symbolic sense (Moola, Faulkner and Schneiderman, 2012), with concerns about a potentially shortened lifespan. This may increase the pressure to achieve significant milestones (e.g., attaining a career, getting married, etc.) within a shortened lifespan (Moola, Faulkner and Schneiderman, 2012), thus overshadowing the need to take part in everyday tasks such as physical activity.

Participation in self-management practices, such as physical activity, is closely related to beliefs regarding the extent to which the condition can be controlled or managed through the behaviour in question, plus the extent to which the individual feels able to perform the behaviour (self-efficacy). Individual differences in perceptions relating their ability to control or manage their condition may influence the extent to which individuals adopt 'active' versus 'passive' coping strategies (Carver et al., 1989). For example, individuals who adopt a fatalistic approach, i.e., believed there is nothing that can be done about CF, tend to be less motivated to adopt positive self-care behaviours such as physical activity (Moola and Faulkner, 2014; Moola, Faulkner and Schneiderman 2012) and utilise dysfunctional, rather than functional coping strategies. However, whilst CF is indeed a chronic condition that cannot be cured, there are many behaviours that can be employed to manage CF. Individuals who report feelings of control over their CF are more likely to adopt positive self-care behaviours (Fereday et al., 2009; Moola and Faulkner, 2014; Shelley et al., 2018) and utilise functional coping strategies.

Social Influences

Social influences on physical activity behaviour can include the impact of family units, peer networks, or cultural norms and values. For young children with CF, parents play a key role. For example, providing physical activity role models (Happ et al., 2013; Moola et al., 2011; Moola, Faulkner and Schneiderman, 2012) teaching children the skills they need to be active (Happ et al., 2013) providing tangible support (Fereday et al., 2009; Shelley et al., 2018), planning, structuring activities and overcoming barriers (Fereday et al., 2009; Happ et al., 2013; Moola and Faulkner, 2014) providing opportunities for physical activity, and providing encouragement and motivation (Happ et al., 2013; Moola, Faulkner and Schneiderman, 2012; Shelley et al., 2018). In contrast, parental support can be detrimental to physical activity behaviour if parents are sedentary (Happ et al., 2013; Moola et al., 2011; Moola, Faulkner and Schneiderman, 2012) or overbearing (Shelley et al., 2018). Within families, there are complex relationships between socio-economic status, activity levels, and sedentary behaviours. Lower income has a positive correlation to light activity, but is inversely related to sedentary time, whereas higher income is associated with more intense, less frequent activity with a notable tendency to engage in bouts of outward-bound 'weekend' activities (Shuval et al., 2017). Furthermore, those of higher socio-economic status are more likely to meet activity guidelines (Shuval et al., 2017).

As young people progress through adolescence, the impact of the family unit reduces, and the impact of peer groups increase. Friendship groups can have a positive impact on physical activity behaviour; either through providing support (Fereday et al., 2009; Shelley et al., 2018), making activity more enjoyable (Fereday et al., 2009), or through acting as positive role models. Several theories help explain the role of peer role models in motivating physical activity behaviour. First, role models can enhance self-efficacy (as outlined in the 'beliefs, attitudes and motivations' subtheme above). Role models can also change perceptions of what others are doing and so lead to pro-physical activity norms; that is the perception that physical activity is approved of and undertaken by others with CF. This means that peers may have a negative impact on physical activity if they promote sedentary activities as the norm.

Theories of social comparison state that individuals determine their own self-worth based on how they compare to others. Individuals can compare themselves to others as a way of fostering self-motivation. Such comparisons can be upwards (comparing to someone better than the self) or downwards (comparisons to someone worse than the self). Both forms of social comparison can be motivational; viewing someone succeeding can be inspirational and lead to the desire to better oneself (Moola et al., 2011; Street et al., 2016) and viewing someone not as good as oneself can make people feel confident in their own abilities (Shelley et al., 2018). However, social comparison can work in reverse, and can lead to negative feelings or inadequacy Street et al., 2016); making adolescents 'stand out' – something they are appear motivated to avoid (Street et al., 2016). This may be exacerbated by negative comments or treatment by others; including teachers and coaches (Fereday et al., 2009; Moola et al., 2011) and members of the public (Street et al., 2016).

Finally, many young people with CF report that physical activity can be used to provide an opportunity for the young people to feel normal through providing a window within which people can be just like everyone else; minimising differences between themselves and those without CF (Street et al., 2016). However, feelings of abnormality may be increased if people are highly self-consciousness (Moola et al., 2011; Moola and Faulkner, 2014; Street et al., 2016); through accentuating the extent to which people feel different or inferior to their peers (Moola et al., 2011; Moola and Faulkner, 2014; Street et al., 2016). Those in the latter group may be more motivated to avoid physical activity than those in the former group.

Environment

The physical environment in which people live will also have an impact on physical activity behaviour (Carlin et al., 2017). Having a garden or outdoor space, access to physical activity programs and equipment within schools, neighbourhood features such as pedestrian and cyclist safety structure (Carlin et al., 2017), good access to local community facilities (e.g., swimming pools, sports centres), and private clubs have been shown to positively influence physical activity (Shelley et al., 2018). Active travel, that is, walking or cycling to school daily can comprise a substantial contribution towards a child's daily physical activity (van Sluijs et al., 2009) with children who regularly walk to school being more active than those who travel by car (van Sluijs et al., 2009). Furthermore, children who have the freedom to play outdoors and/or travel without adult supervision were more active than those who did not (Schoeppe et al., 2012). Living close to the sea or green space (green and blue gym) may also increase participation in physical activity (White et al., 2016); however, the impact of seasons/weather (Tucker and Gilliland, 2007) and concerns about safety (Carver, Timperio and Crawford, 2008) can reduce participation in outdoor activities.

Interventions Targeting Physical Activity for CF – Review of the Evidence

Once potential determinants of behaviour for the population in question have been identified, behaviour change theory can be used to guide the selection of behaviour change techniques most likely to be effective for modifying the determinant and ultimately changing behaviour. Numerous frameworks to support the development of interventions to change behaviour exist (Bartholomew et al., 2016; Michie et al., 2008; Yardley et al., 2015). Critically, in order to ensure engagement and acceptability of the intervention among the target audience, any intervention should be collaboratively developed with those for whom the intervention is developed (Michie et al., 2008; Yardley et al., 2015). The literature regarding the effectiveness of interventions to promote physical activity among individuals with CF is in its infancy, with most research being concerned with the effectiveness of physical activity or exercise for CF; rather than the effectiveness of strategies or approaches aiming to increase participation in physical activity or exercise programs. Whilst there are some promising initiates happening in clinical practice, these are largely without an evidence base as yet. Despite a general lack of consensus regarding the most effective strategies to promote physical activity among young people with CF (Cox and Holland, 2013), some promising approaches are worth a mention. These may be considered as: (1) interventions targeting social influences, (2) interventions targeting motivation, and (3) digital interventions.

Interventions targeting social influences can focus on promoting physical activity at the level of the family or can target social peer groups. Despite a lack of evidence for the effectiveness of interventions targeting the families of young people with CF, there is good evidence that such an approach can be effective for increasing participation in physical activity among young people without CF (Brown et al., 2016). However, as children move through childhood and into adolescence, there is a notable shift from parental influence to peer influence. Interventions in which young people are encouraged to be active with their peers may be more effective at this point (Ginis et al., 2013). There is, as yet, a lack of evidence for the effectiveness of interventions targeting social networks among adolescents with CF. However, the Inspire-CF study is worthy of a mention. Inspire-CF was a randomised controlled trial to explore the effectiveness of weekly personal training sessions on physical activity participation, lung function, and quality of life. Potential mediators of change, e.g., self-efficacy and enjoyment of physical activity, were also measured (Douglas et al., 2018; Ledger et al., 2016). Initial results show promising effects of the intervention on participation in physical activity (Ledger et al., 2016) and mediators of change (Douglas et al., 2018). However, additional research is still needed to confirm these preliminary findings.

Motivational interviewing (MI) is a set of behaviour change techniques, widely used in several behaviour change interventions for disparate populations. It is 'a directive, client centred counselling style for eliciting behaviour change by helping clients to explore and resolve ambivalence' (Rollnick and Miller, 1995). Miller and Rollnick propose seven main principles of MI: (i) motivation to change must be from the patient, not imposed by professionals; (ii) the patient has to articulate and resolve any conflict inherent in changing their behaviour; (iii) persuasion is not an element of MI; (iv) aggression, confrontation, and argumentation are avoided; (v) the role of the professional is to help the patient to resolve conflict; not to teach behavioural strategies; (vi) in MI, readiness to change depends on the interactions between the patient and professional; not a static trait from within the patient; (vii) interactions should be viewed as partnerships as opposed to professional/patient roles. Techniques used in MI include reflective listening, expressing acceptance and affirmation, eliciting and selectively reinforcing the client's own self-motivational statements, and affirming the client's freedom of choice and self-direction (Rollnick and Miller, 1995). There is evidence for the effectiveness of MI for increasing motivation to change behaviour in several contexts; including increasing participation in physical activity among people with chronic health conditions (O'Halloran et al., 2014).

Increasingly, attempts are being made to use the internet to change physical activity behaviour. The internet is beneficial in terms of the number of participants who can be reached, and the flexibility afforded to participants in being able to choose when and where they receive information and utilise the service. This flexibility is vital, allowing adolescents to fit in regular physical activity tracking alongside their treatment regime, school, work, and social life. Additionally, it is estimated that up to 80% of all individuals in the age group 15–44 years have regular access to the internet making the internet a viable route via which to deliver interventions for young people with CF. Online platforms have the unique ability to foster a supportive environment for physical activity to occur whilst removing the risk of cross-infection, as well as removing the fear of social judgement. The adolescents can still receive physical activity support and instruction to enable them to push themselves, enabling to engage in physical activity without the anxiety and embarrassment that comes with activity in public spaces to start with. This has the ability to give them confidence to be physically active, and to reassure them that they are not doing harm (Tomlinson et al., 2019).

Whilst still lacking a conclusive evidence base, a few initiatives deserve a comment. Beam (formally Pactster) provides online exercise classes, delivered by instructors who have CF. The platform allows users to take part in 'live' classes with physiotherapists, instructors, and others with CF, or stream on demand at a time suitable to each individual. The focus of the platform is movement to feel good, focusing on both the physical and mental wellbeing of its users. Similarly, the USA's 'CF Yogi' is an exercise web platform co-founded by a person with CF and a parent of children with CF in partnership with Social Good Fund. It includes livestreamed and recorded fitness videos led by instructors with CF and has community features allowing patients to share progress and fitness goals while avoiding cross-infection risks. An evidence base for the effectiveness of such approaches are still in progress.

Notably, attempts at using online methods are not always successful. Del Corral and colleagues used online gaming to deliver a 6-week training programme of 30–60 minute sessions, 5 days a week, monitored by a virtual personal trainer. However, participation in the intervention did not appear to lead to improvements in any of the outcomes assessed relative to control participants, and long-term adherence to the program was poor. This highlights the need to assess the longevity of the programme; ensuring that any initiatives are capable of sustaining engagement after the novelty has subsided.

Conclusion

In conclusion, changing behaviour is not easy. Throughout this chapter we have highlighted a number of determinants, barriers, and facilitators to physical activity, as well as suggesting some possible approaches to change behaviour. Crucially, attempts to increase physical activity among individuals with CF must take into account the complexity of the behaviour, and the multiple determinants influencing behaviour at multiple levels. Interventions are likely to be more successful if they identify the key barriers (and facilitators) to physical activity for each individual, including those specific to the respiratory condition, as well as understand the social and physical context within which the behaviour will occur.

Key Points

- Behaviour change interventions can target individuals, communities, organisations, and societies.
- Behaviour change is unlikely to occur if people do not have sufficient information, motivation, or the behavioural skills needed to engage in the behaviour.
- Focusing on intrinsic, or autonomous, motivation is likely to lead to sustainable behaviour change.
- Factors such as age, gender, health, beliefs and attitudes, social influences, and the environment all influence how active an individual may be.
- This is particularly important in the context of chronic conditions where fluctuations in health are common.
- It is important to identify which of these influences are limiting physical activity among the individual or population in question.
- A number of interventions targeting physical activity among people with CF have been developed.
- There is a growing evidence for interventions that target families and attempt to develop autonomous motivation for physical activity.
- Digital interventions may also support engagement in activity.

References

Abraham, C., Kools, M. (2011). *Writing health communications: An evidence based guide.* London: Sage.

Amireault, S., Godin, G., Vézina-Im, L.A. (2013). Determinants of physical activity maintenance: a systematic review and meta-analyses, *Health Psychology Review,* 7(1): 55–91. Doi: 10.1080/17437199.2012.701060.

Bandura, A. (1997). *Self-efficacy: The exercise of control.* New York: WH Freeman and Co.

Barr, H.L., Britton, J., Smyth, A.R., Fogarty, A.W. (2011). Association between socio-economic status, sex, and age at death from cystic fibrosis in England and Wales (1959 to 2008): cross sectional study. *British Medical Journal*, 343: d4662. Doi: 10.1136/bmj.d4662.

Bartholomew, E., Markham, C., Ruiter, R., et al. (2016) *Planning health promotion programs: An intervention mapping approach* (4th ed.). Hoboken, NJ: Wiley.

Brawley, L.A., Rejeski, W.J., King, A.C. (2003). Promoting physical activity for older adults: the challenges for changing behaviour. *American Journal of Preventative Medicine*, 25(3): 172–183. Doi: 10.1016/S0749-3797(03)00182-X.

Britten, N. (1994). Patients' ideas about medicines: a qualitative study in a general practice population. *British Journal of General Practice*, 44: 465–468.

Brown, H., Atkin, A., Panter, J., Wong, G., Chinapaw, M.J.M., van Sluijs, E.M.F. (2016). Family based interventions to increase physical activity in children: a systematic review, meta-analysis and realist synthesis. *Obesity Reviews*, 17. Doi: 10.1111/obr.12362.

Carlin, A., Perchoux, C., Puggina, A., Aleksovska, K., Buck, C., Burns, C., Cardon, G., Chantal, S., Ciarapica, D., Condello, G., Coppinger, T., Cortis, C., D'Haese, S. (2017). A life course examination of the physical environmental determinants of physical activity behaviour: a "Determinants of Diet and Physical Activity" (DEDIPAC) umbrella systematic literature review. *PLoS ONE* 12(8). Doi: 10.1371/journal.pone.0182083.

Carver, C., Schieier, M., Weintraub, J. (1989). Assessing coping strategies: a theoretically based approach. *Journal of Personality and Social Psychology*, 56: 267–283. Doi: 10.10377/0022-3514.56.2.267.

Carver, A., Timperio, A., Crawford, D. (2008). Playing it safe: the influence of neighbourhood safety on children's physical activity-a review. *Health and Place*, 14: 217–227. Doi: 10.1016/j.healthplace.2007.06.004.

Cox, N., Holland, A. (2013). Interventions for promoting physical activity in people with cystic fibrosis. *Cochrane Database Systematic Reviews*, 12. Doi: 10.1002/14651858.CD009448.pub2.

Currie, C., Roberts, C., Morgan, A., Smith, R., Settertobulte, W., Samdai, O., Barnekow, V. (2004). *Young people's health in context. Health behaviour in school-aged children (HBSC) study international report from the 2001/2002 survey.* Copenhagen: WHO Regional Office for Europe, 53–161.

Cystic Fibrosis Trust UK. (2020). Life with cystic fibrosis. Accessed December 2020: https://www.cysticfibrosis.org.uk/life-with-cystic-fibrosis.

Darker, C., French D., Eves, F., Sniehotta, F. (2010). An intervention to promote walking amongst the general population based on an extended theory of planned behaviour: a waiting list randomised controlled trial. *Psychology and Health*, 25: 71–88. Doi: 10.1080/08870440902893716.

Deci, E.L., Ryan, M. (1985). *Intrinsic motivation and self-determination in human behavior.* New York: Plenum.

Denford, S., Van Beurden, S., O'Halloran P., Williams C.A. (2020). Barriers and facilitators to physical activity among young people with cystic fibrosis: a systematic review and thematic synthesis of qualitative of research. *BMJ Open*, 10: e035261. Doi: 10.1136/bmjopen-2019-035261.

Denford, S., MackIntosh, K., McNarry, M., Barker, A., Williams, C. (2019). Promotion of physical activity for adolescents with cystic fibrosis: a qualitative study of UK multi-disciplinary cystic fibrosis teams. *Physiotherapy*, 106: 111–118. Doi: 10.1016/j.physio.2019.01.012.

Douglas, H., Bryon, M., Denford, S., Rand, S., Main, E. (2018). Exercise: love it, hate it, or somewhere in-between? Identifying exercise self-efficacy and the impact of personal training in children and young people with CF. Abstract European Cystic Fibrosis Conference, *Journal of Cystic Fibrosis*, 17(Suppl 3): P144.

Elhakeem, A., Cooper, R., Bahn, D., Kuh, D., Hardy, R. (2017). Birth weight, school sports ability and adulthood leisure-time physical activity. *Medicine and Science in Sports and Exercise*, 49: 64–70. Doi: 10.1249/MSS.0000000000001077.

Farooq, A., Martin, A., Janssen, X., Wilson, M. (2020). Longitudinal changes in moderate-to-vigorous-intensity physical activity in children and adolescents: a systematic review and meta-analysis. *Obesity Reviews*, 21:e12953. Doi: 10.1111/obr.12953.

Fereday, J., MacDougall, C., Spizzo, M., Darbyshire, P., Schiller, W. (2009). "There's nothing I can't do–I just put my mind to anything and I can do it": a qualitative analysis of how children with chronic disease and their parents account for and manage physical activity. *BMC Pediatrics*, 9: 1. Doi: 10.1186/1471-2431-9-1.

Ferreira, I., Van Der Horst, K., Wendel-Vos, W., et al. (2007). Environmental correlates of physical activity in youth – a review and update. *Obesity Reviews*, 8: 129–154. Doi: 10.1111/j.1467-789X.2006.00264.x.

Fisher, J., Fisher W. (1992). Changing AIDS-risk behaviour, *Psychological Bulletin*, 111: 455–457. Doi: 10.1037/0033-2909.111.3.455.

Gardener, B., de Bruijn, G., Lally, P. (2011). A systematic review and meta-analysis of applications of the self-report habit index to nutrition and physical activity behaviours. *Annals of Behavioural Medicine*, 42: 174–187. Doi: 10.1007/s12160-011-9282-0.

Gidlow, C., Johnston, L., Crone, D., Ellis, N., James, D. (2006). A systematic review of the relationship between socio-economic position and physical activity. *Health Education Journal*, 65: 338–367. Doi: 10.1177/0017896906069378.

Guthold, R., Stevens, G., Riley, M., Bull, F. (2018). Worldwide trends in insufficient physical activity from 2001 to 2016: a pooled analysis of 358 population-based surveys with 1.9 million participants. *The Lancet Global Health*, 6(10): e1046–1047. Doi: 10.1016/S2214-109X(18)30357-7.

Hagberg, L.A., Lindahl, B., Nyberg, N., Hellenius, M.L. (2009). Importance of enjoyment when promoting physical exercise. *Scandinavian Journal of Medicine and Science in Sports*, 19: 740–747. Doi: 10.1111/j.1600-0838.2008.00844.x.

Happ, M.B., Hoffman, L.A., DiVirgilio, D., Higgins, L.W., Orenstein, D.M. (2013). Parent and child perceptions of a self-regulated, home-based exercise program for children with cystic fibrosis. *Nursing Research*, 62: 305–314. Doi: 10.1097/NNR.0b013e3182a03503.

Jago, R., Salway, R., Emm-Collison, L, et al. (2020). Association of BMI category with change in children's physical activity between ages 6 and 11 years. *International Journal of Obesity*, 44(1)104–113. Doi: 10.1038/s41366-019-0459-0.

Kahneman, D. (2011). *Thinking, fast and slow*. New York: Farrar, Straus and Giroux.

Ledger, S., Wade, A., Douglas, H., et al. (2016). Interim results for INSPIRE-CF: A 24-month RCT evaluating effects of weekly supervised exercise in children with CF. *European Respiratory Society International Congress*. Doi: 10.1183/13993003.congress-2016.OA1493.

Ginis M, K.A., Nigg, C.R., Smith, A. (2013). Peer-delivered physical activity interventions: an overlooked opportunity for physical activity promotion. *Translational Behavioural Medicine*, 3: 434–443. Doi: 10.1007/s13142-013-0215-2.

Michie, S., Johnston, M., Francis, J., Hardeman, W., Eccles, M. (2008). From theory to intervention: mapping theoretical derived behavioural determinants to behaviour change techniques. *Applied Psychology,* 57: 660–680. Doi: 10.1111/j.1464-0597.2008.00341.x.

Montori, V.M., Gafni, A., Charles, C. (2006). A shared decision-making approach between patients with chronic conditions and their clinicians: the case of diabetes. *Health Expectations,* 9(1): 25–36. Doi: 10.1111/j.1369-7625.2006.00359.x.

Moola, F.J., Faulkner, G.E. (2014). 'A tale of two cases:' the health, illness, and physical activity stories of two children living with cystic fibrosis. *Clinical Child Psychology and Psychiatry,* 19: 24–42. Doi: 10.1177/1359104512465740.

Moola, F.J., Faulkner, G.E., Schneiderman. J.E. (2012). "No time to play": perceptions toward physical activity in youth with cystic fibrosis. *Adapted Physical Activity Quarterly,* 29: 44–62. Doi: 10.1123/apaq.29.144.

Moola, F.J., Faulkner, G.E., Kirsh, J.A., Schneiderman, J.E. (2011). Developing physical activity interventions for youth with cystic fibrosis and congenital heart disease: learning from their parents. *Psychology of Sport and Exercise,* 12: 599–608. Doi: 10.1016/j/psychsport.2011.07.001.

Oakley A.D., Booth, M.L., Patterson, J.W. (2001). Relationship of physical activity to fundamental movement skills among adolescents. *Medicine and Science in Sports and Exercise,* 33(11): 1899–1904. Doi: 10.1097/00005768-200111000-00015.

O'Halloran, P.D., Blackstock, F., Shields, N., Holland, A., Iles, R., Kingsley, M., Bernhardt, J., Lannin, N., Morris, M.E. and Taylor, N.F. (2014). Motivational interviewing to increase physical activity in people with chronic health conditions: a systematic review and meta-analysis. *Clinical Rehabilitation,* 28: 1159–1171. Doi: 10.1177/0269215514536210.

Rollnick, S., Miller, W. (1995). What is motivational interviewing? *Behavioural and Cognitive Psychotherapy,* 23:325–344. Doi: 10.1017/S135246580001643X.

Schoeppe, S., Duncan, M., Badland, H., Oliver, M., Curtis, C. (2012). Associations of children's independent mobility and active travel with physical activity, sedentary behaviour, and weight status: a systematic review. *Journal of Science and Medicine in Sport,* 16: 312–319. Doi: 10.1016/j.jsams.2012.11.001.

Selvadurai, H.C., Blimkie, C.J., Cooper, P.J., Mellis, C.M., Van Asperen, P.P. (2004). Gender differences in habitual activity in children with cystic fibrosis. *Archives of Disease in Childhood,* 89: 928–933. Doi: 10.1136/adc.2003.034249.

Sport England (2019). Active Lives Children and Young People Survey. Accessed February 24 2020: https://www.sportengland.org/news/active-lives-children-and-young-people-survey-academic-year-201819-report-published.

Strack, F., Deutsch, R. (2004). Reflective and impulsive determinants of social behaviour. *Personality and Social Psychology Bulletin,* 8: 220. Doi: 10.1207/s15327957pspr0803_1.

Shelley, J., Fairclough, S., Knowles, Z.R., et al. (2018). A formative study exploring perceptions of physical activity monitoring among children and young people with cystic fibrosis and health care professionals. *BMC Pediatrics,* 18: 335. Doi: 10.1186/s12887-018-1301-x.

Shuval, K., Li, Q., Gabriel, K.P., Tchernis, R. (2017). Income, physical activity, sedentary behaviour and the 'weekend warrior' among US adults. *Preventative Medicine,* 103: 91–97. Doi: 10.1016/j.ypmed.2017.07.033.

Street, R., Mercer, J., Mills-Bennett, R., O'Leary, C., Thirlaway, K. (2016). Experiences of physical activity: a phenomenological study of individuals with cystic fibrosis. *Journal of Health Psychology,* 21: 261–270. Doi: 10.1177/1359105314527141.

Swisher, A.K., Erickson, M. (2008). Perceptions of physical activity in a group of adolescents with cystic fibrosis. *Cardiopulmonary Physical Therapy Journal*, 19: 107–113. PMID: 20467507.

Tomlinson, O. Shelley, J., Trott, J., Bowhay, B., Chauhan, R., Sheldon, C. (2019). The feasibility of online video calling to engage patients with cystic fibrosis in exercise training. *Journal of Telemedicine and Telecare*, 26(6): 356–364. Doi: 10.1177/1357633X19828630.

Tucker, P., Gilliland, J. (2007). The effect of season and weather on physical activity: a systematic review. *Public Health*, 121: 909–922. Doi: 10.1016/j.puhe.2007.04.009.

van Sluijs, E.M., Fearne, V., Mattocks C., et al. (2009). The contribution of active travel to children's physical activity levels: cross-sectional results from the ALSPAC study. *Preventive Medicine*, 48: 519–524. Doi: 10.1016/j.ypmed.2009.03.002.

Verplanken, B., Aarts, H. (1999). Habit, attitude, and planned behaviour: is habit an empty construct or an interesting case of goal-directed automaticity, *European Review of Social Psychology*, 10: 101–134. Doi: 10.1080/14792779943000035.

White, M., Pahl, S., Wheeler, B., Fleming, L. (2016). The 'Blue Gym': what can blue space do for you and what can you do for blue space. *Oceans and Human Health*, 69, 5–12. Doi: 10.1017/S0025315415002209.

Yardley, L., Ainsworth, B., Arden-Close, E., Muller, I. (2015). The person-based approach to enhancing the acceptability and feasibility of interventions. *Pilot and Feasibility Studies*, 1(1): 1–7. Doi: 10.1186/s40814-015-0033-z.

6 Exercise in Children and Adolescents with Asthma

Marietta Núñez Cámara and Guillermo Zepeda

Introduction

Asthma is a heterogeneous disease and is the most common chronic disease in children (Asher and Pearce, 2014), characterised by chronic airway inflammation. The typical clinical symptoms are cough, wheezing, breathlessness, and chest tightness that fluctuate in intensity over time and are associated with variable expiratory airflow limitation, triggered by a range of factors including exercise (GINA, 2020).

Children with asthma may have a lower exercise tolerance, as performance can be limited by respiratory symptoms, exercise-induced asthma, and poor fitness that follow avoidance or compromise of physical training (Chandratilleke *et al.*, 2012; Avallone and McLeish, 2013). Consequently, asthma is the most common chronic diseases limiting physical activities and causing disability in children (Newacheck and Halfone, 2000) and children with asthma frequently fail to undertake the levels of physical activity recommended to maintain good health (Desloovere *et al.*, 2010). Avoidance may arise because of misconceptions about exercise and asthma held by patients, their family, schools, or even healthcare providers. Overall, limited performance and abstinence or exclusion from peer group activities will have a negative impact on a child's physical, psychological, and social development (Glazebrook *et al.*, 2006; Westergren *et al.*, 2015).

Successful asthma management must focus on disease control, requiring a multidimensional approach that evaluates both clinical and respiratory functional parameters, including an assessment of symptoms during exercise to determine whether there is any limitation of exercise performance (Gandhi *et al.*, 2013; Lu *et al.*, 2016). High levels of physical activity have a positive impact on the course and severity of the disease. Exercise decreases bronchial hyper-responsiveness and exercise-induced asthma, it increases symptom-free days, improves aerobic capacity, and enhances quality of life (Chandratilleke *et al.*, 2012; Eijkemans *et al.*, 2012; Eichenberger *et al.*, 2013; Wanrooij *et al.*, 2013).

DOI: 10.4324/9781003020462-6

Physical Activity, Obesity, and Asthma

There are associations between asthma, physical inactivity, and obesity, although the strength and causality of relationships remain controversial. In many societies, significant reductions in physical activity have paralleled a dramatic increase in the prevalence of both obesity and asthma (Wanrooij *et al.*, 2013; Lang *et al.*, 2014; McNarry *et al.*, 2014; Leinaar *et al.*, 2016; Lu *et al.*, 2016). Furthermore, physical inactivity and sedentary lifestyle in children and adolescents are associated with the development of risk factors for cardiovascular disease (Al-Mallah *et al.*, 2018; Abrignani *et al.*, 2019). In contrast, fitness is an important marker of global health in children and adolescents, associated with reduced cardiovascular disease risk (Kodama *et al.*, 2009), improved mental health outcomes, and higher self-esteem (Ortega *et al.*, 2008).

A study in Baltimore, U.S.A. that included 137 asthmatics and 106 controls, aged 6–12 years, evaluated physical activity by a questionnaire (Lang *et al.*, 2004). The median time spent in physical activities was significantly lower in asthmatics (odds ratio [OR] 3.0; 95% confidence interval [CI] 1.2–7.5). In a Greek study, 50 asthmatic children and 50 non-asthmatic controls completed a leisure-time exercise questionnaire to define the frequency and intensity of their exercise activities. The findings were that asthmatic children undertook similar light and moderate activities, but significantly fewer vigorous or planned exercise activities compared to controls (Dimitrakaki *et al.*, 2013). A cross-sectional study in the UK of 56 children with asthma and 61 controls attending clinic for non-respiratory conditions found that the asthma cohort had a higher mean body mass index (BMI), a significantly higher incidence of obesity (OR 3.9; 95% CI 1.17–12.9) and lower physical activity levels, evaluated by a questionnaire. Around 60% of both parents and children in the asthma group considered the child's health as a barrier to exercise participation compared to 11% in the control group ($P < 0.001$) (Glazebrook *et al.*, 2006). A study of healthy and newly diagnosed asthmatic children in Denmark used accelerometers to show that uncontrolled asthma is correlated with reduced levels of intense physical activity ($r = 0.35$, $p < 0.05$) (Vahlkvist and Pedersen, 2009).

Lochte *et al.*, (2016) conducted a systematic review of the relationship between low levels of physical activity, determined by sporting and lifestyle questionnaires, and the subsequent development of asthma. This included a meta-analysis of three cohort studies, conducted for up to 11 years; involving 6,037 children aged 7–18 years. Results showed an increased risk of new onset, physician-diagnosed asthma in children with lower physical activity levels (random effects model OR 1.35; 95% CI 0.95–1.84). In another meta-analysis, pooling five longitudinal studies, totalling 85,117 participants, higher baseline physical activity levels appeared to be a protective factor against asthma development (OR = 0.88; 95% CI 0.77–1.01), although further longitudinal studies are needed to elucidate the relative effects of different activity intensities, gender, and whether effects may be different in specific age groups (Eijkemans *et al.*, 2012).

A cross-sectional, web-based, self-reported survey of health risk behaviours in over 72,000 Korean children, aged 13–18 years found that, compared with non-asthmatic adolescents, those with current asthma spent more time undertaking sedentary activities such as watching television. However, there were no differences between asthmatics and non-asthmatics in time spent participating in sporting or vigorous exercise activities. In line with other work, adolescents with atopy, who were male, obese, active smokers or from more affluent families were more likely to report current asthma (Kim *et al.*, 2012). Limitations of self reporting in this work are compensated by its size and cultural characteristics may have influenced engagement in physical activity.

The results of 'The National Youth Fitness Survey' in the U.S. had responses from 665 children aged 6–11 years. Around 17.9% reported a past and 11.4% a current history of asthma. Physical de-conditioning and increased sedentary time were both associated with a current and historical diagnosis of asthma, asthma exacerbations, and asthma symptoms with exercise (Lu *et al.*, 2020).

In recent decades, the prevalence of both asthma and overweight has risen. One meta-analysis of how childhood overweight increases the risk of developing asthma concluded that both high birthweight and mid-childhood overweight increased the risk of subsequent asthma, and for the latter, school age children with BMI ≥ 85th percentile had a 50% increase in the relative risk of developing asthma (RR 1.5; 95% CI 1.2–1.8) (Flaherman and Rutherford, 2006). A more recent meta-analysis corroborated this, finding that the incidence of asthma was increased by 20% in children with BMI ≥ 85th percentile and those with a BMI ≥ 95th had a twofold increased asthma risk (RR 2.02; 95% CI 1.16–3.50). Boys were affected more by this BMI-disease relationship than girls (*Chen et al.*, 2013).

A further meta-analysis of 18 studies including 73,252 children concluded that obesity and overweight are risk factors for asthma (OR 1.3; 95% CI 1.23–1.39) and wheezing (OR 1.9; 95% CI 1.38–2.63) with obesity having the greater affect, but unlike other work, found the association was greater in girls (OR 1.34; 95% CI 1.16–1.56) rather than boys (OR 1.27; 95% CI 1.15–1.4) (Deng *et al.*, 2019). In a systematic review that investigated the temporal and strength of relationship between asthma and overweight in children aged 0–18 years, physical activity was explored as a mediator. Seventy-five studies including cross-sectional, case-control, and longitudinal investigations met eligibility criteria (Leinaar *et al.*, 2016). Although the temporal relationship remains unclear, reduced energy expenditure due to reduced physical activity underpins the association between asthma and obesity. Negative parental or self-perception of exercise ability due to asthma symptoms during exercise was identified as a determinant of reduced physical activity.

There are different mechanisms by which obesity could induce or aggravate asthma. These include dietary factors, gastro-oesophageal reflux, the mechanical effects of obesity and hormonal influences. Additionally, adipose tissue is not inert and influences immunological and inflammatory processes.

In patients genetically predisposed to asthma, the onset of obesity might hasten the development of disease by promoting inflammation (Lu *et al.*, 2016). An inflammatory cascade has been described in obesity that may impact on cardiovascular and respiratory health. This involves a rise in the pool of pro-inflammatory macrophages (M1) in adipose tissue and a fall in anti-inflammatory macrophages (M2) that is associated with an imbalance favouring pro-inflammatory over anti-inflammatory adipocyte cytokines, such as adiponectin which protects against cardiovascular complications of obesity in later life (Vijayakanthi *et al.*, 2016; Orlando *et al.*, 2019). Pro-inflammatory T-helper cell polarisation in obese asthmatic adolescents has been linked to high interleukin 6 (IL-6) levels, produced by adipose tissue macrophages, decreased lung function, and poor asthma control (Fantuzzi, 2005).

Overall, the lack of participation in regular exercise amongst asthmatic patients is related to an increase in obesity, which correlates with poor asthma control, reduces quality of life, and increases health care cost (Kier and Forde, 2011; Avallone and McLeish, 2013; Ahmadizar *et al.*, 2016; Lu *et al.*, 2016; Holderness *et al.*, 2017; Lu *et al.*, 2020).

Exercise-induced Bronchoconstriction and Exercise-induced Asthma

Exercise is an important trigger for asthma symptoms and in some asthmatic children is the dominant feature of the disease. It is important to differentiate between 'exercise-induced asthma' (EIA) and 'exercise-induced bronchoconstriction' (EIB) (Del Giacco *et al.*, 2015). Both can give rise to symptoms of breathlessness, wheezing, cough, chest tightness, and increased mucus production provoked by and limiting exercise activity. EIB, occurring in a substantial proportion of patients with asthma, may be termed EIA, but these individuals have additional symptoms of asthma at times other than following exercise, such as at night or in the early morning and they may suffer exacerbations triggered by viral illnesses or aeroallergen exposure. However, it is important to recognise EIB as an entity in individuals who do not suffer from asthma as there are important differences in management strategy (Aggarwal *et al.*, 2018). There is some consensus in using EIA to indicate asthma symptoms following a bout of heavy exercise and EIB as a physiological term to denote the drop in lung function following exercise and confirmed in a standardised exercise challenge test (Del Giacco *et al.*, 2015).

EIB is defined as acute, transient, and reversible airway narrowing occurring during or after exercise. The diagnosis is based on an objective change in lung function after an exercise or hyperventilation challenge test, irrespective of symptoms. Generally, 5–8 minutes of continuous high-intensity effort is required to develop an exercise-induced bronchoconstriction response, typically requiring a rise in heart rate to 80 or 90% of the maximum predicted. EIB is usually observed 2–5 minutes following the exercise bout, and not during maximum exercise intensity. It peaks at 10 minutes and resolves by

60 minutes. A positive test is defined by a fall in forced expiratory volume in the first second (FEV1) of ≥10% from baseline, where the best of two reproducible forced expiratory manoeuvres is recorded at 5, 10, 15, and 30 minutes post-exercise. The severity of bronchoconstriction is graded as mild (10–25%), moderate (25–50%), or severe (>50%) (Parsons *et al.*, 2013). Eucapnic voluntary hyperpnoea (EVH) is an alternative challenge that simulates the effects of exercise on airways (Anderson *et al.*, 2001), and has been shown to be feasible in the investigation of respiratory difficulties in young athletes (Van der Eycken *et al.*, 2016). EVH requires the subject to breathe a specific gas mixture (21% oxygen, 5% carbon dioxide, and balance nitrogen), at a minute ventilation (VE), of 30–35 times their baseline FEV1 for 6 minutes. FEV1 is measured at intervals and with the same diagnostic criteria for EIB as with an exercise challenge (Hull *et al.*, 2016).

There are two theories promoted to explain the pathophysiology of EIB. The 'osmotic theory' is linked to the inhalation of dry air combined with the increase in minute ventilation, causing dehydration of the respiratory mucosa, increasing the osmolality of airway fluid. In turn this stimulates the release of inflammatory mediators including histamine, prostaglandins, eicosanoids, and leukotrienes, from airway eosinophils and mastocytes leading to bronchial smooth muscle contraction and transient bronchoconstriction. The 'thermic theory' details that airway vasoconstriction occurs in response to the inhalation of dry, cold air and following exercise, rapid reheating produces a rebound vasodilation within and oedema of the airway wall, coupled with a parasympathetic neuronal reflex bronchoconstriction (Weiler *et al.*, 2010; Carlsen *et al.*, 2011; Del Giacco *et al.*, 2015; Anderson, 2006).

The concentration of specific inflammatory cytokines is significantly increased in the exhaled breath condensate of children with EIA, these include monocyte chemotactic protein 1 (MCP 1) and interleukin 16 (IL-16) that may play a role in the pathophysiology, which is in common with the early (MCP-1) and late (IL-16) phases of allergy-mediated bronchoconstriction (Majak *et al.*, 2016). The prevalence of EIB reported in different populations varies depending on study methodologies, healthcare provision, ethnicity, and environmental factors. In the general population, there is a reported prevalence of 5–20%, being higher in children ≤16 years (3–35%) and even higher among elite athletes (30–70%), depending on the kind of the sport, the environment, and the maximum intensity achieved (Batista and Soares 2013; Aggarwal *et al.*, 2018). It has been identified that up to 50% of young elite athletes could suffer from asthma or airway hyper-responsiveness and that there is a need to improve diagnostic pathways in this group (Price *et al.*, 2013; Kippelen, 2016). It is important to emphasise that respiratory symptoms with exercise are poor predictors of EIB, as around one third of asthmatic children who do not report excessive respiratory symptoms during exercise meet the criteria for diagnosing EIB when objectively tested (Parsons *et al.*, 2013; Inci *et al.*, 2017).

EIA is thought to occur in as many as 90% of adult asthmatics and between 20 and 90% of young people with asthma; being more likely if the asthma is severe or poorly controlled. This wide range of prevalence can again be explained by the different study methodologies and diagnostic approaches (Gotshall, 2002), see Figure 6.1. EIA in children aged ≥12 years is more common in those with lower Asthma Control Test (ACT) scores and while low scores were not specific enough to be useful in identifying EIA, high ACT scores may be an effective means of excluding it (Tripodi *et al.*, 2016). Normally, exercise itself is a powerful bronchodilator that can counter pathological processes which impair lung funtion. Classically EIA presents after exercise ceases. However, in adults with EIA, prolonged exercise can trigger bronchoconstriction while exercise is in progress. In children, the processes underpinning EIA may be markedly faster leading to bronchocostriction during exercise. This is called 'breakthrough' EIA (BT-EIA). This earlier and often deeper fall in lung funtion may be considered a more severe form of EIA (Parsons *et al.*, 2013; Lin *et al.*, 2019; van Der Kamp *et al.*, 2019). In one study of 33 asthmatic children, exercising at a sub-maximal level (80% predicted maximum heart rate), about one third of children developed bronchoconstriction at 6–10 minutes while still exercising, and in another third, it developed immediately after exercise (van Leeuwen *et al.*, 2011). Not all children with asthma suffer from EIA, but those who do are even more likely to restrict their physical activities and the sub-group who have the pattern of BT-EIA show a specific avoidance of more moderate and vigourous exercise activity (van Der Kamp *et al.*, 2019).

There are also some important differential diagnoses that can limit exercise performance, the most common being obesity, but other pulmonary and cardiac conditions may need to be considered when there is uncertainty.

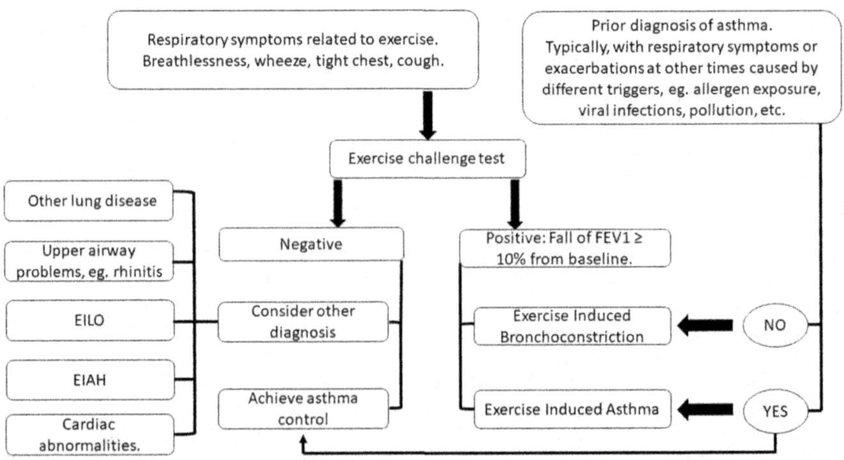

Figure 6.1 Diagnostic pathway for respiratory symptoms associated with exercise.

Two conditions deserve specific mention, firstly, exercise-induced laryngeal obstruction (EILO), characterised by symptoms developing during exercise and usually ceasing on stopping exercise with no benefit from pre-exercise inhaled bronchodilators. This condition is discussed in Chapter 7. Another abnormality is exercise-induced arterial hypoxemia (EIAH) that occurs in well-trained athletes, including adolescents, compromising endurance exercise performance. Limitation of pulmonary gas exchange during exercise leads to arterial desaturation ≥4%. It may result from a blunted alveolar hyperventilatory response or an increased alveolar-arterial oxygen gradient, possibly due to ventilation-perfusion inequality or limited diffusion (Hopkins, 2006).

Differences in the management of EIB and EIA are important to recognise. EIB management should focus on generic preventative strategies and relief of bronchoconstriction. There are many non-pharmacological approaches recommended to reduce the risk of bronchoconstriction which include warming up before exercise to induce a refractory period, techniques to humidify or pre-warm inhaled air and avoiding exposure to air pollutants and allergens. If EIB symptoms continue despite non-pharmacological approaches, pharmacological interventions including short-acting Beta2-agonists (SABA) 15 minutes before exercise, leukotriene receptor antagonists (LTRAs) or chromones can be considered (Aggarwal *et al.*, 2018).

EIA management should be aligned to evidence-based asthma treatment guidelines to achieve asthma control, which may be implemented in addition to EIB recommendations (Aggarwal *et al.*, 2018, Global Initiative for Asthma, 2020). Where there is diagnostic uncertainty, cardiopulmonary exercise testing may be helpful to discriminate between exercise-induced dyspnea and hyperventilation, particularly in older children and adolescents (Weiler *et al.*, 2016; Aggarwal *et al.*, 2018).

Exercise Training – Benefits, Format, and Prescription

Globally, fitness is recognised as an indicator of good health and low cardiorespiratory capacity carries an increased risk of cardiovascular disease and mortality (Clausen *et al.*, 2018). Strategies to improve cardiorespiratory fitness may be of benefit in preventing co-morbidities associated with childhood asthma, such as obesity (Castro-Rodríguez *et al.*, 2001) and mental health disorders (Kier and Forde, 2011; Wanrooij *et al.*, 2013). Physical training improves aerobic capacity, asthma symptoms, quality of life and reduces asthma exacerbations in asthmatic subjects. Although resting spirometric lung function may not improve, bronchial hyper-responsiveness (BHR) may stabilise due to systemic anti-inflammatory effects of training. However, the intensity of physical training studied is variable. Interventional consistency and confirmation of efficacy require that training protocols need to be standardised and defined in terms of type of activity, frequency, duration, and intensity (Welsh *et al.*, 2005; Chandratilleke *et al.*, 2012; Eichenberger *et al.*, 2013; Wanrooij *et al.*, 2013; Candemir *et al.*, 2017; Jaakkola *et al.*, 2019;

McNarry *et al.*, 2019; McNarry *et al.*, 2020). The American College of Sports Medicine advocates that '*the higher the training intensity, the greater the effect,*' which may be true for aerobic capacity, but not necessarily for BHR stabilisation or quality of life (QoL). Standardisation is important if there are to be meaningful evaluations of interventions and factors such as ambient temperature, height above sea level, and temporal relationships to eating and sleep are important to consider in training and testing protocols (American College of Sports Medicine, 1998; Welsh *et al.*, 2005).

Fitness

Aerobic capacity (VO_{2max}) corresponds to an individual's maximum rate of oxygen consumption and is acknowledged as the gold standard for evaluating fitness. A meta-analysis of 6 studies combining 149 asthmatic participants, concluded that exercise training increased VO_{2max} (mean +5.57 $mL \cdot kg^{-1} \cdot min^{-1}$; 95% CI 4.36–6.78). Pooled data from 4 of the studies concluded that there was also an increase in minute ventilation (VE_{max}) mean +6.0 $L \cdot min^{-1}$; 95% CI 1.57–10.43). These improvements were observed irrespective of whether the children had EIA (Chandratilleke *et al.*, 2012). One meta-analysis of the value of physical training in asthmatic children and adolescents, focused on the type of training best suited to improve fitness. The analysis identified that in order to improve aerobic capacity the physical training intensity levels needed to be at the ventilatory threshold, corresponding to the point that the ventilatory rate starts to increase at a faster rate than oxygen consumption (usually at about 50–75% of VO_{2max}), training had to be undertaken for at least 120 minutes per week, divided into two to three sessions in a program lasting at least 3 months (Wanrooij *et al.*, 2013). Overall, the time spent training is positively correlated with the improvement in fitness (Chandratilleke *et al.*, 2012). Swimming training appears to have particular benefit in improving aerobic capacity in asthmatics under 18 years of age, compared to other sports (Huang *et al.*, 1989; Beggs *et al.*, 2013).

Asthma Control

Chandratilleke's systematic review (2012), identified three studies showing improvement in symptoms-free days after exercise training intervention compared to controls. In a larger meta-analysis of randomised control trials involving over 2,000 asthmatic subjects, the exercise training intervention group had significantly more symptom-free days per month than controls (mean +8.9 symptom-free days; 95% CI 8.18–9.61, $p < 0.001$) (Eichenberger *et al.*, 2013). Examining the impact of exercise training on other asthma outcomes, Wanrooij's systematic review, included 13 studies investigating school absenteeism, hospitalisations, and symptom scores. Overall, data was limited but identified a trend towards training reducing the number of emergency attendances and hospitalisations for asthma attacks (Wanrooij *et al.*, 2013).

Quality of Life

Asthma has a negative impact on the QoL in children through several mechanisms. These include non-participation in peer group games and sports for reasons such as the fear of inducing breathlessness confounded by lack of fitness due to inactivity, asthma symptoms related to exercise and poor disease control. Erroneous beliefs about exercise being harmful can become embedded in an individual's psyche (Fanelli *et al.*, 2007), sometimes reinforced by parental or trainer anxiety.

The 'Pediatric Asthma Quality of Life Questionnaire,' (PAQLQ) is a validated tool for children and adolescents aged 7–17 years, which comprehensively explores the impact of a child's asthma on their life, encompassing symptoms, disruptions, or restrictions to social, learning and recreational activities, emotions and aspects of asthma most important to the patient (Juniper *et al.*, 1996). Exercise training improves PAQLQ scores and reduces the level of pharmacological intervention needed for asthma control (Chandratilleke *et al.*, 2012; Wanrooij *et al.*, 2013). In Eichenberger's systematic review asthma QoL improved by 17% more on average in exercise training cohorts compared with controls (Eichenberger *et al.*, 2013).

Resting Spirometric Lung Function and Bronchial Hyperresponsiveness

Exercise training does not appear to reproducibly improve resting spirometric lung function. Most studies, which have involved different sports and training formats, with the exception of swimming, have not identified any significant change in resting measures of airway obstruction including FEV1 and Forced expiratory flow (FEF) 25–75% in asthmatic children (Chandratilleke *et al.*, 2012; Beegs *et al.*, 2013; Wanrooij *et al.*, 2013). However, exercise training can reduce BHR, when assessed by direct challenges of inhaled methacholine or histamine or by indirect exercise challenge tests (Chandratilleke *et al.*, 2012; Wanrooij *et al.*, 2013). In the systematic review by Wanrooij *et al.*, (2013), it was concluded that the magnitude of fall in FEV1 following an exercise challenge test decreased with exercise training interventions. Similarly, in the meta-analysis by Eichenberger *et al.*, (2013), three studies comparing direct BHR challenges before and after exercise training with controls demonstrated a trend for lower BHR after training, the percentage fall in FEV1 lessened significantly by a mean 53%. The stabilisation of BHR may be the consequence of a direct anti-inflammatory effect of exercise. Aerobic exercise training has been associated with a fall in the levels of some circulating pro-inflammatory cytokines such as MPC-1 and IL-6, in parallel with improved QoL scores and reduced asthma exacerbations in moderate to severe asthmatics (França-Pinto *et al.*, 2015), and it is interesting that it is low-to-moderate intensity aerobic exercise that appears to reduce inflammation and potentially airway remodelling in asthmatics (Del Giacco and Garcia-Larsen, 2016).

Generally, physical training in asthmatics is well tolerated, with no adverse effects identified (Chandratilleke *et al.*, 2012; Eichenberger *et al.*, 2013; Wanrooij *et al.*, 2013), although to train at the desired intensity, children need to have adequate asthma control with appropriate pharmacological therapy. Individualisation of exercise prescriptions, which provide options and variations, can help with motivation and adherence, although make standardisation more difficult (Wanrooij *et al.*, 2013). Consequently, exercise should be discussed and promoted as an integral part of the management of children with asthma and as such, it has been shown to be a cost-effective intervention (Global Initiative for Asthma, 2020).

Swimming and Asthma

Swimming requires some specific consideration as it is generally well tolerated by stable asthmatic patients and comes with notable benefits although awareness of certain hazards is important. In common with other sports, studies of swimming training have demonstrated benefits in terms of improved asthma symptom control, but there is evidence for greater improvements in fitness and, unlike other sports, improvements in resting lung function and ventilation techniques in asthmatic patients (Fitch *et al.*, 1976; Wang and Hung, 2009; Beggs *et al.*, 2013; Lahart and Metsios, 2018). A Cochrane library meta-analysis of 8 studies in well-controlled asthmatics aged 5–18 years involved swimming training schedules over 6–12 weeks, typically being 30–90 minutes 2–3 times a week with one study training for 30 minutes 6 times a week (Beggs *et al.*, 2013). The analysis concluded that the mean increase in VO_{2max} achieved by swimming training was 9.67 $mL \cdot kg^{-1} \cdot min^{-1}$; (95% CI 5.84–13.51; $n = 32$), representing a remarkable 25% increase from baseline, a much greater increase than measured in other types of physical training in children without asthma (5–15%) or children with asthma (9%). In 4 of the studies ($n = 113$), the mean difference in resting FEV1% predicted was 8.07% higher after swimming training (95% CI 3.59–12.54). Epidemiological studies have suggested that the swimming pool environment, which is warm, humid, and usually cleansed by disinfection by products, such as chlorine, may pose a risk for triggering or even developing asthma and other allergic diseases, especially when physically exerting in such environments (Clearie *et al.*, 2010). Much controversy about this prevails (Uyan *et al.*, 2009; Weisel *et al.*, 2009; Bougault and Boulet, 2012, 2013; Andersson *et al.*, 2018; Kanikowska *et al.*, 2018).

Chlorine is the most common disinfectant used in swimming pools, and when combined with nitrogenous compounds (dirt, sweat, and urine), chloramines and other disinfection by-products (DBPs) are generated, especially nitrogen trichloride (NCl_3), which remain aerosolised above the water surface and can damage airway epithelium when inhaled (Uyan *et al.*, 2009). Strategies to reduce the formation of chloramines in swimming pools include actions to reduce the introduction of organic nitrogen compounds into pool water, such as bathing feet and showering with soap and water before entering the pool, wearing a swimming cap, using swimsuits reserved exclusively for swimming and removal of makeup. Vigilance in monitoring NCl_3 levels has shown that when kept below 0.3 mg·m^{-3}, there are no acute effects on lung function and so are considered safe (Kippelen *et al.*, 2012).

Despite the pathophysiological mechanisms described in which chronic exposure to DBPs in swimming training can induce epithelial airway injury (Pedersen *et al.*, 2008), evidence does not support any causative association between swimming and asthma development. A meta-analysis including 5,851 subjects did not identify any association between swimming and the development of asthma in children ≤16 years (OR 1.084; 95% CI 0.89–1.31) (Valeriani *et al.*, 2017). A 10-year prospective longitudinal study of 5,738 children found no association between chlorinated swimming pool exposure and asthma and in contrast, found that swimming was associated with an increase in lung function and a reduction in the risk of asthma symptoms, especially in children with pre-existing respiratory conditions (Font Rivera *et al.*, 2011).

In the Cochrane review by Beggs *et al.*, (2013), the chlorination status of the pool was unknown in four of the eight studies, two used non-chlorinated pools, one used an indoor chlorinated pool, and one a well-ventilated chlorinated pool. Overall, there was no evidence that swimming training caused adverse effects on asthma control in young people, although vigilance is advised in relation to DBP level control and the schedule and intensity of pool training (see Chapter 7).

Conclusion

Exercise should be recommended routinely for children with asthma, as part of their comprehensive management, as there are many benefits including improved disease control, fitness, QoL, and mental health while co-morbidities such as obesity can be reduced. The relationships between physical activity levels, obesity, and asthma are complex and intertwined, and more work is required to understand the associations in order to inform strategies to reduce morbidity.

Exercise intolerance in asthmatic children needs careful and systematic assessment to identify the cause, which can include poorly controlled disease, EIA, poor fitness secondary to inactivity, and conditions which masquerade as and co-exist with asthma, such as EILO. Physicians should be attentive to these conditions, supported by appropriate investigations, as respiratory symptoms alone are not specific.

Effective exercise training programs for children with asthma are most likely to be sustained when personalised and adjusted to individual capabilities. Programs need to include aerobic training where low to moderate activity may have anti-inflammatory effects and activity beyond the ventilatory threshold can increase fitness; however, the precise schedules, in terms of intensity, frequency, and duration that are best suited to improve outcomes are yet to be determined. There is no evidence of adverse effects caused by exercise training in asthmatic children, but good disease control is a prerequisite. Swimming training has been shown to have a positive impact on asthmatic children and adolescents, improving aerobic capacity and is the only sport that appears to increase resting lung function.

Key Points

- Low levels of physical activity and obesity are independent risk factors for asthma development in children.
- Poor fitness and reduced activity levels in children with asthma can impact negatively on disease control, QoL, BMI, and mental health.
- EIB is underestimated and arises in non-asthmatics, its diagnosis and severity grading require an exercise challenge test with formal lung function testing.
- EIA is the presence of EIB in a patient with an asthma diagnosis and is associated with asthma symptoms in response to non-exertional triggers.
- Exercise training for young asthmatics improves asthma control, fitness, QoL, and reduces bronchial hyper-reactivity while swimming is the only activity identified to improve resting lung function.

References

Abrignani, M.G., Luca, F., Favilli, S., Benvenuto, M., Rao, C.M., Di Fusco, S.A., Gabrielli, D. and Gulizia, M.M. (2019) Lifestyles and cardiovascular prevention in childhood and adolescence. *Pediatric Cardiology*, 40(6), 1113–1125. Doi 10.1007/s00246-019-02152-w.

Aggarwal, B., Mulhirigama, A., Berend, N. (2018) Exercise-induced bronchoconstriction: Prevalence, pathophysiology, patients' impact, diagnosis and management. *Primary Care Respiratory Medicine*, 28(1), 31. Doi 10.1038/s41533-018-0098-2.

Ahmadizar, F., Vijverberg, S., Arets, H., de Bour, A., et al. (2016) Childhood obesity in relation to poor asthma control and exacerbation: A meta-analysis. *European Respiratory Journal*, 48, 1063–1073. Doi 10.1183/13993003.00766-2016.

Al-Mallah, M.H., Sakr, S., Al-Qunaibet, A. (2018) Cardiorespiratory fitness and cardiovascular disease prevention: An update. *Current Atherosclerosis Reports*, 20(1). Doi 10.1007/s11883-018-0711-4.

American College of Sports Medicine (1998) The recommended quantity and quality of exercise for developing and maintaining cardio-respiratory and muscular fitness, and flexibility in healthy adults. *Medicine and Science in Sports and Exercise*, 30(6), 975–991. Doi 10.1097/00005768-199806000-00032.

Anderson, S. (2006) How does exercise cause asthma attacks? *Current Opinion in Allergy and Clinical Inmunology*, 6, 37–42. Doi 10.1097/01.all.0000199797.02423.78.

Anderson, S.D., Argyros, G.J., Magnussen, H., Holzer, K. (2001) Provocation by eucapnic voluntary hyperpnoea to identify exercise induced bronchoconstriction. *British Journal of Sports Medicine*, 35(5), 344–347. Doi 10.1136/bjsm.35.5.344.

Andersson, M., Backman, H., Nordberg, G., Hagenbjörk, A., et al. (2018) Early life swimming pool exposure and asthma onset in children: A case-control study. *Environmental Health*, 17. Doi 10.1186/s12940-018-0383-0.

Asher, I., Pearce, N. (2014) Global burden of asthma among children. *International Journal of Tuberculosis and Lung Disease*, 18(11), 1269–1278. Doi 10.5588/ijtld.14.0170.

Avallone, K., McLeish, A. (2013) Asthma and aerobic exercise: A review of the empirical literature. *Journal of Asthma*, 50(2). Doi 10.3109/02770903.2012.759963.

Batista, C., Soares, J.M. (2013) Are former athletes more prone to asthma? *Journal of Asthma*. Doi 10.3109/02770903.2013.776075.

Beggs, S., Foong, Y.C., Le Hong, C., Noor, D., et al. (2013) Swimming training for asthma in children and adolescents aged 18 years and under. Cochrane Database of Systematic Reviews. *The Cochrane Library*, 7, CD009607. Doi 10.1002/14651858.CD009607.pub4.

Bougault, V., Boulet, L. (2012) Is there a potential link between indoor chlorinated pool environment and airway remodeling/inflammation in swimmers? *Expert Reviews Respiratory Medicine*, 6(5), 469–471. Doi 10.1586/ers.12.51.

Bougault, V., Boulet, L. (2013) Airways disorders and the swimming pool. *Immunology and Allergy Clinics of North America*, 33, 395–408. Doi 10.1016/j.iac.2013.02.008.

Candemir, I., Ergun, P., Kaymaz, D. (2017) Efficacy of a multidisciplinary pulmonary rehabilitation outpatient program on exacerbations in overweight and obese patients with asthma. *The Central European Journal of Medicine*, 129, 655–664. Doi 10.1007/s00508-017-1258-z.

Carlsen, K.H., Hem, E., Stensrud, T. (2011) Asthma in adolescent athletes. *British Journal of Sports Medicine*, 45, 1266–1271. Doi 10.1136/bjsports-2011-090591.

Castro-Rodríguez, J., Holberg, C., Morgan, W., Wright, A., et al. (2001) Increased incidence of asthma-like symptoms in girls who become overweight or obese during the school years. *American Journal of Respiratory and Critical Care Medicine*, 163, 1344–1349. Doi 10.1164/ajrccm.163.6.2006140.

Chandratilleke, M. G., Carson, K. V., Picot, J., Brinn, M. P., Esterman, A. J., & Smith, B. J. (2012) Physical training for asthma. *The Cochrane Library*, (5). Doi 10.1002/14651858.CD001116.pub3.

Chen, Y., Dong, Lin, K., Lee, L. (2013) Gender difference of childhood overweight and obesity in predicting the risk of incident asthma: A systematic review and meta-analysis. *Obesitiy Reviews*, 14, 222–231. Doi 10.1111/j.1467-789X.2012.01055.x.

Clausen, J. S., Marott, J. L., Holtermann, A., Gyntelberg, F., & Jensen, M. T. (2018) Midlife cardiorespiratory fitness and the long-term risk of mortality. *Journal of the American College of Cardiology*, 72(9). Doi 10.1016/j.acc.2018.06.045.

Clearie, K. L., Vaidyanathan, S., Williamson, P. A., Goudie, A., Short, P., Schembri, S., & Lipworth, B. J. (2010) Effects of chlorine and exercise on the unified airway in adolescent elite Scottish swimmers. *Allergy*, 65, 269–273. Doi 10.1111/j.1398-9995.2009.02173.x.

Del Giacco, S.R., Firinu, D., Bjermer, L., Carlsen, K.H. (2015) Exercise and asthma: An overview. *European Clinical Respiratory Journal,* 2(1), 27984. Doi 10.3402/ecrj.v2.27984.

Del Giacco, S., Garcia-Larsen, V. (2016) Aerobic exercise training reduces bronchial hyper-responsiveness and serum pro-inflammatory cytokines in patients with asthma. *Evidence Based Medicine*. Doi 10.1136/ebmed-2015-110260.

Deng, X., Ma, J., Yuan, Y., Zhang, Z., & Niu, W. (2019) Association between overweight or obesity and the risk for childhood asthma and wheeze: An updated meta-analysis on 18 articles and 73 252 children. *Pediatric Obesity*. Doi 10.1111/ijpo.12532.

Desloovere, P., Bull, F., Khasnabis, C., Elsheik, E., M. Ciecierska. (2010) Global recommendations on physical activity for health. Chapter 4: Age group 5-17 years old. *WHO: 15.*

Dimitrakaki, V., Porpodis, K., Bebetsos, E., Zarogoulidis, P., Papaiwannou, A., Tsiouda, T., Tsioulis, H. and Zarogoulidis, K. (2013) Attitudes of asthmatic and nonasthmatic children to physical exercise. *Patient Preference and Adherence*, 7, 81–88. Doi 10.2147/PPA.S40577.

Eichenberger, P., Diener, S., Kofmehl, R., Spengler, C. (2013) Effects of exercise training on airway hyperreactivity in asthma: A systematic review and meta-analysis. *Sports Medicine*, 43, 1157–1170. Doi 10.1007/s40279-013-0077-2.

Eijkemans, M., Mommers, M., Jos, M. T., Thijs, C., & Prins, M. H. (2012) Physical activity and asthma: A systematic review and meta-analysis. *PloS ONE*, **7**(12). Doi 10.1371/journal.pone.0050775.

Eisenberg, S.R., Jelalian, E., Farrow, M., Kopel, S.J., Vehse, N., Mitchell, P., Dunsiger, S. & Koinis-Mitchell, D. (2019) Perceptions of asthma and exercise, and associations with weight status and asthma morbidity in urban children. *Academic Pediatrics*, 20(1), 55–62. Doi 10.1016/j.acap.2019.07.001.

Fanelli, A., Cabral, A. L., Neder, J. A., Martins, M. A., & Carvalho, C. R. (2007) Exercise training on disease control and quality of life in asthmatic children. *Medicine and Science in Sports and Exercise*, 39, 1474–1480. Doi 10.1249/mss.0b013e3180d099ad.

Fantuzzi, G. (2005) Adipose tissue, adipokines and inflammation. *Journal of Allergy and Clinical Immunology*, 115(5), 911–919. Doi 10.1016/j.jaci.2005.02.023.

Fitch, K., Morton, A., Blansky, B. (1976) Effects of swimming training on children with asthma. archives of disease in childhood. *British Medical Journal*, 51, 190–194. Doi 10.1136/adc.51.3.190.

Flaherman, V., Rutherford, G. (2006) A meta-analysis of of the effect of high weight on asthma. *Archives of Disease in Childhood*, 91, 334–339. Doi 10.1136/adc.2005.080390.

Font-Ribera, L., Villanueva, C. M., Nieuwenhuijsen, M. J., Zock, J. P., Kogevinas, M., & Henderson, J. (2011) Swimming pool attendance, asthma, allergies, and lung function in the Avon. Longitudinal Study of Parents and Children Cohort. *American Journal of Respiratory and Critical Care Medicine*, 183, 582–588. Doi 10.1164/rccm.201005-0761OC.

França-Pinto, A., Mendes, F.A., de Carvalho-Pinto, R.M., Agondi, R.C., Cukier, A., Stelmach, R., Saraiva-Romanholo, B.M., Kalil, J., Martins, M.A., Giavina-Bianchi, P. & Carvalho, C.R. (2015) Aerobic training decreases bronchial hyper-responsiveness and systemic inflammation in patients withmoderate or severe asthma: A randomised controlled trial. *Thorax*, 70:732–9. Doi 10.1136/thoraxjnl-2014-206070.

Gandhi, P.K., Kenzik, K.M., Thompson, L.A., DeWalt, D.A., Revicki, D.A., Shenkman, E.A. & Huang, I.C., (2013) Exploring factors influencing asthma control and asthma specific health related quality of life among children. *Respiratory Research*, 14(26). Doi 10.1186/1465-9921-14-26.

Glazebrook, C., McPherson, A. C., Macdonald, I. A., Swift, J. A., Ramsay, C., Newbould, R., & Smyth, A. (2006) Asthma as a barrier to children's physical activity: Implications for body mass index and mental health. *Pediatrics*, 118(6), 2443–2449. Doi 10.1542/peds.2006-1846.

Global Initiative for Asthma (2020) Strategy for Asthma Management and Prevention. Available at: http://www.ginasthma.org.

Gotshall, R. (2002) Exercise-induced bronchoconstriction. *Drugs*, 62(12), 1725–1739. Doi 10.2165/00003495-200262120-00003.

Holderness, H., Chin, N., Ossip, D. (2017) Physical activity, restrictions in activity, and body mass index among urban children with persistent asthma. *Annals of Allergy, Asthma and Immunology*. Doi 10.1016/j.anai.2017.01.014.

Hopkins, S.R. (2006) Exercise induced arterial hypoxemia: The role of ventilation-perfusion inequality and pulmonary diffusion limitation. *Advances in Experimental Medicine and Biology*, 588, 17–30. Doi 10.1007/978-0-387-34817-9_3.

Huang, S. W., Veiga, R., Sila, U., Reed, E., & Hines, S. (1989) Effect of swimming in asthmatic children: Participants in a swimming program in the city of Baltimore. *Journal of Asthma*, 26 (2), 117–121. Doi 10.3109/02770908909073240.

Hull, J., Ansley L., Price O., Dickinson J., Bonini M. (2016) Eucapnic voluntary hyperpnea: Gold standard for diagnosing exercise-induced bronchoconstriction in athletes? *Sports Medicine*, 46:1083–1093. Doi 10.1007/s40279-016-0491-3.

Inci, D., Guggenheim, R., Altintas, D. U., Wildhaber, J. H., & Moeller, A. (2017) Reported exercise-related respiratory symptoms and exercise-induced bronchoconstriction in asthmatic children. *Journal of Clinical Medicine Research*, 9, 410–415. Doi 10.14740/jocmr2935w.

Jaakkola, J. J., Aalto, S. A., Hernberg, S., Kiihamäki, S. P., & Jaakkola, M. S. (2019) Regular exercise improves asthma control in adults: A randomized controlled trial. *Scientific Reports*, 9. Doi 10.1038/s41598-019-48484-8

Juniper, E., Guyatt, G., Feeny, D., Ferrie, P. (1996) Measuring quality of life in children with asthma. *Quality of Life Research*, 5, 35–46. Doi 10.1007/BF00435967.

Kanikowska, A., Napiórkowska-Baran, K., Graczyk, M., Kucharski, M. (2018) Influence of chlorinated water on the development of allergic diseases – An overview. *Annals of Agricultural and Envionmental Medicine*, 25(4), 651–655. Doi 10.26444/aaem/79810.

Kier, C., Forde, S. (2011) Childhood overweight and obesity and their association with asthma. *Journal of Asthma and Allergy Educators*, 2(3), 119–125. Doi 10.1177/2150129710384503.

Kim, J.W., So, W.J., Kim, Y.S. (2012) Association between asthma and physical activity in Korean adolescents: The 3rd Korea Youth Risk Behavior Web-based Survey (KYRBWS-III). *European Journal of Public Health*, 22(6), 864–868. Doi 10.1093/eurpub/ckr175.

Kippelen, P., Fitch, K.D., Anderson, S.D., Bougault, V., Boulet, L.P., Rundell, K.W., Sue-Chu, M. & McKenzie, D.C. (2012) Respiratory health of elite athletes-preventing airway injury: A critical review. *British Journal of Sports and Medicine*, 46, 471–476. Doi 10.1136/bjsports-2012-091056

Kippelen, P. (2016) Is there a need to improve asthma diagnosis in young athletes?. *Expert Review of Respiratory Medicine*. Doi 10.1080/17476348.2016.1219657.

Kodama, S., Saito, K., Tanaka, S., Maki, M., Yachi, Y., Asumi, M., Sugawara, A., Totsuka, K., Shimano, H., Ohashi, Y. & Yamada, N. (2009) Cardiorespiratory fitness as a quantitative predictor of all-cause mortality and cardiovascular events in healthy men and women: A meta-analysis. *JAMA*, 301(19), 2024–2035. Doi 10.1001/jama.2009.681.

Lahart, M., Metsios, G. (2018) Chronic physiological effects of swim training interventions in non-elite swimmers: A systematic review and meta-analysis. *Sports Medicine*, 48. Doi 10.1007/s40279-017-0805-0.

Lang, D., Butz, A., Duggan, A., Serwint, J. (2004) Physical activity in urban school-aged children with asthma. *Pediatrics*, 113(4), e331–336. Doi 10.1542/peds.113.4.e341

Lang, J. (2014) Exercise, obesity, and asthma in children and adolescents. *Jornal de Pediatria (Rio J)*, 90 (3); 215–217. Doi 10.1016/j.jped.2014.01.002.

Leinaar, E., Alamian, A., Wang, L. (2016) A systematic review of the relationship between asthma, overweight, and the effects of physical activity in youth. *Annals of Epidemiology*, 26(7), 504–510. Doi 10.1016/j.annepidem.2016.06.002.

Lin, L. L., Huang, S. J., Ou, L. S., Yao, T.C., Tsao, K. C., Yeh, K. W., & Huang, J. L. (2019) Exercise-induced bronchoconstriction in children with asthma. *Journal of Microbiology, Immunology and Infections*, 52, 471–479. Doi 10.1016/j.jmii.2017.08.013.

Lochte, L., Nielsen, K., Petersen, P., Platts-Mills, T. (2016) Childhood asthma and physical activity: A systematic review with meta-analysis and Graphic Appraisal Tool for Epidemiology assessment. *BMC Pediatrics*, 16 (50). Doi 10.1186/s12887-016-0571-4.

Lu, K., Forno, E., Radom-Aizik, S., Cooper, D. (2020) Low fitness and increased sedentary time are associated with worse asthma—The National Youth Fitness Survey. *Pediatric Pulmonology*, 55(5), 1116–1123. Doi 10.1002/ppul.24678.

Lu, K. D., Manoukian, K., Radom-Aizik, S., Cooper, D. M., & Galant, S. P. (2016) Obesity, asthma, and exercise in child and adolescent health. *Pediatric Exercise Science*, 28, 264–274. Doi 10.1123/pes.2015-0122.

Majak, P., Jerzyńska, J., Bojo, M., Brzozowska, A., Koczkowska, M., Sielski, P., Stelmach, W., Stelmach, R., Janas, A. & Stelmach, I. (2016) Cytokine profiling in exhaled breath condensate after exercise challenge in asthmatic children with post-exercise symptoms. *Archives of Medical Science*, 12(4), 778–784. Doi 10.5114/aoms.2015.48547.

McNarry, M., Boddy, L., Stratton, G. (2014) The relationship between body mass index, aerobic performance and asthma in a pre-pubertal, population-level cohort. *European Journal of Applied Physiology*, 114(2), 243–249. Doi 10.1007/s00421-013-2772-y.

McNarry, M.A., Lewis, M.J., Wade, N., Davies, G.A., Winn, C., Eddolls, W.T.B., Stratton, G.S. & Mackintosh, K.A. (2019) Effect of asthma and six-months high-intensity interval training on heart rate variability during exercise in adolescents. *Journal of Sports Sciences*, 37(19); 2228–2235. Doi 10.1080/02640414.2019.1626115.

McNarry, M. A., Winn, C. O., Davies, G. A., Eddolls, W. T., & Mackintosh, K. A. (2020) Effect of high-intensity training and asthma on the 2 kinetics of adolescents. *Medicine & Science in Sports and Exercise*, 52(6), 1322–1329. Doi 10.1249/MSS.0000000000002270.

Newacheck, P., Halfone, N. (2000) Prevalence, impact, and trends in childhood disability due to asthma. *Archives of Pediatrics and Adolescent Medicine*, 154, 287–293. Doi 10.1001/archpedi.154.3.287.

Orlando, A., Nava, E., Giussani, M., Genovesi, S. (2019) Adiponectin and cardiovascular risk. From pathophysioly to clinic: Focus on children and adolescents. *International Journal of Molecular Sciences*, 20(13); 3228. Doi 10.3390/ijms20133228.

Ortega, F.B., Ruiz, J.R., Castillo, M.J., Sojstrom, M. (2008) Physical fitness in childhood and adolescence: A powerful marker of health. *International Journal of Obesity (London)*, 32(1), 1–11. Doi 10.1038/sj.ijo.0803774.

Parsons, J.P., Hallstrand, T.S., Mastronarde, J.G., Kaminsky, D.A., Rundell, K.W., Hull, J.H., Storms, W.W., Weiler, J.M., Cheek, F.M., Wilson, K.C. & Anderson, S.D. (2013) An official American Thoracic Society clinical practice guideline: Exercise-induced bronchoconstriction. *American Journal of Respiratory and Critical Care Medicine*, 187(9), 1016–1027. Doi 10.1164/rccm.201303-0437ST.

Pedersen, L., Lund, T. K., Barnes, P. J., Kharitonov, S. A., & Backer, V. (2008) Airway responsiveness and inflammation in adolescent elite swimmers. *American Academy of Allergy, Asthma and Immunology*. Doi 10.1016/j.jaci.2008.04.041.

Price, O. J., Ansley, L., Menzies-Gow, A., Cullinan, P., & Hull, J. H. (2013) Airway dysfunction in elite athletes-an occupational lung disease? *Allergy*, 68, 1343–1352. Doi 10.1111/all.12265.

Tripodi, S., Barreto, M., Rienzo-Businco, D., Grossi, O., Sfika, I., Ragusa, G., Campisano, M. & Miceli-Sopo, S. (2016) Asthma control test and bronchial challenge with exercise in pediatric asthma. *Frontiers in Pediatrics*, 4, 16. Doi 10.3389/fped.2016.00016.

Uyan, Z.S., Carraro, S., Piacentini, G., Baraldi, E. (2009) Swimming pool, respiratory health, and childhood asthma: Should we change our beliefs? *Pediatric Pulmonology*, 44, 31–37. Doi 10.1002/ppul.20947.

Vahlkvist, S., Pedersen, S. (2009) Fitness, daily activity and body composition in children with newly diagnosed, untreated asthma. *Allergy*, 64, 1649–1655. Doi 10.1111/j.1398-9995.2009.02081.x.

Valeriani, F., Protano, C., Vitali, M., Romano-Spica, V. (2017) Swimming attendance during childhood and development of asthma: Meta-analysis. *Pediatrics International*, 59, 614–621. Doi 10.1111/ped.13230.

Van der Eycken, S., Schelpe, A., Marijsse, G., Dilissen, E., Troosters, T., Vanbelle, V., Aertgeerts, S., Dupont, L.J., Peers, K., Bullens, D.M. and Seys, S.F. (2016). Feasibility to apply eucapnic voluntary hyperventilation in young elite athletes. *Respiratory Medicine*, 111, 91–93. Doi 10.1016/j.rmed.2015.12.012.

van der Kamp, M.R., Thio, B.J., Tabak, M., Hermens, H.J., Driessen, J.M.M. & van der Palen, J.A.M. (2019) Does exercise induce bronchoconstriction affect physical activity patterns in asthmatic children? *Journal of Clinical Child Health*. Doi 10.1177/1367493519881257.

van Leeuwen, J.C., Driessen, J.M., De Jongh, F.H., Van Aalderen, W.M. & Thio, B.J. (2011) Monitoring pulmonary function during exercise in children with asthma. *Archives of Disease in Childhood*, 96, 664–668. Doi 10.1136/adc.2010.209411.

Vijayakanthi, N., Greally, J., Rastogi, D. (2016) Pediatric obesity related asthma: The role of metabolic dysregulation. *Pediatrics*, 137 (5): e20150812. Doi 10.1542/peds.2015-0812.

Wang, J.S., Hung, W.P. (2009) The effects of a swimming intervention for children with asthma. *Respirology, Asian Pacific Society of Respirology*, 14, 838–842. Doi 10.1111/j.1440-1843.2009.01567.x.

Wanrooij, V., Willeboordse, M., Dompeling, E., van de Kant, K. (2013) Exercise training in children with asthma: A systematic review. *British Journal of Sports Medicine*, 48(13); 1024–1031. Doi 10.1136/bjsports-2012-091347.

Weiler, J.M., Anderson, S.D., Randolph, C., Bonini, S., Craig, T.J., Pearlman, D.S., Rundell, K.W., Silvers, W.S., Storms, W.W., Bernstein, D.I. & Blessing-Moore, J. (2010) Pathogenesis, pre- valence, diagnosis and management of exercise-induced bronchoconstriction: A practice parameter. *Annals of Allergy, Asthma and Immunology*, 115, S483–S523. Doi 10.1016/j.anai.2010.09.021.

Weiler, J.M., Brannan, J.D., Randolph, C.C., Hallstrand, T.S., Parsons, J., Silvers, W., Storms, W., Zeiger, J., Bernstein, D.I., Blessing-Moore, J. & Greenhawt, M. (2016) Exercise induced bronchoconstriction update. *The Journal of Allergy and Clinical Immunology*, 138(5), 1292–1295. Doi 10.1016/j.jaci.2016.05.029.

Weisel, C.P., Richardson, S.D., Nemery, B., Aggazzotti, G., Baraldi, E., Blatchley III, E.R., Blount, B.C., Carlsen, K.H., Eggleston, P.A., Frimmel, F.H. & Goodman, M. (2009) Childhood asthma and environmental exposures at swimming pools: State of the Science and Research Recommendations. *Environmental Health Perspectives*, 117, 500–507. Doi 10.1289/ehp.11513.

Welsh, L., Kemp, J., Roberts, R. (2005) Effects of physical conditioning on children and adolescents with asthma. *Sports Medicine*, 35 (2), 127–141. Doi 10.2165/00007256-200535020-00003.

Westergren, T., Ommundsen, Y., Lødrup Carlsen, K. C., Carlsen, K. H., Mowinckel, P., Fegran, L., & Berntsen, S. (2015) A nested case-control study: Personal, social and environmental correlates of vigorous physical activity in adolescents with asthma. *Journal of Asthma*, 52(2), 155–161. Doi 10.3109/02770903.2014.955190.

7 Competitive Sports and Respiratory Illness

Guillermo Zepeda and Marietta Núñez Camara

Introduction

Competitive sports have maintained their centrality in human culture since antiquity; the first Olympic Games were staged in 776 BC. In order to enhance fitness and performance, young athletes often train several times a day or for prolonged periods at high intensity, significantly exceeding the minimum activity levels recommended for children and adolescents to maintain health by the World Health Organization (WHO, 2010). The demands placed on their cardiopulmonary and locomotor systems are much greater than those required in typical recreational activities. Such physiological stresses and the situations in which they arise explain why athletes are more prone to suffering from respiratory disorders (Carlsen and Kowalski, 2008; Halvorsen *et al.*, 2017; Mountjoy *et al.*, 2015). When young athletes present with respiratory symptoms that may be limiting their performance, clinicians need to be aware of the common diagnoses encountered. These include exercise-induced asthma (EIA), exercise-induced bronchoconstriction (EIB), exercise-induced laryngeal obstruction (EILO), gastro-oesophageal reflux (GORD), and both allergic and non-allergic rhinitis. Problems can co-exist but need to be identified and managed both generally and individually to support athletic performance and ensure that potentials are achieved (Campisi *et al.*, 2019). Preventative and relief treatments need to be prescribed within the confines of regulations stipulated by regulatory bodies.

Initial Considerations

Apart from the health benefits of exercise, competitive sport is a significant economic enterprise. In 2004, global sporting events were estimated to have generated revenues in excess of 550 billion Euros (Andreff, 2008). Children are introduced to competitive sports in schools and clubs and when they perform well, may be directed towards ever increasing levels of competition, where the rewards of success such as kudos amongst peers, travel,

DOI: 10.4324/9781003020462-7

and sponsorship are significant motivators for training, reinforced by family encouragement.

The youngest recorded winner of an Olympic medal was Dimitrios Loundras, a Greek gymnast, aged 10 years, who won a bronze medal in the parallel bars in Athens in 1896 (IOC, 2004). Present regulations governing whether children can enter high-competition tournaments depend on individual International Sport Federations. The International Tennis Federation (ITF) organises tournaments from the age of 13 years (ITF, 2020), whilst in professional level football, tests to enter the minor divisions can start from the age of 6 years (Real Madrid, 2020). The Youth Olympic Games for 15–18 year olds were established in 2010 (Youth Olympic Games, 2020). Ensuring that competing young athletes are healthy is not only an important safety precaution, but also ensures that individual performance is not compromised. Some medical societies now recommend that young athletes undergo medical evaluations (Fritsch *et al.,* 2017), and precision healthcare has become integral in the preparation of athletes to compete. For instance, 247 teenage Italian athletes participated in the 2010 Youth Olympic Games and were required to undergo a detailed pre-participation health evaluation that included a personal and family medical history, physical examination, electrocardiogram, echocardiogram, bicycle ergometer exercise test, spirometry, blood and urine investigations (Adami *et al.*, 2019). Asymptomatic pathologies were detected in 12%, although none of these prevented them from participating.

Many young athletes train or compete away from home, so safeguarding their welfare is paramount. At the 2018 Youth Olympic Games in Argentina, a survey revealed high perception levels of harassment and abuse; out of 1,254 competitors, a worrying 34% responded that abuse or harassment was likely or very likely to occur in their sport, only 63% responded that they knew where to ask for help (Mountjoy *et al.*, 2020). Although this may appear irrelevant, psychological stress can influence symptom perception in respiratory illness.

The Aetiology and Pathogenesis of Respiratory Diseases in Athletes

Several proposed mechanisms account for a higher prevalence of respiratory problems in athletes, although these are primarily based on research in adults. They can be divided into internal or functional factors and external or environmental factors, recognising that, in practice, these often interact simultaneously in their contribution to respiratory disease. There is potential for airway damage to arise throughout the respiratory tract, but smaller airways appear particularly affected. Injury is followed by efficient repair mechanisms, but with repeated and sometimes prolonged exposures, these mechanisms may be outstripped, leading to structural remodelling and functional changes, including goblet cell hyperplasia and bronchial hyperresponsiveness (Bougault *et al.*, 2012; Couto *et al.*, 2018). It is not known whether more lengthy sporting careers starting in early childhood carry a greater risk of such long-term changes. Children have anatomically narrower airways and a relatively high resistance to nasal airflow before puberty, causing a greater proportion of inspired air to bypass the protective functions of the nose (Bennett *et al.*, 2007). It is not known whether these anatomical factors could influence the evolution of airway inflammation in younger athletes. Furthermore, inflammatory responses in children may be different to that in adults, undermining the extrapolation of adult research when investigating airway inflammation in children (Jeljeli *et al.*, 2019).

Internal or Functional Factors

Internal or functional factors relate to the direct pathophysiological consequences of prolonged intense exercise that may aggravate or trigger medical comorbidities.

Resting minute ventilation (VE) in adults is 6–8 $L \cdot min^{-1}$, but in athletes this can increase to 200 $L \cdot min^{-1}$. The degree of hypernoea will depend on the type of sport undertaken; being much higher in endurance and high-intensity activities than in field events, although training to improve fitness invariably involves physiological stress. VE rates above 30 $L \cdot min^{-1}$ are associated with a progressive increase in the proportion of inspired air that enters the lungs via the mouth rather than the nose, which has a role in warming, humidifying, and filtering inspired air. This short-cut exposes airways to greater volumes of dry, unfiltered, and cold air, with an increased potential for allergens and other inhaled particles to be carried into and deposited inside the airways (Anderson and Tocias, 2000). The presence of rhinitis will intensify the consequences of inhaled air by-passing the nasal passages.

Airway Injury

Traditionally, thermal and osmotic mechanisms have been proposed to explain epithelial injury during intense exercise. However, it is important to acknowledge that other factors contribute, not least, the high-shearing forces and transmural pressure gradients generated during severe hyperpnoea which can put epithelial cells at risk of detachment (Kippelen and Anderson, 2012a).

The cooling of airways by high airflow causes vasoconstriction of airway microvasculature followed by rebound vasodilation and hyperaemia in the minutes after exercise (Rundell *et al.*, 2011; Kippelen *et al.*, 2018). Cooling can also disrupt tight junctions between cells threatening mucosal integrity (Bolger *et al.*, 2011; Kippelen *et al.*, 2012b).

When the inhaled air is dry, particularly if the nasal airway is by-passed, evaporation of lung surface liquid increases mucus viscosity, impeding ciliary function and mucociliary transport. Epithelial cells dehydrate, increasing intra-cellular osmolarity and reducing cell volume. These processes contribute to epithelial damage provoking the release of inflammatory cytokines and mediators which lead to the inward migration of neutrophil and eosinophil inflammatory cells. Histamine, prostaglandin D and cysteinyl leukotrienes, released from stimulated airway mast cells and eosinophils, cause smooth muscle contraction and oedema leading to obstruction (Hallstrand, 2012). Clara cell secretory protein (CC16) levels, an anti-inflammatory marker of epithelial injury, increase after exercise in both serum and urine. The number of shed epithelial cells in induced sputum following exercise correlates with the levels of inflammatory markers. Why bronchoconstriction usually develops after exercise may be explained by opposing protective mechanisms that are active during activity, such as cysteinyl leukotriene receptor desensitisation and increased protective prostaglandins, possibly PGE2 (Larsson *et al.*, 2013). Secretory IgA protects airway mucosa against infection and levels decline in association with exercise induced epithelial injury, signalling an increased risk of symptomatic inflammation, including from 'viral reactivation' (Yamauchi *et al.*, 2011). Indeed, viral infections are common amongst athletic teams and can have an impact on their performance (Valtonen *et al.*, 2019). Systemic pro-inflammatory cytokines such as IL-6 rise following exercise induced metabolic stress and muscle damage and is counteracted by a rise in anti-inflammatory cytokines including IL-10 during recovery. The level of these responses map to symptoms of fatigue but it is not clear whether these have any relationship to airway inflammation. Although the type of sport, and the environment in which it is undertaken, accounts for variability in airway injury in athletes, genetically determined variations in the pattern of cytokine response may play a role. Unsurprisingly, those with demonstrable EIB or with illnesses such as asthma, appear more vulnerable (Gleeson and Pyne, 2016).

Autonomic Nervous System Activity and Lung Function

Bronchoconstriction and increased airway mucus production may result from parasympathetic (cholinergic) innervation, and cooling may directly stimulate cholinergic receptors, while sympathetic (adrenergic) innervation has the opposite effect. In endurance athletes an increased parasympathetic tone has been observed, partly explaining lower resting heart rates, reduced sweating and slower salivary flow rates compared to controls (Couto *et al.*, 2018). It is hypothesised that increased parasympathetic tone is a counter mechanism compensating for the frequent and sustained sympathetic activity associated with heavy exercise training (Stang *et al.*, 2016).

Allergic Sensitisation

Bronchial hyper responsiveness is known to increase with age, but the incidence of allergic sensitisation in elite athletes appears disproportionately high. Whilst they may be more attuned to functional changes, there is some evidence for a true increase in allergic sensitisation amongst athletes through their careers (Knöpfli *et al.*, 2007; Gleeson and Pyne, 2016). It is hypothesised that epithelial injury increases permeability and facilitates allergic sensitisation to inhaled allergens in athletes who are genetically susceptible to allergic disease (Bernard, 2007). Once sensitised, continued exposure triggers allergic airway inflammation and bronchoconstriction, compromising lung function and exercise performance (Georas and Rezaee, 2014).

Endocrine Effects

Female sex hormones can reduce mucociliary clearance and immune responsiveness, potentially influencing respiratory symptoms and explaining the female predominance of some conditions (Campisi *et al.*, 2019). Oestradiol in particular has been implicated and levels will fluctuate depending on the menstrual cycle or hormonal contraception taken (Raghavan and Jain, 2016).

External or Environmental Factors

Environments in which sports are conducted may be associated with specific chemical or physical irritants, as is the case with chlorinated swimming pools, very cold, low humidity ski courses and less obvious hazards such as combustion fumes in indoor venues. More generally, event or training locations may be prone to air pollution or high aeroallergen levels (Rundell, 2003; Cutrufello *et al.*, 2012; Mountjoy *et al.*, 2015).

Swimming Pool Disinfectants

The use of chlorine and bromine-based disinfectants are important in guarding against harmful bacterial contamination but generate numerous disinfectant by-products (DBPs) including carbonaceous and more toxic nitrogenous compounds such as chloramines (Ilyas *et al.*, 2018). Chloramines form when chlorine-based products react with organic compounds in pool water. DBPs remain aerosolised within a 10-cm thick layer of air above the water surface that may be harmful when inhaled (Gałązka-Franta *et al.*, 2016). Neutrophilic and eosinophilic inflammation can be identified throughout the upper and lower airways of swimmers and serum CC16 increases significantly during exposure (Cavaleiro Rufo *et al.*, 2018). Chloramines, including trichloramine, not only cause direct tissue irritation, but as membrane penetrating oxidants, react rapidly with cell proteins, disrupting tight junctions and increasing epithelial permeability, thus potentially promoting allergic sensitisation. Toxicity relates to the concentration and duration of exposure and so competitive swimmers are more likely to suffer than recreational ones. Swimmers exposed to trichloramine >0.37 $mg{\cdot}m^{-3}$ suffer significantly more upper airway and eye irritation than those swimming in lower concentrations, emphasising the importance of monitoring and optimising disinfectant levels (Wastensson and Eriksson, 2020). Adequate ventilation of swimming pools helps to prevent the problem. The replacement of chlorine with alternative methods of disinfection such as ozone, ultraviolet radiation, salt, and silver or copper ions requires more investigation (Kanikowska *et al.*, 2018).

Pollution

Exercising in polluted environments inevitably exposes airways, peripheral lung structures, and through diffusion, increases the number of pollutants in the systemic circulation than would occur when breathing at rest (Gałązka-Franta *et al.*, 2016). Pollutant exposure during exercise can impair cardiovascular function and exercise performance (Giorgini *et al.*, 2016). Children playing ice hockey in arenas cleaned by machines emitting nitrogen dioxide have been shown to suffer increased asthma symptoms (Thunqvist *et al.*, 2002). In another study, exposure to high levels of pollutants was shown to reduce aerobic capacity in healthy athletes (Kargarfard *et al.*, 2015). In a systematic review and meta-analysis, acute exposure to ozone and traffic pollution, during exercise, found that only peak expiratory flow was significantly decreased, although an increased risk of airway inflammation, decrements in pulmonary function, hypertension, and microvascular function were reported in some studies (Qin *et al.*, 2019). The authors concluded that exercising in the presence of pollution increased the risk of health problems and impaired exercise performance. Consequently, the performance benefits of training may be offset by the harmful effects of inhaled pollutants and the precise effects of cumulative exposure needs further study (Fitch, 2016).

Globally, air pollution in specific locations is reported in real time by the Air Quality Indices (AQI). Key pollutants measured are particulate matter (PM10 and PM2.5; diameters of 2.5–10 µm and ≤2.5 µm, respectively), ozone (O_3), nitrogen oxides (NOx), sulphur dioxide (SO_2), and carbon monoxide (CO), although ammonia, lead, and ultrafine PMs are included in some monitoring. Ranges for each pollutant map to a scale of health concern, with 6 levels. These pollutants harm airways, particularly the oxides which react to form free radicals that directly damage airway epithelium, triggering the release of inflammatory cytokines. Pollutants impair cilial function and weakening anti-microbial and regulatory immune responses (Cao *et al.*, 2020; Glencross *et al.*, 2020). Exposure to pollution invariably involves a mixture of substances and the relative contribution of specific air pollutants or combinations in triggering or exacerbating respiratory conditions is difficult to decipher. Smog is dense, humid, and polluted air, rich in PMs and it is well established that it has detrimental effects on both healthy people and those with respiratory disease. Modelling determines that training in the presence of smog would pose a significant hazard to performance and long-term health (Han, 2019).

Surprisingly, smoking amongst Olympic athletes, who are a paradigm of healthy living, has been reported as high as 18% in one study (Bonini *et al.*, 2015).

Cold Air

Strenuous exercise in cold air which has low humidity is typical of winter sports environments and will aggravate the effects of increased ventilation described above. Elite cross-country skiers, irrespective of co-morbid asthma, have evidence of chronic airway inflammation (Larsson *et al.*, 1998). Exhaled breath condensates from winter sports athletes have pro-inflammatory cytokine profiles, such as elevated tumour necrosis factor (TNF)-α levels, that correlate with exercise symptoms and spirometry abnormalities (Kurowski *et al.*, 2018). Acknowledging the combined effect of environmental factors influencing athletic performance, a novel field study of parkrun performance determined that ozone levels, cold and low humidity appeared to have a detrimental impact (Hodgson *et al.*, 2020).

Allergens

Acknowledging that allergic sensitisation may be more prevalent in athletes, the accurate diagnosis, early treatment to control allergic disease, and allergen avoidance measures may be important. Once sensitised, geography, climatic season, altitude, industrial and agricultural practices will influence the allergen profile of air in specific locations. Pollen counts can be tracked and predicted, allowing decisions to be made about treatments and training schedules (Atchley and Smith, 2020).

Cough

Cough is a common symptom in the general population, often made worse by exercise, but in athletes, it is particularly prevalent, prompting clinic attendance with health concerns, disrupting rest, compromising training, and undermining performance. Cough may be a feature of all the conditions discussed in this chapter, so distinguishing between these while ruling out other respiratory or non-respiratory causes requires a structured evaluation, recognising subtle differences in cough characteristics and the pattern of associated symptoms. Confirmatory investigations then inform treatment choices and responses need to be appraised to help avoid misdiagnoses (Boulet and Turmel, 2019; GINA, 2020).

Asthma and Competitive Sports

Chapter 6 in this book describes how exercise affects children with asthma and defines both EIA and EIB. Neither should be diagnosed based on symptoms alone. The distinction is important as different pathophysiological

Table 7.1 The Treatment Goals for Exercise-Induced Asthma (EIA) and Exercise-Induced Bronchoconstriction (EIB)

Treatment Goals for EIA and EIB
Achieve good symptom control.
Reduction the risk of an asthma attack.
Maintain good lung function.
Train and compete without compromise of performance.
Good school attendance.

mechanisms may be responsible that require different approaches to management (Couto *et al.*, 2018). EIA describes symptoms of bronchoconstriction triggered by exercise in those with a diagnosis of asthma. EIB can arise in athletes without a diagnosis of asthma and requires objective evidence of bronchoconstriction with an exercise challenge test or surrogate eucapnic voluntary hyperpnoea (EVH) (Parsons *et al.*, 2013; Hull *et al.*, 2016). Specific sport exercise testing, such as rowing or skiing in the field, have been described, but are logistically challenging and more difficult to standardise than those in laboratory settings (Atchley and Smith, 2020).

The prevalence of EIA in athletes is estimated to be between 12 and 45% (Bonini *et al.*, 2015; Näsman *et al.*, 2018). Asthma prevalence amongst elite swimmers is especially high; reported to be 22% in Olympic open water swimmers and 26% in synchronised swimmers (Mountjoy *et al.*, 2015).

EIB has been estimated to affect 19.2% in a general adolescent population (Johansson *et al.*, 2015), and 30–70% in athletes, depending on the type of sport practiced (Boulet and O'Byrne, 2015). One study identified EIB in 17% of nonathletic controls, 29% of cold weather athletes, and 60% of swimmers (Bougault *et al.*, 2010). The wide ranges of prevalence reported for both EIA and EIB are partly explained by differing methodologies, study population heterogeneity, and subject recruitment bias (Bonini and Silvers, 2018). Nevertheless, it is evident that athletes, especially swimmers, endurance skiers, and cyclists, suffer a greater prevalence of both EIA and EIB than the general population.

The management of EIB and EIA is helped by identifying goals (Table 7.1), encouraging general measures and stratifying pharmacological interventions that are different for EIA and EIB (Boulet and O'Byrne, 2015), see Table 7.2. Treatments must comply with regulations and athletes must provide authorisation by regulatory agencies for any prescription drugs used (IOC, 2008).

Allergic and Non-allergic Rhinitis

Rhinitis is defined as an inflammation of the lining of the nose and is characterised by symptoms including a runny nose (rhinorrhoea), postnasal drip, which can trigger coughing, nasal blockage, sneezing, and itching of the nose (Bousquet *et al.*, 2008), it is frequently accompanied by eye watering and conjunctival irritation which may impair vision and hand-eye coordination.

Table 7.2 Pharmacological Treatment of EIB and EIA

Regular medical supervision
To promote understanding of the condition, rationale for treatments and risks of side effects.
Support with written personalised treatment plan.
Review and ensure appropriate inhaler techniques.
Support and motivate adherence.
Ensure awareness of drug and dosing regulations.
Up-to-date immunisations against respiratory diseases (influenza)
Advice against smoking/smoking cessation.
Management of EIB[a]
SABA[b] 15–20 minutes before exercise and relief (first choice)
SAMA before exercise
LTRA (montelukast) or sodium cromoglycate/nedrocromil sodium (second choice) before exercise
Management of EIA
Follow asthma guidelines (GINA)
Promote reliever treatment, SABA[b] before exercise and as needed for relief
Stratify preventer therapies using the lowest dose to achieve control. ICS (first choice). LTRA (second choice)
If control is not achieved with ICS, options include the addition of another controller such as a LABA or LTRA, alternatively a 'step up' in ICS can be considered

[a]High heterogeneity in individual responses reported.
[b]Tolerance to and side effects of SABA need consideration.

Abbreviations: SABA = short-acting β2 agonist; SAMA = short acting anti-muscarinic drugs; LTRA = leukotriene-receptor antagonist; ICS = inhaled corticosteroids; LABA = long-acting β2 agonist.

Symptoms can disrupt sleep, interfere with taste and appetite, and cause headache, especially if associated with sinusitis (Bougault *et al.*, 2010a). This can have a very negative impact on both quality of life and exercise performance.

The 'Allergic rhinitis and its impact on Asthma' study (ARIA), reminds us that allergic rhinitis occurs as a result of IgE-mediated inflammation following allergen exposure, diagnostically supported by evidence of allergic sensitisation (aeroallergen specific skin prick tests or IgE assays) and can be classified by symptom pattern (intermittent or persistent) and severity (mild, moderate, or severe) (Bousquet *et al.*, 2008). High exhaled fraction of nitric oxide (FeNO) correlates with increased symptom severity in children and may also predict response to treatments targeting allergic inflammation (Wang *et al.*, 2017). Allergic rhinitis alone can cause symptoms sufficient to impair exercise performance. In one study, 57% of children and adolescents with the condition reported respiratory symptoms limiting their exercise, which were not associated with the 37% who had EIB on exercise challenge tests. Furthermore, different methodologies for the latter only had moderate agreement (Rodrigues Filho *et al.*, 2018).

Non-allergic rhinitis is generally dominated by chronic nasal obstruction and rhinorrhoea perpetuated by the physical and chemical characteristics of inhaled air (Tran *et al.*, 2011). However, rather than there being two distinct types of rhinitis, there is likely to be a significant overlap and non-allergic rhinitis may predispose to allergic sensitisation, as described above.

In one report investigating young athletes, 12% of elite swimmers and 18% of track and field athletes suffered from allergic rhinitis while non-allergic rhinitis diagnosed in 33% of swimmers and 13% of track and field athletes (Surda *et al.*, 2018). In another study, 74% of swimmers reported rhinitis symptoms that persisted for up to two weeks after training stopped (Bougault *et al.*, 2010b).

In swimmers, nose clips will help prevent repeated douching of nasal airways by pool water. Saline douches can be used to clear secretions in rhinitis and may facilitate the deposition of topical drug treatments (Tran *et al.*, 2011). Preventative pharmacological treatments centre on topical nasal corticosteroids, with day-to-day symptoms helped by non-sedating antihistamines. (Bousquet *et al.*, 2008). Cysteinyl leukotriene receptor antagonists (LTRA) are useful for allergic rhinitis.

Exercise-induced Larynx Obstruction (EILO)

EILO is defined as a transitory, inappropriate narrowing of the larynx and surrounding structures specifically occurring during intense exercise, leading to discomfort and breathing difficulty. It is distinct from induced laryngeal obstruction, ILO which may be associated with emotional factors, chemical and allergic triggers (Halvorsen *et al.*, 2017). EILO can masquerade as asthma (McFadden and Zawadski, 1996), although characteristically it is refractory to inhaled rescue and preventative asthma medications (Røksund *et al.*, 2017). Cross-specialty international consensus discourages terms such as 'vocal cord dysfunction' or 'paradoxical movement of the vocal cords' (Christensen *et al.*, 2015).

EILO prevalence is estimated to be 2–3% in the general population (Boulet and Turmel, 2019), but 35% in elite athletes, especially women (Nielsen *et al.*, 2013). Although one study, in non-athletic adolescents, found no gender disparity (Johansson *et al.*, 2015).

Various mechanisms have been suggested to account for the abnormal narrowing of the larynx during exercise. Normally the vocal cord abduction is coupled with diaphragmatic contraction during inspiration and the former is heightened in strenuous exercise to help reduce turbulence as flow increases. In EILO, the laryngeal aperture narrows and the supraglottic structures fold inwards, without necessarily any adduction of the vocal cords, and turbulent airflow leads to symptoms. The pressure gradient across the larynx may account for the aerodynamic infolding of less rigid structures including the aryepiglottic folds. Laryngeal irritability and neuronally mediated hyper-reactivity of the laryngeal musculature may play a role, contributed to or perpetuated by exercise-induced airway inflammation, especially in cold, dry, or polluted settings, post-nasal drip due to rhinitis (Peters *et al.*, 2003), acid reflux (Woolnough *et al.*, 2013), higher centre emotional influences on respiratory control, and possibly hormonal factors. No doubt, in individuals, aetiology is likely to be multifactorial (Campisi *et al.*, 2019).

Symptoms develop during exercise and increase in parallel with exercise intensity, stopping when exercise ceases. Symptoms described by patients include shortness of breath, cough, a feeling of throat tightness, noisy breathing, and chest pain. The respiratory noise generated in EILO is stridulous, on inspiration, distinguishable from expiratory wheezing in EIB (Panchasara *et al.*, 2015, Halvorsen *et al.*, 2017). Patients, parents, and even sporting trainers may not be able to discriminate them. Recordings and ultimately witnessing an episode will be diagnostically helpful. A resting clinical examination is usually normal and so a careful clinical history and assessment is needed to avoid misdiagnosing the condition (Shay *et al.*, 2019). Continuous laryngoscopy during exercise (CLE) is the definitive diagnostic investigation, and requires a flexible nasendoscope in situ during the test (Halvorsen *et al.*, 2017). The severity can be visually classified using a scoring system (Walsted *et al.*, 2017). It allows a direct view of the upper airway during exercise and although formats such as treadmill running or cycle ergometry are used, testing whist the athlete undertakes their chosen sport is desirable and has been achieved in rowing and climbing (Panchasara *et al.*, 2015; Halvorsen *et al.*, 2017).

The optimum treatment for EILO has yet to be determined and further prospective controlled studies are urgently needed to inform best management although heterogeneity in the diagnosis of EILO means that such studies are logistically challenging. Progress, however, is anticipated after the publication of international consensus recommendations on terminology, diagnosis, and management of the condition and associated problems (Halvorsen *et al.*, 2017; Røksund *et al.*, 2017). Treatment aims are to enable effective training, ensure performance potentials are realised for athletes, and enhance their quality of life. The removal of laryngeal irritants (e.g., caffeine, untreated reflux) alongside breathing and laryngeal control techniques delivered by a physiotherapist or speech and language therapist form the cornerstone of therapy, underpinned by reassurance that the condition is not dangerous. The use of biofeedback from CLE may help in gaining control over laryngeal dysfunction. Young athletes who have stopped playing sports due to their fear of becoming breathless with this condition are likely to benefit from psychological intervention (McFadden and Zawadski, 1996). Studies of pharmacological interventions including inhaled anticholinergics and tricyclic antidepressants do not support their use (Halvorsen *et al.*, 2017).

Co-morbidities, such as EIB, asthma, rhinitis, and GORD, can co-exist, need to be identified, and treated. Rarely, in the most severe cases, surgical intervention such as supraglotoplasty has been reported with good outcome (Mehlum *et al.*, 2016).

Gastro-oesophageal Reflux Disease (GORD)

Although not well studied in athletes, some sports may predispose to GORD, including running, activities involving recumbent postures, and straining with high workloads that cause a rise in intra-abdominal pressure (Ter Steege *et al.*, 2008). Ingestion of large volumes of sports drinks, particularly if carbonated, may aggravate reflux symptoms. Patients with GORD have reduced laryngopharyngeal sensitivity, which may render them more prone to aspiration and cough (Phua *et al.*, 2005). However, where laryngeal dysfunction has been shown to be associated with GORD, acid suppression with proton pump inhibitors did not show clinical benefit (Woolnough *et al.*, 2013) and studies investigating associations between GORD and EILO have been inconclusive.

Non-pharmacological Interventions

General measures and forward planning to ameliorate or avoid the physical or allergenic triggers of airway inflammation are important. The promotion of nasal breathing and pre-exercise warm-ups, consisting of short bursts (15–30 seconds) of activity alternating with rests (60–90 seconds) and then post-exercise 'warm-downs' may help reduce EIA symptoms (Morton and Fitch, 2011).

Heat-and-moisture-exchanging devices (HMEs) may be worn by winter sports athletes to prevent airways damage and EIB, especially those competing in endurance events (Hanstock *et al.*, 2020). Even appliances to dilate and improve airflow through the nose in adolescents have been shown to reduce perceived breathlessness and improve aerobic capacity in adolescent athletes (Ferreira *et al.*, 2020). In controlled trials, some limited benefit has been reported for several nutritional interventions in athletes to preserve mucosal integrity and counter the symptoms of exercise-induced epithelial injury; these include vitamins A and D, antioxidants, bovine colostrum, and probiotics (Gleeson and Pyne, 2016).

Event logistics need to consider the increased transport and energy generators required to host events, as spikes in air pollution well above accepted air quality may arise (Bunds *et al.*, 2019). Personal monitors to record precise timing and levels of exposure to pollutants, such as polycyclic aromatic hydrocarbons, may help understand the impact of pollution on general and individual athletic performance. Such technology could guide the scheduling of training and competition to avoid local pollution peaks (Reche *et al.*, 2020). Similarly, seasonal variation in performance in sensitised athletes has been described, paving the way for early preventative treatments to be started (Komarow and Postolache, 2005).

World Anti-doping Agency (WADA) and Global Drug Reference Online (Global DRO)

Anti-doping regulations are provided by WADA, bringing global consistency to rules governing drug use in competitive sports. It is updated annually and informs trainers and athletes of all ages about their obligations to comply with dose limits of specific medications and avoid prohibited substances when both training and competing (WADA, 2020). The information is available in many languages and in age-appropriate format, accessible via the Global DRO, providing specific information on products sold throughout the developed world (Global DRO, 2020).

Exceptional circumstances allow prohibited drugs to be used by athletes if they obtain a Therapeutic Use Exemption (TUE) authorisation that is issued by the international anti-doping agency (WADA, 2020), see Table 7.3.

Future Research

There are many unanswered questions relating to the respiratory health of young athletes and the way in which different sports, training schedules, and environmental factors may cause problems. International consensus statements have helped to refine the understanding and diagnosis of specific conditions. However, more work is required to determine the true prevalence of respiratory illnesses in young athletes and further explore how they evolve. Standardised diagnostic pathways will facilitate randomised controlled trials to determine the value of preventative strategies and interventions.

Conclusion

Young athletes are motivated by the kudos and celebrity of winning as well as the financial rewards of success. They become role models and promote engagement in exercise which has important health benefits across society. However, training and participation in competitive sport is associated with a high prevalence of respiratory disorders. Susceptibility relates to the pathophysiological consequences of high-intensity and endurance exercise, coupled with environmental factors, individual predispositions, and co-morbidities. Important increments in performance may depend on precision medicine where accurate diagnoses depend on structured clinical assessments and inform therapeutic interventions that need to be open to scrutiny and must comply with regulation. Many of the respiratory problems encountered appear to increase in prevalence with age, which may reflect the intensity levels of competition, cumulative time spent training, and intrinsic differences in paediatric versus adult physiology, immunology, and psychology. More needs to be learnt about the relevant processes involved in the development

Table 7.3 Common Drugs Used in Respiratory Medicine and WADA status (WADA 2020; Global DRO 2020)

Drug	*Status*	*Considerations*
Inhaled β2- agonists		
Albuterol/salbutamol	Permitted	The maximum daily doses are 1,600 μg. A urinary concentration greater than 1,000 $ng{\cdot}mL^{-1}$ is considered by the WADA to be an 'adverse analytical finding' unless the athlete proves the drug was used therapeutically.
Formoterol	Permitted	The maximum daily doses are 54 μg. A urinary concentration greater than 40 $ng{\cdot}mL^{-1}$ is considered by the WADA to be an 'adverse analytical finding' unless the athlete proves the drug was used therapeutically.
Salmeterol	Permitted	
Terbutaline	Prohibited	
Inhaled anticholinergics	Permitted	
Glucocorticoids		
Inhaled	Permitted	
Nasal	Permitted	
Oral	Prohibited	These agents are prohibited during competition only
Injected	Prohibited	These agents are prohibited during competition only
Leukotriene antagonists (Montelukast)	Permitted	FDA warned about central nervous system effects of using these drugs.
Sodium cromoglicate and nedocromil sodium	Permitted	
Omalizumab	Permitted	
Antihistamines		
Sedating	Permitted	
Non-sedating	Permitted	
Proton pump inhibitors	Permitted	
Pseudoephedrine	Permitted	The maximum daily doses are 240 mg. The urinary concentration of pseudoephedrine should not be >150 $\mu g{\cdot}mL^{-1}$. Athletes must stop taking pseudoephedrine at least 24 hours before competition.

Abbreviations: WADA = World Anti-doping Agency. Global DRO = Global Reference Online. FDA = Food and Drug Administration.

of respiratory illnesses in young athletes and what the longer-term outcomes and consequences are. Generic preventative strategies may help ameliorate symptoms whilst awareness and a better understanding of the processes at bay amongst athletes and their coaches will help individuals achieve their athletic goals.

Key Points

- Young athletes suffer a high incidence of respiratory illnesses including EIA, EIB, EILO, and rhinitis. Prevalence may differ depending on the type of sport performed and the environment in which it takes place.
- The development of respiratory problems in young athletes warrants further study to understand the processes at bay and determine long-term outcomes. This will help inform preventative and management strategies.
- Symptoms alone may be misleading and comprehensive clinical assessments have become part of athletic team support structures in order to diagnose and treat conditions appropriately and verify that medications comply with regulations.

References

Adami, P., Squeo, M., Quattrini, F., Di Paolo, F., Pisicchio, C., DiGiacinto, B., Lemme, E., Maestrini, V. and Pelliccia, A. (2019). Pre-participation health evaluation in adolescent athletes competing at Youth Olympic Games: proposal for a tailored protocol. *British Journal of Sports Medicine*, 53, 1111–1116. Doi 10.1136/bjsports-2018-099651.

Anderson, S.D. and Tocias, A.G. (2000). Dry-air and hyperosmolar challenge in asthma and rhinitis, in Busse W. and Holgate S. (eds). *Asthma and Rhinitis.* Oxford, UK: Blackwell Science Ltd, pp. 1449.

Andreff, W. (2008). Globalization of the sports economy. *Rivisti di diritto ed economia dello Sport*, 4 (3), 13–32.

Atchley, T.J. and Smith, D.M. (2020). Exercise-induced bronchoconstriction in elite or endurance athletes: pathogenesis and diagnostic considerations. *Annals of Allergy, Asthma and Immunology*, 125(1), 47–54. Doi 10.1016/j.anai.2020.01.023.

Bennett, W.D., Zeman, K.L. and Jarabek, A.M. (2007). Nasal contribution to breathing and fine particle deposition in children versus adults. *Journal of Toxicology and Environmental Health, Part A*, 71(3), 227–237. Doi 10.1080/15287390701598200.

Bernard, A. (2007). Chlorination products: emerging links with allergic diseases. *Current Medicinal Chemistry*, 14(16), 1771–1782. Doi 10.2174/092986707781058940.

Bolger, C., Tufvesson, E., Anderson, S.D., Devereux, G., Ayres, J.G., Bjermer, L. and Kippelen, P. (2011). Effect of inspired air conditions on exercise-induced bronchoconstriction and urinary CC16 levels in athletes. *Journal of Applied Physiology*, 111(4), 1059–1065. Doi 10.1152/japplphysiol.00113.2011.

Bonini, M., Gramiccioni, C., Fioretti, D., Ruckert, B., Rinaldi, M., Akdis, C., Todaroe, A., Palangea, P., Carlsen, K.H., Pelliccia, A., Rasi, G. and Bonini, S. (2015). 'Asthma, allergy and the Olympics: a 12-year survey in elite athletes'. *Current Opinions in Allergy and Clinical Immunology,* 15, 184–192. Doi 10.1097/ACI.0000000000000149.

Bonini, M. and Silvers, W. (2018). Exercise-induced bronchoconstriction: background, prevalence, and sport considerations. *Immunology and Allergy Clinics of North America*, 38(2), 205–214. Doi 10.1016/j.iac.2018.01.007.

Bougault, V., Loubaki, L., Joubert, P., Turmel, J., Couture, C., Laviolette, M. and Boulet, L.P. (2012). Airway remodeling and inflammation in competitive swimmers training in indoor chlorinated swimming pools. *Journal of Allergy and Clinical Immunology*, 129(2), 351–358. Doi 10.1016/j.jaci.2011.11.010.

Bougault, V., Turmel, J. and Boulet, L.P. (2010a). Bronchial challenges and respiratory symptoms in elite swimmers and winter sport athletes: airway hyperresponsiveness in asthma: its measurement and clinical significance. *Chest*, 138(2), 31–37. Doi 10.1378/chest.09-1689.

Bougault, V., Turmel, J. and Boulet, L.P. (2010b). Effect of intense swimming training on rhinitis in high-level competitive swimmers. *Clinical and Experimental Allergy*, 40(8), 1238–1246. Doi 10.1111/j.1365-2222.2010.03551.x.

Boulet, L.P. and Turmel, J. (2019). Cough in exercise and athletes. *Pulmonary Pharmacology and Therapeutics*, 55, 67–74. Doi 10.1016/j.pupt.2019.02.003.

Boulet L.P. and O'Byrne P. (2015). Asthma and exercise-induced bronchoconstriction in athletes. *New England Journal of Medicine*, 372, 641–8. Doi 10.1056/NEJMra1407552.

Bousquet, J., Khaltaev, N., Cruz, A.A., Denburg, J., Fokkens, W.J., Togias, A. and Agache, I. (2008). Allergic rhinitis and its impact on asthma (ARIA). *Allergy*, 63, 8–160. Doi 10.1111/j.1398-9995.2007.01620.x.

Bunds, K.S., Casper, J.M., Frey, H.C. and Barrett, M. (2019). Air pollution at college football games: developing a methodology for measuring air pollutant exposure in a sport event microenvironment. *Event Management*, 23(3), 399–412. Doi 10.3727/152599518X15403853721484.

Campisi, E.S., Schneiderman, J.E., Owen, B., Moraes, T.J. and Campisi, P. (2019). Exercise-induced laryngeal obstruction: quality initiative to improve assessment and management. *International Journal of Pediatric Otorhinolaryngology*, 127, 109677. Doi 10.1016/j.ijporl.2019.109677.

Cao, Y., Chen, M., Dong, D., Xie, S. and Liu, M. (2020). Environmental pollutants damage airway epithelial cell cilia: implications for the prevention of obstructive lung diseases. *Thoracic Cancer*, 11(3), 505–510. Doi 10.1111/1759-7714.13323.

Carlsen, K.H. and Kowalski, M.L. (2008). Asthma, allergy, the athlete and the Olympics. *Allergy*, 63 383–386. Doi 10.1111/j.1398-9995.2008.01630.x.

Cavaleiro Rufo, J., Paciência, I., Silva, D., Martins, C., Madureira, J., Oliveira Fernandes, E., Padrão, P., Moreira, P., Delgado, L. and Moreira, A. (2018). Swimming pool exposure is associated with autonomic changes and increased airway reactivity to a beta-2 agonist in school aged children: a cross-sectional survey. *PLoS ONE*, 13(3), e0193848. Doi 10.1371/journal.pone.0193848.

Christensen, P.M., Heimdal, J.H., Christopher, K.L., Bucca, C., Cantarella, G., Friedrich, G., Halvorsen, T., Herth, F., Jung, H., Morris, M.J., Remacle, M., Rasmussen, N. and Wilson, J.A. (2015). ERS/ELS/ACCP 2013 international consensus conference nomenclature on inducible laryngeal obstructions. *European Respiratory Review*, 24(137), 445–50. Doi 10.1183/16000617.00006513.

Couto, M., Kurowski, M., Moreira, A., Bullens, D.M.A., Carlsen, K.H., Delgado, L., Kowalski, M.L. and Seys, S.F. (2018). Mechanisms of exercise-induced bronchoconstriction in athletes: current perspectives and future challenges. *Allergy*, 73(1), 8–16. Doi 10.1111/all.13224.

Cutrufello, P. T., Smoliga, J. M. and Rundell, K.W. (2012). Small things make a big difference: particulate matter and exercise. *Sports Medicine*, 42(12), 1041–1058. Doi 10.1007/BF03262311.

Ferreira, C.H.S., Dinardi, R.R., da Cunha Ibiapina, C. and de Andrade, C.R. (2020). Nasal function and cardio-respiratory capacity of adolescent with external nasal dilator. *International Journal of Pediatric Otorhinolaryngology*, 110430. Doi 10.1016/j.ijporl.2020.110430.

Fitch, K. (2016). Air pollution, athletic health and performance at the Olympic Games. *Journal of Sports Medicine and Physical Fitness*, 56, 922–932. PMID: 25786594.

Fritsch, P., Pozza, E., Ehringer-Schetitska, D., Jokinen, E., Herceg-Cavrak, V., Hidvegi, E., Oberhoffer, R., and Petropoulos, A. (2017). Cardiovascular pre-participation screening in young athletes: recommendations of the Association of European Paediatric Cardiology. *Cardiology in the Young*, 27, 1655–1660. Doi 10.1017/S1047951117001305.

Gałązka-Franta, A., Jura-Szołtys, E., Smółka, W. and Gawlik, R. (2016). Upper respiratory tract diseases in athletes in different sports disciplines. *Journal of Human Kinetics*, 53, 99–106. Doi 10.1515/hukin-2016-0014.

Georas, S. and Rezaee, F. (2014). Epithelial barrier function: at the front line of asthma immunology and allergic airway inflammation. *Journal of Allergy and Clinical Immunology*, 134(3), 509–520. Doi 10.1016/j.jaci.2014.05.049.

Giorgini, P., Rubenfire, M., Bard, R.L., Jackson, E.A., Ferri, C. and Brook, R.D. (2016). Air pollution and exercise. *Journal of Cardiopulmonary Rehabilitation and Prevention*, 36(2), 84–95. Doi 10.1097/HCR.0000000000000139.

Gleeson, M. and Pyne, D.B. (2016). Respiratory inflammation and infections in high-performance athletes. *Immunology and Cell Biology*, 94(2), 124–131. Doi 10.1038/icb.2015.100.

Glencross, D.A., Ho, T.R., Camina, N., Hawrylowicz, C.M. and Pfeffer, P.E. (2020). Air pollution and its effects on the immune system. *Free Radical Biology and Medicine*, 151, 56–68. Doi 10.1016/j.freeradbiomed.2020.01.179.

Global Initiative for Asthma (2020). Global strategy for asthma management and prevention. Available at: https://ginasthma.org/wp-content/uploads/2020/04/GINA-2020-full-report_-final-_wms.pdf (Accessed: May 24 2020).

Global Drug Reference Online (2020). Available at: https://www.globaldro.com/Home (Accessed: May 24 2020).

Hallstrand, T.S. (2012). New insights into to pathogenesis of exercise-induced bronchoconstriction. *Current Opinion in Allergy and Clinical Immunology*, 12(1), 42–48. Doi 10.1097/ACI.0b013e32834ecc67.

Halvorsen T., Walsted, E.S., Bucca, C., Bush, A., Cantarella, G., Friedrich, G., Herth, F.J.F., Hull, J.H., Jung, H., Maat, R., Nordang, L., Remacle, M., Rasmussen, N., Wilson, J.A. and Heimdal, J.H. (2017). Inducible laryngeal obstruction: an official joint European Respiratory Society and European Laryngological Society statement. *European Respiratory Journal*, 50, 1602221. Doi 10.1183/13993003.02221-2016.

Han, X. (2019). Modeling and analysis of the impact of smog pollution on the training effect of intensive sports. *Ekoloji*, 28(108), 1783–1787.

Hanstock, H.G., Ainegren, M. and Stenfors, N. (2020). Exercise in sub-zero temperatures and airway health: implications for athletes with special focus on heat-and-moisture-exchanging breathing devices. *Frontiers in Sports and Active Living*, 2, 34. Doi 10.3389/fspor.2020.00034.

Hodgson, J.R., Elliott, S., Chapman, L., Hudson, C. and Pope, F.D. (2020). The influence of meteorology and air quality on parkrun athletic performance. https://orcid.org/0000-0003-4227-533.

Hull, J., Ansley, L., Price, O., Dickinson, J. and Bonini, M. (2016). Eucapnic voluntary hyperpnea: gold standard for diagnosing exercise-induced bronchoconstriction in athletes? *Sports Medicine*, 46, 1083–1093. Doi 10.1007/s40279-016-0491-3.

Ilyas, H., Masih, I. and van der Hoek, J.P. (2018). An exploration of disinfection by-products formation and governing factors in chlorinated swimming pool water. *Journal of Water and Health*, 16(6), 861–892. Doi 10.2166/wh.2018.067.

International Olympic Committee. (2004). From the youngest to the oldest. Available at: https://www.olympic.org/news/from-the-youngest-to-the-oldest (Accessed: July 20, 2020).

International Olympic Committee. (2008) 'Consensus Statement on Asthma in Elite Athletes'. Available at: https://stillmed.olympic.org/media/Document%20 Library/OlympicOrg/IOC/Who-We-Are/Commissions/Medical-and-Scientific-Commission/EN-IOC-Consensus-Statement-on-Asthma-in-Elite-Athletes.pdf#_ga=2.106221575.505712876.1591030208-67467564.1591030208 (Accessed: May 24, 2020).

International Tennis Federation. (2020). World tennis tour junior regulations. Available at: https://www.itftennis.com/media/3894/2020-junior-circuit-regulations-updated-14-august-2020.pdf (Accessed: Sep 1, 2020).

Jeljeli, M., Guérin-El Khourouj, V., Pédron, B., Gressens, P., Sibony, O. and Sterkers, G. (2019). Ontogeny of cytokine responses to PHA from birth to adulthood. *Pediatric Research*, 86(1), 63–70. Doi 10.1038/s41390-019-0383-y.

Johansson, H., Norlander, K., Berglund, L., Janson, C., Malinovschi, A., Nordvall, L., Nordang, L., Emtner, M. (2015). Prevalence of exercise-induced bronchoconstriction and exercise-induced laryngeal obstruction in a general adolescent population. *Thorax*, 70, 57–63. Doi 10.1136/thoraxjnl-2014-205738.

Kanikowska, A., Napiórkowska-Baran, K., Graczyk, M. and Kucharski, M.A. (2018). Influence of chlorinated water on the development of allergic diseases – An overview. *Annals of Agricultural and Environmental Medicine*, *25*(4), 651–655. Doi 10.26444/aaem/7981.

Kargarfard, M., Shariat, A., Shaw, B., Shaw, I., Lam, E., Kheiri, A., et al. (2015). Effects of polluted air on cardiovascular and haematological parameters after progressive maximal aerobic exercise. *Lung*, 193(2), 275–281. Doi 10.1007/s00408-014-9679-1.

Kippelen, P. and Anderson, S.D. (2012a). Airway injury during high-level exercise. *British Journal of Sports Medicine*, 46, 385–390. Doi 10.1136/bjsports-2011-090819.

Kippelen, P., Fitch, K.D., Anderson, S.D., Bougault, V., Boulet, L.P., Rundell, K.W., Sue-Chu, M., McKenzie, D.C. (2012b). Respiratory health of elite athletes – preventing airway injury: a critical review. *British Journal of Sports Medicine*, 46, 471–476. Doi 10.1136/bjsports-2012-091056.

Kippelen, P., Anderson, S.D. and Hallstrand, T.S. (2018). Mechanisms and biomarkers of exercise-induced bronchoconstriction. *Immunology and Allergy Clinics*, 38(2), 165–182. Doi 10.1016/j.iac.2018.01.008.

Knöpfli, B.H., Luke-Zeitoun, M., von Duvillard, S.P., Burki, A., Bachlechner, C. and Keller, H. (2007). High incidence of exercise-induced bronchoconstriction in triathletes of the Swiss national team. *British Journal of Sports Medicine*, 41(8), 486–491. Doi 10.1136/bjsm.2006.030569.

Komarow, H.D. and Postolache, T.T. (2005). Seasonal allergy and seasonal decrements in athletic performance. *Clinics in Sports Medicine*, 24(2), 35–50. Doi 10.1016/j.csm.2004.12.006.

Kurowski, M., Jurczyk, J., Olszewska-Ziaber, A., Jarzebska, M., Krysztofiak, H. and Kowalski, M.L. (2018). A similar pro/anti-inflammatory cytokine balance is present in the airways of competitive athletes and non-exercising asthmatics. *Advances in Medical Sciences*, 63, 79–86. Doi 10.1016/j.advms.2017.07.004.

Larsson, J., Anderson, S.D., Dahlén, S.E. and Dahlén, B. (2013). Refractoriness to exercise challenge: a review of the mechanisms old and new. *Immunology and Allergy Clinics*, 33(3), 329–345. Doi 10.1016/j.iac.2013.02.004.

Larsson, K., Tornling, G., Gavhed, D., Muller-Suur, C. and Palmberg, L. (1998). Inhalation of cold air increases the number of inflammatory cells in the lungs in healthy subjects. *European Respiratory Journal*, 12(4), 825–830. Doi 10.1183/09031936.98.12040825.

McFadden, Jr, E.R. and Zawadski, D.K. (1996). Vocal cord dysfunction masquerading as exercise-induced asthma. a physiologic cause for "choking" during athletic activities. *American Journal of Respiratory and Critical Care Medicine*, 153(3), 942–947. Doi 10.1164/ajrccm.153.3.8630577.

Mehlum, C.S., Walsted, E.S., Godballe, C. and Backer, V. (2016). Supraglottoplasty as treatment of exercise induced laryngeal obstruction (EILO). *European Archives of Oto-rhino-laryngology*, 273(4), 945–951. Doi10.1007/s00405-015-3823-2.

Morton, A.R. and Fitch, K.D. (2011). Australian association for exercise and sports science position statement on exercise and asthma. *Journal of Science and Medicine in Sport*, 14, 312–316. Doi10.1016/j.jsams.2011.02.009.

Mountjoy, M., Fitch, F., Boulet, L.P., Bougault, V., Van Mechelen, W. and Verhagen, E. (2015). Prevalence and characteristics of asthma in the aquatic disciplines. *Journal of Allergy and Clinical Immunology*, 136, 588–594. Doi 10.1016/j.jaci.2015.01.041.

Mountjoy, M., Vertommen, T., Burrows, K. and Greinig, S. (2020). SafeSport: safeguarding initiatives at the Youth Olympic Games 2018. *British Journal of Sports Medicine*, 54, 176–182. Doi 10.1136/bjsports-2019-101461.

Näsman, A., Irewall, T., Hållmarker, U., Lindberg, A. and Stenfors, N. (2018). Asthma and asthma medication are common among recreational athletes participating in endurance sport competitions. *Canadian Respiratory Journal*. Doi 10.1155/2018/3238546.

Nielsen, E.W., Hull, J.H. and Backer, V. (2013). High prevalence of exercise-induced laryngeal obstruction in athletes. *Medicine and Science in Sports and Exercise*, 45(11), 2030–2035. Doi 10.1249/MSS.0b013e318298b19a.

Panchasara, B., Nelson, C., Niven, R., Ward, S. and Hull, J.H. (2015). Lesson of the month: rowing-induced laryngeal obstruction: a novel cause of exertional dyspnoea: characterised by direct laryngoscopy. *Thorax*, 70:95–97. Doi 10.1136/thoraxjnl-2014-205773.

Parsons, J.P., Hallstrand, T.S., Mastronarde, J.G., Kaminsky, D.A., Rundell, K.W., Hull, J.H., Storms, W.W., Weiler, J.M., Cheek, F.M., Wilson, K.C. and Anderson, S.D. (2013). An official American Thoracic Society clinical practice guideline: exercise-induced bronchoconstriction. *American Journal of Respiratory and Critical Care Medicine*, 187(9), 1016–1027. Doi 10.1164/rccm.201303-0437ST.

Peters, E.J., Hatley, T.K., Crater, S.E., Phillips, C.D., Platts-Mills, T.A. and Borish, L. (2003). Sinus computed tomography scan and markers of inflammation in vocal cord dysfunction and asthma. *Annals of Allergy, Asthma and Immunology*, 90(3), 316–322. Doi 10.1016/S1081-1206(10)61800-5.

Phua, S.Y., McGarvey, L.P.A., Ngu, M.C. and Ing, A.J. (2005). Patients with gastro-oesophageal reflux disease and cough have impaired laryngopharyngeal mechanosensitivity. *Thorax*, 60(6), 488–491. Doi 10.1136/thx.2004.033894.

Qin, F., Yang, Y., Wang, S.T., Dong, Y.N., Xu, M.X., Wang, Z.W. and Zhao, J.X. (2019). Exercise and air pollutants exposure: a systematic review and meta-analysis. *Life Sciences*, 218, 153–164. Doi 10.1016/j.lfs.2018.12.036.

Raghavan, D. and Jain, R. (2016). Increasing awareness of sex differences in airway diseases. *Respirology*, 21(3), 449–459. Doi 10.1111/resp.12702.

Real Madrid FC. (2020). Pruebas de acceso. Available at: https://www.realmadrid.com/futbol/cantera/pruebas-acceso (Accessed: Sept 01, 2020).

Reche, C., Viana, M., Van Drooge, B.L., Fernández, F.J., Escribano, M., Castaño-Vinyals, G., Nieuwenhuijsen, M., Adami, P.E. and Bermon, S. (2020). Athletes' exposure to air pollution during world athletics relays: a pilot study. *Science of the Total Environment*, 717, 137161. Doi 10.1016/j.scitotenv.2020.137161.

Rodrigues Filho, A., Rizzo, J.Â., Gonçalves, A.V., Correia Junior, M.A.V., Sarinho, E.S.C. and Medeiros, D. (2018). Exercise-induced bronchospasm in children and adolescents with allergic rhinitis by treadmill and hyperventilation challenges. *Respiratory Medicine*, 138, 102–106. Doi 10.1016/j.rmed.2018.04.001.

Røksund, O.D., Heimdal, J.H., Clemm, H., Vollsæter, M., Halvorsen, T. (2017). Exercise inducible laryngeal obstruction: Diagnostics and management. *Paediatric Respiratory Review*, 21, 86–94. Doi 10.1016/j.prrv.2016.07.003.

Rundell, K.W. (2003). High levels of airborne ultrafine and fine particulate matter in indoor ice arenas. *Inhalation Toxicology*, 15(3), 237–250. Doi 10.1080/08958370304502.

Rundell, K.W., Anderson, S.D., Sue-Chu, M., Bougault, V. and Boulet, L.P. (2011). Air quality and temperature effects on exercise-induced bronchoconstriction. *Comprehensive Physiology*, 5(2), 579–610. Doi 10.1002/cphy.c130013.

Shay, E.O., Sayad, E. and Milstein, C.F. (2019). Exercise-induced laryngeal obstruction (EILO) in children and young adults: from referral to diagnosis. *Laryngoscope*. Doi 10.1002/lary.28276.

Stang, J., Stensrud, T., Mowinckel, P. and Carlsen, K.H. (2016). Parasympathetic activity and Bronchial hyperresponsiveness in athletes. *Medicine and Science in Sports and Exercise*, 48(11), 2100–2107. Doi 10.1249/MSS.0000000000001008.

Surda, P., Putala, M., Siarnik, P., Walker, A., Bernic, A. and Fokkens, W. (2018). Rhinitis and its impact on quality of life in swimmers. *Allergy*, 73, 1022–1031. Doi 10.1111/all.13359.

Ter Steege, R.W., Van Der Palen, J. and Kolkman, J.J. (2008). Prevalence of gastrointestinal complaints in runners competing in a long-distance run: an internet-based observational study in 1281 subjects. *Scandinavian Journal of Gastroenterology*, 43(12), 1477–1482. Doi 10.1080/00365520802321170.

Thunqvist, P., Lilja, G., Wickman, M. and Pershagen, G. (2002). Asthma in children exposed to nitrogen dioxide in ice arenas. *European Respiratory Journal*, 20(3), 646–650. Doi 10.1183/09031936.02.00266302.

Tran, N., Vickery, J. and Blaiss, M. (2011). Management of rhinitis: allergic and non-allergic. *Allergy Asthma and Immunology Research*, 3(3), 148–156. Doi 10.4168/aair.2011.3.3.148.

Valtonen, M., Waris, M., Vuorinen, T., Eerola, E., Hakanen, A.J., Mjosund, K., Grönroos, W., Heinonen, O.J. and Ruuskanen, O. (2019). Common cold in Team Finland during 2018 Winter Olympic Games (PyeongChang): epidemiology, diagnosis including molecular point-of-care testing (POCT) and treatment. *British Journal of Sports Medicine*, 53 (17), 1093–1098. Doi 10.1136/bjsports-2018-100487.

Walsted, E.S., Hull, J.H., Hvedstrup, J., Maat, R. and Backer, V. (2017). Validity and reliability of grade scoring in the diagnosis of exercise-induced laryngeal obstruction. *ERJ Open Research*, 3, 00070–2017. Doi 10.1183\\23120541.00070-2017.

Wastensson, G. and Eriksson, K. (2020). Inorganic chloramines: a critical review of the toxicological and epidemiological evidence as a basis for occupational exposure limit setting. *Critical Reviews in Toxicology*, 50(3), 219–271. Doi 10.1080/10408444.2020.1744514.

Wang, P., Wang, G., Ge, W., Tang, L., Zhang, J. and Ni, X. (2017). Nasal nitric oxide in allergic rhinitis in children and its relationship to severity and treatment. *Allergy, Asthma and Clinical Immunology*, 13, 20. Doi10.1186/s13223-017-0191-z.

Woolnough, K., Blakey, J., Pargeter, N. and Mansur, A. (2013). Acid suppression does not reduce symptoms from vocal cord dysfunction, where gastro-laryngeal reflux is a known trigger. *Respirology*, 18(3), 553–554. Doi10.1111/resp.12058.

World Anti-Doping Agency. (2020). '2021 World Anti-Doping Code'. Available at: https://www.wada-ama.org/sites/default/files/resources/files/2021_code.pdf (Accessed: May 24, 2020).

World Health Organization. (2010) 'Global recommendations on physical activity for health'. Available at: https://apps.who.int/iris/bitstream/handle/10665/44399/9789241599979_eng.pdf?sequence=1 (Accessed: May 24, 2020).

Yamauchi, R., Shimizu, K., Kimura, F., Takemura, M., Suzuki, K., Akama, T., Kono, I. and Akimoto, T. (2011). Virus activation and immune function during intense training in rugby football players. *International Journal of Sports Medicine*, 32(5), 393–398. Doi 10.1055/s-0031-1271674.

Youth Olympic Games. (2020). Available at: https://www.olympic.org/youth-olympic-games (Accessed: July 1, 2020).

8 Tailoring Physical Activity and Exercise Prescription in Children with Respiratory Diseases

Daniel Stevens

Introduction

There has been a major global increase in the prevalence of chronic health conditions among children and adolescents; with non-communicable disease in the young predicted to be one of the leading causes of death in 2020 (Burns, Sadof and Kamat, 2007). The 2007 U.S. National Survey of Children's Health showed that 13.6% of children aged 0–17 years surveyed had at least one current chronic condition excluding obesity, while 8.7% had two more chronic conditions (Department of Health and Human Services, 2015). Children and adolescents with respiratory disease make-up one of the world's major chronic disease groups consisting of a diverse set of conditions including asthma, cystic fibrosis (CF), bronchiectasis, sleep apnoea, and interstitial lung disease. Asthma is the most common respiratory disease affecting approximately 16 million children worldwide (Tesse et al., 2018), categorised with reversible airway obstruction, airway inflammation, and increased airway responsiveness, while CF is the most common life-threatening disease in children with 95% mortality due to respiratory failure (Elborn, 2016). More common than CF, bronchiectasis contributes significantly to respiratory morbidity especially among more socially and economically disadvantaged groups (Goyal et al., 2016), and is characterised by irreversible dilation of one or more bronchi and decreased lung function (O'Donnell, 2008).

Recently, there has been a major shift in focus on the potential benefits of physical activity and exercise training in children living with respiratory and other chronic diseases. Indeed, the emerging concept of 'exercise is medicine' that can be used in a dose-dependent manner, similarly to pharmaceutical drugs, to positively impact health outcomes for individuals with chronic disease, is gaining increasing traction (Lee et al., 2012). Physical activity and exercise are terms often used interchangeably but have different characteristics. Physical activity is a complex set of behaviours encompassing any bodily movement that results in energy expenditure above the resting level (Armstrong and Van Mechelen, 2008), while exercise training refers to bodily movement that is planned and repetitive in nature that is often performed with the intention of improving a particular component of physical fitness.

DOI: 10.4324/9781003020462-8

The emphasis of physical activity is generally to discern health benefits or prevent the development of chronic disease, while exercise training is generally performed to improve human performance by purposefully improving a component of fitness, for example, speed, strength, aerobic fitness (Pieles et al., 2014). However, by training and enhancing body systems consequently, health benefits can also be derived from the latter.

In healthy children, those free of chronic disease, there is strong evidence confirming the physiological benefits of an active lifestyle such as improved cardiovascular fitness, musculoskeletal health, and elements of decreased cardiometabolic risk factors including reduced adiposity, blood lipids, blood glucose levels, and blood pressure (Janssen and LeBlanc, 2010). Physical activity has also been shown to influence the psychological health of young persons. Children that are more physically active tend to exhibit increased self-esteem, increased perception of wellbeing, and lower levels of anxiety and stress (Tomporowski, Lambourne and Okumura, 2011). Moreover, the benefits of physical activity are not only discerned during childhood and adolescence by reducing the risk for conditions such as diabetes, obesity, and cardiovascular disease, but increased participation in physical activity during this period in the lifespan has been shown to reduce future risk of chronic disease in adulthood (Raitakan et al., 1994; Twisk et al., 1997). Therefore, encouraging and engaging in physical activity early in the lifespan is critically important to promote lifelong health and well-being.

Given the evidence showing the positive association between physiological and psychological health and increased participation in physical activity in children and its transition into adulthood, multiple agencies including The Canadian Society for Exercise Physiology (CSEP) (Tremblay et al., 2011; Tremblay et al., 2016; Tremblay et al., 2017), the American College of Sport Medicine (ACSM) (Garber et al., 2011) and the World Health Organization (World Health Organization, 2010) have published physical activity guidelines. For young persons aged 5–17 years, current guidelines recommend participating in at least 60 minutes of daily moderate-to-vigorous intensity physical activity (Tremblay et al., 2011). Furthermore, a clear relationship between volume of physical activity and greater health benefits has been indicated (Janssen and LeBlanc, 2010).

In children with respiratory disease, there is also evidence showing physical activity and exercise training offers a treatment with the potential to improve functional capacity (cardiorespiratory fitness), manage/control symptoms, and improve quality of life (Joschtel et al., 2018); however, despite wide acceptance from the medical community is still underused in most healthcare systems across the globe (Pieles et al., 2014). This is further confounded by the fact that although the published guidelines indicate the volume of physical activity for healthy children (those free of chronic disease) (Tremblay et al., 2016, 2017), paediatric disease-specific guidelines are lacking. Therefore, clinicians may be uncertain about the prescription of physical activity they should prescribe to their paediatric patients. Indeed, similarly to pharmacological medicine, the dose of physical activity (i.e., the frequency, type, intensity, and duration) may be dependent on the type of chronic disease the child has and the severity. Furthermore, clinicians may also be unsure of the process in which to prescribe physical activity to their young patient. For example, clinicians may be unsure of the precautions that should be taken to sure safe participation in physical activity, and how best to promote physical activity as a treatment for the child. Clinicians may also require more guidance for the prescription of effective and enjoyable physical activity, and possible referral recommendations to an exercise and/or physical activity/exercise specialist.

Asthma

Asthma is the most common respiratory disease in children with an estimated global prevalence of 14%; and is characterised by chronic inflammation of the airways, airway hyper-responsiveness, and reversible airflow limitation (Global Initiative for Asthma, 2018). Symptoms often include shortness of breath, cough, and wheezing. Greater bronchial hyper-reactivity in asthma is associated with viral infections, cigarette smoke, inhaled allergens, emotional stress, environmental factors, and exercise (Philpott, Houghton and Luke, 2010). In 90% of asthmatics, an increase in ventilation during exercise is a trigger for bronchoconstriction (Randolph and Weiler, 2014). However, exercise is rarely the only trigger, making 'exercise-induced bronchoconstriction' better terminology to describe the condition. Exercise-related dyspnoea is often mistakenly diagnosed as exercise-induced bronchoconstriction; however, bronchial hyper-responsiveness is not associated with exercise-related dyspnoea (Seear, Wensley and West, 2005). Asthma can vary considerably in its severity, however, it is important to note that asthma can be controlled for all levels of disease severity. If well controlled, exercise tolerance should not be a limiting factor for participating in physical activity. While some children with asthma may be less physically active due to fears of exercise-induced bronchoconstriction, it has been shown that their physical activity levels do not differ from healthy aged matched peers (Cassim et al., 2016). It is useful for clinicians to note that children with a new diagnosis of asthma tend to present with lower levels of fitness including exercise capacity (Vahlkvist and Pedersen, 2009), and are more likely to be obese (Lu et al., 2016) which may further exacerbate exercise tolerance.

Clinicians need to be mindful of the potential risks and precautions when prescribing physical activity and exercise to children with asthma. As ventilation increases with more vigorous exercise, the onset of exercise-induced bronchoconstriction is greater, therefore, prescribing lower exercise intensities may be safer and allow for ventilation to better cope with the intensity of the activity. However, there is some evidence to show that high-intensity intermittent exercise is well-tolerated in children with asthma; this form of exercise includes brief intervals of high-intensity exercise followed by recovery intervals that may allow ventilation to recover (Counil et al., 2003). The environment in which physical activity is prescribed also requires consideration. Certain activities can expose individuals to dry, cool air (Zeitoun et al., 2004), and environmental allergens and pollutants that may trigger symptoms. In running and winter sports, asthmatic individuals have reported an increase in symptoms (Bar-Yishay et al., 1982), while breathing humid, warm air typically exposed to when swimming may be protective (Inbar et al., 1980). However, there is potential risk from exaggerated parasympathetic tone and chlorine-related airway irritation that may trigger bronchoconstriction (Bar-Or and Inbar, 1992). While asthma-related deaths in individuals younger than 20 years of age have been reported in both competitive and recreational sports, such incidences are rare (Becker et al., 2004).

Physical activity and exercise have been shown to have physical and psychosocial benefits for asthmatic children and can be used to effectively control symptoms. Indeed, a decrease in exercise hours per week increases bronchial hyper-responsiveness (Nystad, Stigum and Carlsen, 2001); but regular participation in exercise training has shown to result in fewer hospital visits, less medication usage, decrease in wheezing, and better quality of life (Basaran et al., 2006; Bonsignore et al., 2008; Fanelli et al., 2007; Neder et al., 1999; Welsh, Kemp and Roberts, 2005). However, despite the evidence for improving asthma control, regular exercise has not been associated with improvements in lung function (Ram, Robinson and Black, 2000). Currently, there are no recommendations for exercise in the National Asthma Education and Prevention Guidelines for the Diagnosis and Management of Asthma or the Global Initiative for Asthma guidelines (Lucas and Platts-Mills, 2005). Therefore, it is challenging for clinicians to prescribe exercise prescriptions for children with asthma using evidence-based guidelines. The intensity of exercise is an important consideration, as it is directly related to the ventilatory response that may trigger bronchoconstriction. Furthermore, the environment also needs to be considered, as some settings are less asthmogenic than others. Generally, aerobic exercise is well-tolerated in asthmatic children and is unlikely to lead to adverse events if well-controlled and medication is available (Eves and Davidson, 2011). Presently, there is little data on the acute and chronic effects of anaerobic exercise and resistance training in children with asthma and warrants further research. From the available evidence, it is suggested that children with asthma have a lower anaerobic capacity compared to healthy children (Counil et al., 1997), and that anaerobic training induces mild airway obstruction (Boas, Danduran and McColley, 1999).

Asthmatic children should be encouraged to keep an accurate account of symptoms, trigger exposures, treatments, and course of recovery from episodes of bronchoconstriction (Philpott, Houghton and Luke, 2010). Such information would assist the clinician in making a more informed and effective exercise prescription plan for the asthmatic child. Given the present lack of recommended guidelines for exercise in asthmatic children, those with well-controlled asthma and who take medication prior to physical activity can be encouraged to follow their own current national or global physical activity guidelines (Davies et al., 2019; Department of Health and Children and Health Service Executive, 2009; Tremblay et al., 2011, 2016); Piercy et al., 2018; World Health Organization, 2010). Those who are deconditioned and have poor control of their asthmatic symptoms can start at a lower intensity and shorter duration and gradually progress to meet the guidelines. Despite the lack of evidence for anaerobic training, it is hypothesised that increased ventilation during this form of exercise is more likely to induce an asthmatic response. Anaerobic exercise, however, that allows ventilation to recover, such as high-intensity intermittent training, may be tolerated in this patient group (Counil et al., 2003). More evidence is needed to determine the safety and benefits of anaerobic exercise for children with asthma before any clear recommendations can be made.

Cystic Fibrosis and Bronchiectasis

CF is an autosomal recessive disease caused by mutations in the CF transmembrane conductance regulator protein, a complex chloride channel located in all exocrine tissues (Orenstein and Higgins, 2005). Abnormal chloride transport leads to viscous secretions in the pulmonary, gastrointestinal, endocrine, and reproductive system, and greater salt loss in sweat. However, pulmonary disease is the most common cause of morbidity and mortality. Disease severity is variable and progressive, individually affecting exercise tolerance in children with CF. Importantly, higher levels of aerobic fitness in children with CF are associated with a slower deterioration in lung function and greater survival rates (Nixon et al., 1992; Pianosi, LeBlanc and Almudevar, 2005; Schneiderman-Walker et al., 2000). This is salient when considering physical activity and exercise prescription in this patient group, as such programmes can improve exercise tolerance especially those with poor aerobic fitness (Andréasson et al., 1987; Gulmans et al., 1999; Turchetta et al., 2004). Other benefits derived from physical activity and exercise interventions include enhanced lung mucous clearance specifically during intense exercise (Zach, Oberwaldner and Hausler, 1982; Zach, Purrer and Oberwaldner, 1981), improved strength and endurance of the respiratory muscles from swimming, walking, and jogging (Asher et al., 1982), and strength training may improve fat-free mass, weight gain, muscle strength, and lung function (forced expiratory volume in one second) (Orenstein et al., 2004; Selvadurai et al., 2002). Children with CF have also reported improvements in quality of life through participating in physical activity and exercise interventions (Barak et al., 2005; Klijn et al., 2004). Although few, randomised controlled exercise interventions in children and adolescents with CF have been performed in both in-hospital (Klijn et al., 2004; Santana-Sosa et al., 2014; Selvadurai et al., 2002; Sosa et al., 2012) and home-based settings (Del Corral et al., 2018; Orenstein et al., 2004; Schneiderman-Walker et al., 2000). These randomised controlled exercise interventions are summarised in Table 8.1.

Table 8.1 Randomised Controlled Exercise Interventions in Paediatric Cystic Fibrosis

	Methods	*Results*	*Conclusions*
(Schneiderman-Walker et al., 2000)	72 participants (7–19 years) were randomly assigned to a 3-year home aerobic training group or control group (usual physical activity participation)	Participants in the control group demonstrated a greater annual decline in lung function over the study period compared to those in the aerobic training group.	Lung function declined more slowly in the exercise group than the control group over the study period, suggesting a potential benefit of regular aerobic exercise. Compliance with the home exercise was good and corresponded with a self-reported positive attitude towards exercise.
(Selvadurai et al., 2002)	Participants (n = 66; 8–16 years) were randomised into three groups: aerobic training; resistance training; and control (standard chest physiotherapy).	Participants in the aerobic training group showed significantly greater peak aerobic capacity, activity levels, and quality of life than those in the resistance training group who demonstrated significantly better weight gain (total mass and fat free mass), lung function, and leg strength. No significant improvements were shown in the control group.	A combination of both aerobic and resistance training may be best to improve overall outcomes in children with cystic fibrosis.
(Klijn et al., 2004)	20 participants (13.6 ± 1.3 years) were randomly assigned to either a training programme consisting of anaerobic exercises or a control group maintaining their normal daily activities.	Participants in the anaerobic training group showed significant improvements in aerobic and aerobic performance and quality of life. However, after a 12-week follow-up period only anaerobic performance and quality of life were significantly higher compared to pre-training levels. No improvements were shown in the control group.	Anaerobic training has measureable effects on both aerobic (although not sustained) and anaerobic performance, and health-related quality of life in children with cystic fibrosis. Anaerobic training may be considered an important component of therapeutic exercise programs for these young patients.

(Orenstein et al., 2004)	67 participants (8–18 years) were randomised to either a 1-year home-based, semi-supervised, upper-body strength training program or a similarly structured aerobic training program of the same duration.	Participants in the strength-training programme increased 1 rep max for bicep curls significantly more than the aerobic training group. However, this difference was not significant when controlling for an increase in height. Both training conditions were associated with a significant increase in strength and physical work capacity.	Home-based, semi-supervised, upper-body strength and aerobic training over a 1-year period can improve both strength and physical work capacity.
(Sosa et al., 2012)	11 participants (6 boys; 10 ± 2 years) were randomly assigned to an 8-week intrahospital combined circuit and aerobic training programme, and 11 participants (7 boys; 11 ± 3 years) were assigned to a control group.	In the intervention group, both cardiorespiratory fitness and strength increased significantly during the training period. While cardiorespiratory fitness decreased significantly over a 4-week detraining period, strength did not decrease significantly. No significant changes were observed in the control group. Lung function, weight, body composition, functional mobility, and quality of life did not change significantly during the training period in either group.	A combined, short-term, circuit and aerobic training programme performed in a hospital setting can induce improvements in cardiorespiratory fitness and muscle strength of children with cystic fibrosis.

(*continued*)

Table 8.1 (*Continued*)

	Methods	*Results*	*Conclusions*
(Santana-Sosa et al., 2014)	Male participants (10 ± 1 years) were randomly allocated to a control (standard therapy) group or intervention group consisting of a combined programme of inspiratory muscle training and aerobic and strength exercises.	A significant interaction (group×time) effect for inspiratory muscle strength, cardiorespiratory fitness, and five-repetition maximum strength (leg-press, bench-press, seated row) was shown in the intervention group only. Inspiratory muscle strength and leg-press were also maintained after a 4-week detraining period in the intervention group.	An 8-week combined resistance and aerobic (whole muscle), and inspiratory muscle training induced significant benefits in important health outcomes in young cystic fibrosis patients.
(Del Corral et al., 2018)	39 participants were randomised to a control group (n = 20; age 11 ± 6 years) or a training group (n = 19; 13 ± 3 years) consisting of 6-weeks using a Nintendo Wii™ platform.	Group×time interaction ANOVAs showed that using the Nintendo Wii™ platform derived significant group differences in exercise capacity, 6-minute walk test farthest walking distance, modified shuttle walk test distance, and muscular strength. These all being greater in the training group compared to controls.	A home-based programme using active video games can improve exercise capacity, muscular strength and quality of life in the short-term in children and adolescents with cystic fibrosis. The effects of muscular performance and quality of life derived through active video gaming were sustained over 12-months.

While exercise in young people with stable CF is generally well-tolerated and safe, some precautions should be considered. Cardiac dysfunction may be present in CF patients with more severe lung disease (forced expiratory volume in one second less than 50% predicted), these patients are reported to have lower stroke volumes or cardiac output during submaximal exercise than those with mild lung disease; and maximal heart rate during exercise is often lower than in healthy children (Perrault et al., 1992). Children with CF should be cautious when engaging in physical activity in warm environments due to a low tolerance to heat stress (Bar-Or et al., 1992; Orenstein et al., 1983). Compared to healthy children, children with CF need to be more mindful of replacing their fluid loss and electrolytes when participating in physical activity due to higher concentrations of sodium in their sweat (Orenstein et al., 1983), lose more fluid and underestimate their fluid needs (Bar-Or et al., 1992). Prolonged exercise (1.5–3 hours) may also lead to hyponatremic dehydration in children with CF and ingesting flavored sodium chloride-containing drinks (50 $mmol{\cdot}L^{-1}$) above thirst levels is recommended for prevention (Kriemler et al., 1999). CF-related diabetes may also make hypoglycemia and dehydration a potential concern during prolonged physical activity and additional carbohydrate supplementation may be considered (Mcniven Temple, Bar-Or and Riddell, 1995).

In more severe CF lung disease, it is advisable to monitor variables such as heart rate and oxygen saturation during physical activity to ensure children are exercising within safe physiological limits. While there is presently no clear definition of significant oxygen desaturation (Urquhart, Montgomery and Jaffé, 2005), guidelines suggest that oxygen saturation in children should be maintained at or above 92% (Balfour-Lynn, Primhak and Shaw, 2005). Monitoring oxygen saturation during exercise may present challenges, however, new technologies worn on the wrist can record oxygen saturation levels as well as other physiological variables such as heart rate. Indeed, before prescribing an exercise programme it is advisable that children with CF undergo a cardiopulmonary exercise test that allows the identification of maximal heart rate, levels at which oxygen desaturation and ventilatory limitation occurs, exercise-related bronchoconstriction, and response to therapy so that the safest programme can be designed (Hebestreit et al., 2015).

Although, presently, there is a lack of or conflicting data to support any specific physical activity recommendations, clinicians may consider prescribing aerobic (cardiorespiratory-based exercise) or anaerobic-type exercise (short bouts of intense physical activity interspersed with periods of recovery) depending on the child's preference. Indeed, children with CF should be encouraged to participate in physical activity but consultation within their interprofessional health care team, including an exercise physiologist (specialist) is highly recommended. There is evidence to show that exercising at a moderate intensity (~70% of maximum heart rate) can improve lung function and aerobic capacity in CF (Van Doorn, 2010). Therefore, exercising at or above this threshold is probably required to derive any physiological benefits. Clinicians may wish to consider current physical activity guidelines (Tremblay et al., 2011, 2016) as benchmarks, however, these should be modified depending on the physical condition of the child and severity of lung disease. Anaerobic activities offer a more natural form of physical activity shown in children and can include team field sports. There is evidence to show that this form of physical activity is safe for children with CF (Klijn et al., 2004; Stevens et al., 2011; Stevens, Oades and Williams, 2015) and can improve both aerobic and anaerobic performance (Klijn et al., 2004). However, consideration of the duration of recovery periods following intense bouts of exercise is needed. Individualised physical activity programmes that include a resistance component are recommended and should also be considered. Resistance training for children and adolescents with CF has been shown to be safe and yield physical benefits such as improvements in upper and lower body strength (Orenstein et al., 2004). Given the compromised digestive system in CF resulting in malnutrition and muscle wasting (Marcotte et al., 1986) increases in muscular strength is a clinically meaningful outcome. A moderate intensity workload has been proposed as 70% of one-repetition maximum for different exercises at 3–5 sets of 10 repetitions (Selvadurai et al., 2002). Resistance training should be progression with a gradual increase in weight and repetitions. It is strongly recommended that any resistance training involving weights or machines should be done under the supervision of a qualified exercise professional.

Bronchiectasis is described as an abnormal irreversible dilation of the airways, related to airway infection and inflammation (Wurzel and Chang, 2017). The prevalence of this chronic lung disease ranges from 0.2 to 15 cases per 100,000 and is particularly high among socially disadvantaged populations, such as Indigenous communities of Australia, New Zealand, Alaska, and Canada (Hall et al., 2017; McCallum and Binks, 2017). Despite current guidelines for the treatment and management of bronchiectasis recommending participation in regular physical activity as a means of improving aerobic fitness and health related quality of life (Chang et al., 2015), physical activity data in this young population is limited compared to other respiratory diseases. Therefore, little is known about how active children living with bronchiectasis are or how many are meeting current physical activity guidelines. Consequently, the lack of data makes it difficult to make informed decisions regarding physical activity prescriptions for children living with bronchiectasis. A study assessing the physical activity behaviour of children with bronchiectasis showed that the vast majority were found to be insufficiently active for health benefits with only 6% meeting recommended guidelines of 60 minutes per day of moderate to vigorous physical activity, in contrast to 42% of healthy children in the study sample (Joschtel et al., 2019). The study also reported that children with bronchiectasis accumulated 48 minutes per day of moderate to vigorous physical activity, with boys demonstrating marginally higher levels of moderate to vigorous daily physical activity than girls. These data highlight the need for programmes to promote physical activity in this young patient group. Such programmes should be tailored to the child, however, more data is required before informed evidence-based decisions can be made regarding physical activity prescription in this specific chronic lung disease.

Counselling and Identifying Barriers and Facilitators

The *Exercise is Medicine*© (Lobelo, Stoutenberg and Hutber, 2014) initiative has created resources to assist clinicians with an action guide for prescribing physical activity to patients. However, the resources are general and do not apply to specific chronic diseases. Furthermore, the recommendations have been designed more towards adult patients rather than paediatric. Nevertheless, the guidelines may provide a starting point for clinicians working with paediatric populations who plan to use physical activity in the child's treatment plan. Using best evidence, the resources include advice on safety screening (Riebe et al., 2015) and counselling on physical activity in general practice (Elley et al., 2003). Until more specific evidence-based recommendations are available for the prescription of physical activity for paediatric populations, clinicians may wish to consider adapting existing recommendations. The '5 As' (Ask, Assess, Advise, Agree, and Assist) has been adapted to provide a minimal intervention for obesity counselling in primary care (Vallis et al., 2013) and could provide a useful model for physical activity prescription (Table 8.2).

Identifying barriers to physical activity participation is central to tailoring its prescription for children with chronic disease. Qualitative research has been conducted in young patients with CF to better understand how physical activity is perceived. Such information can be used in the tailoring of specific physical activity programmes. 'Fun' and 'enjoyment' are indicated to be central for sustained physical activity participation, (Denford et al., 2019, 2020; Moola, Faulkner and Schneiderman, 2012; Swisher and Erickson, 2008) and should place emphasis in programme design for young children with respiratory disease. Exacerbated symptoms of respiratory disease during and post-physical activity may also pose an additional barrier. Sensations of discomfort such as muscle soreness, fatigue, joint pain, and

Table 8.2 The '5 As'

Ask	Permission to discuss inactivity, be non-judgmental, and explore the child's readiness for change.
Assess	Current physical activity behaviour and explore drivers and complications of physical inactivity.
Advise	The child and parents about the health risks of inactivity, the benefits of being physically active, and the need for a long-term strategy.
Agree	On realistic goals, expectations, behavioural changes, and specific details of the treatment plan.
Assist	In identifying and addressing barriers, providing resources and finding and consulting with appropriate health care providers, and arrange regular follow-up.

breathlessness aggravate negative perceptions of physical activity (Happ et al., 2013; Shelley et al., 2018). Feelings of self-consciousness towards physical activity also need to be addressed in its prescription. Young patients can feel exposed and vulnerable (Moola and Faulkner, 2014), despondent (Moola et al., 2011), and anxious to avoid physical activity (Moola et al., 2011). The burden of the disease also requires consideration with a time-consuming treatment regime encroaching on time that could be spent participating in physical activity (Happ et al., 2013; Moola et al., 2011; Moola, Faulkner and Schneiderman, 2012). An open dialogue between the clinician and the young patient and their family that addresses motivators, facilitators, and barriers for physical activity is recommended for creating an effective physical activity programme. The present chapter has provided a brief overview of physical activity counselling; however, a more comprehensive discussion on this topic is provided in Chapter 5.

New Digital Technologies and Telehealth/Medicine

Digital technologies that monitor disease progression and programme adherence during interventions are emerging. Such technologies enable the clinician to determine if the patient's condition is related to disease progression, attributable to poor treatment adherence, or a combination of the two. In chronic obstructive pulmonary disease and asthma, strategies that include text messaging reminders and web-based and mobile applications to monitor and record symptoms, and programme adherence have been investigated (Blakey et al., 2018; Chan et al., 2015). Given the importance of physical activity in the management and treatment of respiratory disease, the use of digital technologies to support such interventions has gained interest. Fitness trackers can provide useful information to both the clinician and patient on the frequency, duration, and intensity of exercise. The use of fitness trackers to promote physical activity in adult CF has been investigated, however, the results of this randomised controlled trial found no significant differences in terms of exercise tolerance, pulmonary function, or patient reported outcomes between a group using a fitness tracker with a personalised exercise prescription and social media platform to another group with exercise prescription alone (Bishay et al., 2018). Table 8.3 shows ongoing studies using digital technologies to promote physical activity in paediatric respiratory disease such as CF.

The utilisation of social media and wed-based platforms for the promotion of physical activity in respiratory disease is also starting to be realised. A closed Facebook group has been used for a small interventional study to promote a 30-day exercise challenge to increase daily physical activity (Smith and Gouick, 2015). In the U.K., 'Beam,' a programme initially developed by the CF Trust provides online exercise classes instructed by individuals living with CF (Beam for Cystic fibrosis, 2020. Available: https://beamfeelgood.com/on-demand/cystic-fibrosis). While in the U.S., 'CFYOGI' is an exercise

Table 8.3 Ongoing Studies Using Digital Technologies to Promote Physical Activity in Paediatric Respiratory Disease

Study	*Description*
ACTIVATE-CF (Hebestreit et al., 2018)	A randomised controlled trial using an online interface that allows individuals with cystic fibrosis to log their exercise activities and pedometer step counts. Participants will also receive three-monthly counselling sessions encouraging three hours of exercise per week. Forced expiratory volume in one second is being used as the primary outcome used to determine study efficacy.
Steps Ahead: Optimising Physical Activity and Health in Adults with Cystic Fibrosis (NCT03672058, 2018)	A randomised controlled trial comparing the combined use of Fitbit exercise trackers with an online activity monitoring system (Fitabase) and individualised feedback on activity levels and progress, with the use of a standard Fitbit alone. The study will use steps per day and forced expiratory volume in one second as the primary study outcomes.
Project Fizzyo (Raywood et al., 2019)	Designed to capture information on adherence to airway clearance devises in cystic fibrosis. Fizzyo device data will be transmitted and sent automatically to a tablet computer synchronised with the airway clearance device. Video games have also been developed while using the airway clearance device and will be introduced at different intervals of the study to assess the impact of gaming on adherence.
ActionPACT (Cox et al., 2019)	A randomised controlled trial to test a web-based application (ActivOnline) to promote physical activity. The trial will also investigate the influence of the technology-based intervention during the period immediately following hospital discharge on aerobic fitness, pulmonary function, quality of life, anxiety and depression, sleep quality, and healthcare utilisation. It is hypothesised that the web-based intervention will increase uptake and participation in physical activity following hospital admission for respiratory exacerbation compared with standard care that will lead to improvements in these outcomes.

web platform cofounded by a person living with CF and a parent of children with CF in partnership with social Good Fund. The online platform includes live-streams and recorded fitness videos led also by instructors with CF. It also allows patients to share progress and fitness goals while avoiding risk of cross-infection (CFYOGI. Yoga for cystic fibrosis 2018, 2019. Available at: https://cfyogi.org/).

Telehealth/medicine could hold promise in the prescription and promotion of physical activity and exercise for children with respiratory disease. Telemedicine refers to the use of electronic communication and information technologies to provide and support clinical care at a distance; while telehealth includes activities such as education for healthcare professionals, community health education, public health, research, and administration of health services (Shaw et al., 2001). Telemonitoring utilises clinical equipment and technological devices, and surveys within the patient's home, which are subsequently transmitted in real time or in a retrospective manner to the clinician (McLean et al., 2011; Polisena et al., 2010). Access may be difficult for families of children with respiratory conditions not located near or in large cities where, in most cases, specialist centres or major hospitals are located, therefore, telemedicine has the potential to provide such families with specialist services (Shaw, 2009; Smith, Elkin and Partridge, 2009). In respiratory diseases, telehealth has been promoted as a potential method for reducing human recourses and the fiscal burden on healthcare systems (Bartoli et al., 2009; Paré, Jaana and Sicotte, 2007). Telemonitoring interventions in respiratory disease have also been able to identify early changes in a patient's condition allowing for timely changes in treatment and possible prevention of pulmonary exacerbation (Paré, Jaana and Sicotte, 2007).

Quality of life and exercise tolerance has been shown to be optimised by multi-disciplinary health care programmes (Lacasse et al., 2007), especially when including an exercise or physical activity component (Kruis et al., 2013). These programmes, however, are advised to be more individually tailored and accessible by the patient when they need it most (Agusti and MacNee, 2013; Bourbeau and Saad, 2013). Thus, new technological advances in healthcare could supply this need through the telemonitoring of physical activity and symptoms, and provide timely treatment and changes to the patient's management plan in daily life. Indeed, despite the reported benefits of regular participation in physical activity, uptake and adherence to such programmes in CF is poor (White, Stiller and Haensel, 2007). This problem may be exacerbated by the limited range of methods presently trialed to promote participation in physical activity (Cox, Alison and Holland, 2013), and telehealth may offer an accessible and feasible solution. Studies have shown that the monitoring of symptoms and making objective measures such as spirometry via telehealth are feasible in individuals with CF (Bella et al., 2009; Grzincich et al., 2010; Jarad and Sund, 2011; Sarfaraz, Sund and Jarad, 2010). It must be recognised, however, that many studies investigating the effectiveness of telehealth applications in CF have mainly been small, feasibility trials with limited external validity with the age and disease severity of the participants varying widely (Cox et al., 2012). Presently, there is insufficient evidence to derive any robust conclusions on the effectiveness of telehealth/medicine interventions in children with respiratory disease and large powered studies are needed to determine its potential. The reach and cost-benefit of using digital forms of technology to promote physical activity in this clinical population also needs to be considered to make its implementation more attractive to various healthcare systems. As well as the privacy and security of the technology used to deliver the remote service.

Conclusion

While physical activity and exercise is recommended in the management and treatment of paediatric respiratory disease, there is a lack of disease-specific guidelines for clinicians to follow. Moreover, except for asthma and CF, there is an absence of studies evaluating the efficacy of physical activity and exercise training programmes in other paediatric lung diseases. Despite the recommendation of exercise in the clinical guidelines for the treatment and management of respiratory disease (Chang et al., 2015), more studies in other respiratory conditions, such as bronchiectasis, are needed. In children with bronchiectasis, there are data, albeit limited, which show physical activity is reduced. However, the potential of physical activity and exercise programmes to improve health outcomes in this specific lung disease is not known. This makes it challenging for clinicians to make informed decisions regarding safe and effective doses of physical activity and exercise for children with bronchiectasis. Pathophysiological differences do not suit a 'one size fits all' approach to physical activity prescription, and exercise programmes ideally should be tailored to evidence based on the specific lung disease.

A further challenge for clinicians, particularly those working with young CF patients, is a recent systematic review reported limited evidence for both the short- and long-term benefits of aerobic, anaerobic, or a combination of both forms of exercise (Radtke et al., 2017). Methodological and recruitment challenges make these interventional studies difficult to conduct especially when considering adherence and drop out. However, participation in physical activity is safe for children with respiratory disease (Ruf et al., 2010) and is already offered as part of standard care for most individuals with CF. Therefore, despite its limited evidence, physical activity should be encouraged and individual variability within studies should be recognised. Although international guidelines do not include paediatric disease-specific recommendations, moderate to vigorous physical activity of 60 minutes per day may be used as a benchmark until comprehensive disease-specific guidelines that consider frequency, intensity, and duration (dose) become available. Such guidelines should also include the type of exercises/sports and safety considerations. To promote adherence and enjoyment, physical activity counselling is recommended to tailor the physical activity programme and improve efficacy. With the child and their family, the clinician should set realistic and achievable goals, and determine motivators, barriers, and enablers before any physical activity programme is designed.

Recently, social media platforms are being utilised as a vehicle to provide virtual instructor lead exercise classes (e.g., Beam for Cystic fibrosis and CFYOGI) providing an exciting interactive means of promoting physical activity in the home. Such programmes have the potential to create a virtual community among participants to support and encourage each other. For young participants with CF, virtual exercise classes also afford the opportunity to exercise with their peers without the risk of cross-infection. Currently, there are ongoing studies (Hebestreit et al., 2018; NCT03672058, 2018) or studies in development (Cox et al., 2019; Raywood et al., 2019) that will use online interfaces for participants to record and monitor their physical activity behaviour. These results will be of interest to those working to promote physical activity in individuals with CF. It must be noted, besides CF, that there are a lack of initiatives to promote physical activity in other paediatric respiratory diseases, and a focus on other pulmonary conditions is needed. Telehealth/medicine may play a valuable future role in providing physical activity to children with respiratory diseases. The concept is presently in its infancy, however, extrapolating from other telehealth/medicine studies could offer an effective (Piazza-Waggoner et al., 2006) and cost-effective (Raza et al., 2009) service. However, it must be recognised that many studies investigating the use of telehealth/medicine applications have mainly been small, feasibility trials with poor generalisability and more investigation into its efficacy to deliver effective physical activity programming are needed. With the increasing accessibility and development of new technologies, it is an exciting time to be working in the field of physical activity promotion as potential new methods and opportunities develop.

Key Points

- Presently, there is a lack of specific guidelines for physical activity and exercise prescription in children with respiratory disease.
- Current physical activity guidelines for children may be used as a benchmark in the absence of disease-specific guidelines. However, precautions and contradictions to exercise must be considered.
- Physical activity counselling should be encouraged in which the clinician discusses with the child and their family realistic and achievable goals, and determine motivators, barriers, and enablers.
- The use of telehealth/medicine may offer an effective and cost-efficient platform to deliver physical activity and exercise prescription. However, more evidence as to its effectiveness in children with respiratory disease is needed.
- Ongoing or developing studies that use an online interface for children with respiratory disease to monitor and record their physical activity may show promise and future direction for its delivery.

References

Agusti, A. and MacNee, W. (2013) 'The COPD control panel: Towards personalised medicine in COPD', *Thorax*. 68(7):687–690. doi: 10.1136/thoraxjnl-2012-202772.

Andréasson, B., Jonson, B., Kornfält, R., Nordmark, E.V.A. and Sandström, S. (1987) 'Long-term effects of physical exercise on working capacity and pulmonary function in cystic fibrosis', *Acta Paediatrica Scandinavica*. 76(1):70–75. doi: 10.1111/j.1651-2227.1987.tb10417.x.

Armstrong, N. and Van Mechelen, W. (2008) *Paediatric exercise science and medicine.* Oxford: Oxford University Press.

Asher, M. I., Pardy, R. L., Coates, A. L., Thomas, E., & Macklem, P. T. (1982) 'The effects of inspiratory muscle training in patients with cystic fibrosis', *American Review of Respiratory Disease.* 126(5):855–859. doi: 10.1164/arrd.1982.126.5.855.

Balfour-Lynn, I.M., Primhak, R.A. and Shaw, B.N.J. (2005) 'Home oxygen for children: who, how and when?', *Thorax.* 60(1):76–81. doi: 10.1136/thx.2004.031211.

Bar-Or, O. *et al.* (1992) 'Voluntary dehydration and heat intolerance in cystic fibrosis', *The Lancet.* 21:696–699. doi: 10.1016/0140-6736(92)90597-V.

Bar-Or, O. and Inbar, O. (1992) 'Swimming and asthma: Benefits and deleterious effects', *Sports Medicine: Evaluations of Research in Exercise Science and Sports Medicine.* 14(6):397–405. doi: 10.2165/00007256-199214060-00006.

Bar-Yishay, E., Gur, I., Inbar, O., Neuman, I., Dlin, R. A., & Godfrey, S. (1982) 'Differences between swimming and running as stimuli for exercise-induced asthma', *European Journal of Applied Physiology and Occupational Physiology.* 48(3):387–397. doi: 10.1007/BF00430229.

Barak, A., Wexler, I.D., Efrati, O., Bentur, L., Augarten, A., Mussaffi, H., Avital, A., Rivlin, J., Aviram, M., Yahav, Y. and Kerem, E. (2005) 'Trampoline use as physiotherapy for cystic fibrosis patients', *Pediatric Pulmonology.* 39(1):70–73. doi: 10.1002/ppul.20133.

Bartoli, L., Zanaboni, P., Masella, C., & Ursini, N. (2009) 'Systematic review of telemedicine services for patients affected by chronic obstructive pulmonary disease (COPD)', *Telemedicine and e-Health.* 15(9):877–883. doi: 10.1089/tmj.2009.0044.

Basaran, S., Guler-Uysal, F., Ergen, N., Seydaoglu, G., Bingol-Karakoç, G., & Ufuk Altintas, D. (2006) 'Effects of physical exercise on quality of life, exercise capacity and pulmonary function in children with asthma', *Journal of Rehabilitation Medicine.* 38(2):130–135. doi: 10.1080/16501970500476142.

Becker, J. M., Rogers, J., Rossini, G., Mirchandani, H., & D'alonzo, G. E. (2004) 'Asthma deaths during sports: report of a 7-year experience', *Journal of Allergy and Clinical Immunology.* 113(2):264–267. doi: 10.1016/j.jaci.2003.10.052.

Bella, S., Murgia, F., Tozzi, A. E., Cotognini, C., & Lucidi, V. (2009) 'Five years of telemedicine in cystic fibrosis disease', *Clinica Terapeutica.* 160(6):457–460. PMID: 20198287.

Bishay, L. C., E. Nelson, K. Williams, J. Greenberg, A. Gould, I. Bailey, E. Moulis, D. Goldman, G. S. Sawicki, & A. Z. Uluer. (2018) 'Effect of a wearable fitness tracker on exercise tolerance for adults with cystic fibrosis: a pilot randomized clinical trial', *Pediatric Pulmonology.* 53(S2):S148–S456. doi: 10.1002/ppul.24152.

Blakey, J. D., Bender, B. G., Dima, A. L., Weinman, J., Safioti, G., & Costello, R. W. (2018) 'Digital technologies and adherence in respiratory diseases: the road ahead', *European Respiratory Journal.* 52:1801147. doi: 10.1183/13993003.01147-2018.

Boas, S.R., Danduran, M.J. and McColley, S.A. (1999) 'Energy metabolism during anaerobic exercise in children with cystic fibrosis and asthma', *Medicine and Science in Sports and Exercise.* 31(9):1242–1249. doi: 10.1097/00005768-199909000-00003.

Bonsignore, M.R., La Grutta, S., Cibella, F., Scichilone, N., Cuttitta, G., Interrante, A., Marchese, M., Veca, M., Virzi, M., Bonanno, A. & Profita, M. (2008) 'Effects of exercise training and montelukast in children with mild asthma', *Medicine and Science in Sports and Exercise.* 40(3):405–412. doi: 10.1249/MSS.0b013e31815d9670.

Bourbeau, J. and Saad, N. (2013) 'Integrated care model with self-management in chronic obstructive pulmonary disease: From family physicians to specialists', *Chronic Respiratory Disease*. 10(2):99–105. doi: 10.1177/1479972312473844.

Burns, J.J., Sadof, M. and Kamat, D. (2007) 'The adolescent with a chronic illness: Epidemiology, developmental issues and health care provision', *World Health Organization*. doi: 10.1136/adc.2003.045377.

Cassim, R., Koplin, J. J., Dharmage, S. C., Senaratna, B. C., Lodge, C. J., Lowe, A. J., & Russell, M. A. (2016) 'The difference in amount of physical activity performed by children with and without asthma: A systematic review and meta-analysis', *Journal of Asthma*. 53(9):882–892. doi: 10.1080/02770903.2016.1175474.

Chan, A. H., Stewart, A. W., Harrison, J., Camargo Jr, C. A., Black, P. N., & Mitchell, E. A. (2015) 'The effect of an electronic monitoring device with audiovisual reminder function on adherence to inhaled corticosteroids and school attendance in children with asthma: a randomised controlled trial', *The Lancet Respiratory Medicine*. 3(3):210–219. doi: 10.1016/S2213-2600(15)00008-9.

Chang, A.B., Bell, S.C., Torzillo, P.J., King, P.T., Maguire, G.P., Byrnes, C.A., Holland, A.E., O'Mara, P. & Grimwood, K. (2015) 'Chronic suppurative lung disease and bronchiectasis in children and adults in Australia and New Zealand', *Medical Journal of Australia*. 202(3):130. doi: 10.5694/mja14.00287.

del Corral, T., Cebrià i Iranzo, MÀ, López-de-Uralde-Villanueva, I., Martínez-Alejos, R., Blanco, I., Vilaró, J. (2018) 'Effectiveness of a home-based active video game programme in young cystic fibrosis patients', *Respiration*. 95(2):87–97. doi: 10.1159/000481264.

Counil, F. P., Varray, A. L. A. I. N., Karila, C., Hayot, M., Voisin, M., & Prefaut, C. (1997) 'Wingate test performance in children with asthma: aerobic or anaerobic limitation?', *Medicine and Science in Sports and Exercise*. 29(4):430–435. doi: 10.1097/00005768-199704000-00002.

Counil, F. P., Varray, A., Matecki, S., Beurey, A., Marchal, P., Voisin, M., & Préfaut, C. (2003) 'Training of aerobic and anaerobic fitness in children with asthma', *Journal of Pediatrics*. 142(2):179–184. doi: 10.1067/mpd.2003.83.

Cox, N. S., Alison, J. A., Rasekaba, T., & Holland, A. E. (2012) 'Telehealth in cystic fibrosis: a systematic review', *Journal of Telemedicine and Telecare*. 18(2):72–78. doi: 10.1258/jtt.2011.110705.

Cox, N.S., Eldridge, B., Rawlings, S., Dreger, J., Corda, J., Hauser, J., Button, B.M., Bishop, J., Nichols, A., Middleton, A. & Ward, N. (2019) 'A web-based intervention to promote physical activity in adolescents and young adults with cystic fibrosis: protocol for a randomized controlled trial', *BMC Pulmonary Medicine*. 19:253. doi: 10.1186/s12890-019-0942-3.

Cox, N.S., Alison, J.A. and Holland, A. (2013) 'Interventions for promoting physical activity in people with cystic fibrosis', *Cochrane Database of Systematic Reviews*. 13(12). doi: 10.1002/14651858.cd009448.pub2.

Davies, D. S. C., Atherton, F., McBride, M., & Calderwood, C. (2019) 'UK Chief Medical Officers' Physical Activity Guidelines', *Department of Health and Social Care*.

Denford, S., Hill, D. M., Mackintosh, K. A., McNarry, M. A., Barker, A. R., & Williams, C. A. (2019) 'Using photo-elicitation to explore perceptions of physical activity among young people with cystic fibrosis', *BMC Pulmonary Medicine*. 19(220). doi: 10.1186/s12890-019-0985-5.

Denford, S., van Beurden, S., O'Halloran, P., & Williams, C. A. (2020) 'Barriers and facilitators to physical activity among children, adolescents, and young adults with cystic fibrosis: a systematic review and thematic synthesis of qualitative research', *BMJ Open*. 10(20). doi: 10.1136/bmjopen-2019-035261.

Department of Health and Children and Health Service Executive (2009) 'The national guidelines on physical activity for Ireland', *Children*.

Department of Health and Human Services (2015) *U.S. Department of Health and Human Services, Health Resources and Services Administration, Maternal and Child Health Bureau. Child Health USA 2014, Women's Health USA 2013.*

Elborn, J.S. (2016) 'Cystic fibrosis', *The Lancet*. 19(388):2519–2531. doi: 10.1016/S0140-6736(16)00576-6.

Elley, C. R., Kerse, N., Arroll, B., & Robinson, E. (2003) 'Effectiveness of counselling patients on physical activity in general practice: cluster randomised controlled trial', *British Medical Journal*. 326(7393):793. doi: 10.1136/bmj.326.7393.793.

Eves, N.D. and Davidson, W.J. (2011) 'Evidence-based risk assessment and recommendations for physical activity clearance: Respiratory disease', *Applied Physiology, Nutrition and Metabolism*. 36(1):S80–S100. doi: 10.1139/H10-087.

Fanelli, A., Cabral, A. L., Neder, J. A., Martins, M. A., & Carvalho, C. R. (2007) 'Exercise training on disease control and quality of life in asthmatic children', *Medicine and Science in Sports and Exercise*. 39(9):1474–1480. doi: 10.1249/mss.0b013e3180d099ad.

Garber, C.E., Blissmer, B., Deschenes, M.R., Franklin, B.A., Lamonte, M.J., Lee, I.M., Nieman, D.C. & Swain, D.P. (2011) 'Quantity and quality of exercise for developing and maintaining cardiorespiratory, musculoskeletal, and neuromotor fitness in apparently healthy adults: Guidance for prescribing exercise', *Medicine and Science in Sports and Exercise*. 43(7):1334–1359. doi: 10.1249/MSS.0b013e318213fefb.

Global Initiative for Asthma (2018) *2018 GINA Report: Global Strategy for Asthma Management and Prevention 2018, Global Initiative for Asthma*. doi: 10.1002/uog.8947.

Goyal, V., Grimwood, K., Marchant, J., Masters, I. B., & Chang, A. B. (2016) 'Pediatric bronchiectasis: No longer an orphan disease', *Pediatric Pulmonology*. 51(5):450–469. doi: 10.1002/ppul.23380.

Grzincich, G., Gagliardini, R., Bossi, A., Bella, S., Cimino, G., Cirilli, N., Viviani, L., Iacinti, E. & Quattrucci, S. (2010) 'Evaluation of a home telemonitoring service for adult patients with cystic fibrosis: a pilot study', *Journal of Telemedicine and Telecare*. 16(7):359–362. doi: 10.1258/jtt.2010.091006.

Gulmans, V. A. M., De Meer, K., Brackel, H. J. L., Faber, J. A. J., Berger, R., & Helders, P. J. M. (1999) 'Outpatient exercise training in children with cystic fibrosis: physiological effects, perceived competence, and acceptability', *Pediatric Pulmonology*. 28(1):39–46. doi: 10.1002/(sici)1099-0496(199907)28:1<39::aid-ppul7>3.3.co;2-8.

Hall, K.K., Chang, A.B., Anderson, J., Arnold, D., Goyal, V., Dunbar, M., Otim, M. & O'Grady, K.A.F. (2017) 'The incidence and short-term outcomes of acute respiratory illness with cough in children from a socioeconomically disadvantaged urban community in Australia: a community-based prospective cohort study', *Frontiers in Pediatrics*. 5:228. doi: 10.3389/fped.2017.00228.

Happ, M. B., Hoffman, L. A., Higgins, L. W., DiVirgilio, D., & Orenstein, D. M. (2013) 'Parent and child perceptions of a self-regulated, home-based exercise program for children with cystic fibrosis', *Nursing Research*. 62(5):305–314. doi: 10.1097/NNR.0b013e3182a03503.

Hebestreit H, Arets HG, Aurora P, Boas S, Cerny F, Hulzebos EH, Karila C, Lands LC, Lowman JD, Swisher A, Urquhart DS. & European Cystic Fibrosis Exercise Working Group. (2015) 'Statement on exercise testing in cystic fibrosis', *Respiration*. 90(4):332–51. doi: 10.1159/000439057.

Hebestreit, H., Lands, L.C., Alarie, N., Schaeff, J., Karila, C., Orenstein, D.M., Urquhart, D.S., Hulzebos, E.H., Stein, L., Schindler, C. & Kriemler, S. (2018) 'Effects of a partially supervised conditioning programme in cystic fibrosis: an international multi-centre randomised controlled trial (ACTIVATE-CF): Study protocol', *BMC Pulmonary Medicine.* 18(1):31. doi: 10.1186/s12890-018-0596-6.

Inbar, O., Dotan, R., Dlin, R. A., Neuman, I., & Bar-Or, O. (1980) 'Breathing dry or humid air and exercise-induced asthma during swimming', *European Journal of Applied Physiology and Occupational Physiology.* 44(1):43–50. doi: 10.1007/BF00421762.

Janssen, I. and LeBlanc, A.G. (2010) 'Systematic review of the health benefits of physical activity and fitness in school-aged children and youth', *International Journal of Behavioral Nutrition and Physical Activity.* 7:40. doi: 10.1186/1479-5868-7-40.

Jarad, N.A. and Sund, Z.M. (2011) 'Telemonitoring in chronic obstructive airway disease and adult patients with cystic fibrosis', *Journal of Telemedicine and Telecare.* 16(3):120–127. doi: 10.1258/jtt.2010.100309.

Joschtel, B., Gomersall, S. R., Tweedy, S., Petsky, H., Chang, A. B., & Trost, S. G. (2018) 'Effects of exercise training on physical and psychosocial health in children with chronic respiratory disease: a systematic review and meta-analysis', *BMJ Open Sport and Exercise Medicine.* 4(1). doi: 10.1136/bmjsem-2018-000409.

Joschtel, B., Gomersall, S. R., Tweedy, S., Petsky, H., Chang, A. B., & Trost, S. G. (2019) 'Objectively measured physical activity and sedentary behaviour in children with bronchiectasis: a cross-sectional study', *BMC Pulmonary Medicine.* 19(7). doi: 10.1186/s12890-018-0772-8.

Klijn, P. H., Oudshoorn, A., van der Ent, C. K., van der Net, J., Kimpen, J. L., & Helders, P. J (2004) 'Effects of anaerobic training in children with cystic fibrosis: a randomized controlled study', *Chest.* 125(4):1299–1305. doi: 10.1378/chest.125.4.1299.

Kriemler, S., Wilk, B., Schurer, W., Wilson, W. M., & Bar-Or, O. (1999) 'Preventing dehydration in children with cystic fibrosis who exercise in the heat', *Medicine and Science in Sports and Exercise.* 31(6):774–779. doi: 10.1097/00005768-199906000-00003.

Kruis, A. L., Smidt, N., Assendelft, W. J., Gussekloo, J., Boland, M. R., Rutten-van Mölken, M., & Chavannes, N. H. (2013) 'Integrated disease management interventions for patients with chronic obstructive pulmonary disease', *Cochrane Database of Systematic Reviews.* 10(10). doi: 10.1002/14651858.CD009437.pub2.

Lacasse, Y., Wong, E., Guyatt, G. H., King, D., Cook, D. J., & Goldstein, R. S. (2007) 'Meta-analysis of respiratory rehabilitation in chronic obstructive pulmonary disease a Cochrane systematic review', *Europa Medicophysica.* 43(4): 475–485. PMID: 18084170.

Lee, I. M., Shiroma, E. J., Lobelo, F., Puska, P., Blair, S. N., Katzmarzyk, P. T., & Lancet Physical Activity Series Working Group. (2012) 'Effect of physical inactivity on major non-communicable diseases worldwide: an analysis of burden of disease and life expectancy', *The Lancet.* 380(9838):219–229. doi: 10.1016/S0140-6736(12)61031-9.

Lobelo, F., Stoutenberg, M. and Hutber, A. (2014) 'The exercise is medicine global health initiative: a 2014 update', *British Journal of Sports Medicine.* 48(22):1627–1233. doi: 10.1136/bjsports-2013-093080.

Lu, K. D., Manoukian, K., Radom-Aizik, S., Cooper, D. M., & Galant, S. P. (2016) 'Obesity, asthma, and exercise in child and adolescent health', *Pediatric Exercise Science.* 28(2):264–274. doi: 10.1123/pes.2015-0122.

Lucas, S.R. and Platts-Mills, T.A.E. (2005) 'Physical activity and exercise in asthma: relevance to etiology and treatment', *Journal of Allergy and Clinical Immunology.* 115(5): 928–934. doi: 10.1016/j.jaci.2005.01.033.

Marcotte, J.E., Canny, G.J., Grisdale, R., Desmond, K., Corey, M., Zinman, R., Levison, H. and Coates, A.L. (1986) 'Effects of nutritional status on exercise performance in advanced cystic fibrosis', *Chest*. 90(3):375–379. doi: 10.1378/chest.90.3.375.

McCallum, G.B. and Binks, M.J. (2017) 'The epidemiology of chronic suppurative lung disease and bronchiectasis in children and adolescents', *Frontiers in Pediatrics*. 5:27. doi: 10.3389/fped.2017.00027.

McLean, S., Nurmatov, U., Liu, J. L., Pagliari, C., Car, J., & Sheikh, A. (2011) 'Telehealthcare for chronic obstructive pulmonary disease', *Cochrane Database of Systematic Reviews*. 6(7). doi: 10.1002/14651858.cd007718.pub2.

Mcniven Temple, M.Y., Bar-Or, O. and Riddell, M.C. (1995) 'The reliability and repeatability of the blood glucose response to prolonged exercise in adolescent boys with IDDM', *Diabetes Care*. 18(3):326–332. doi: 10.2337/diacare.18.3.326.

Moola, F. J., Faulkner, G. E., Kirsh, J. A., & Schneiderman, J. E. (2011) 'Developing physical activity interventions for youth with cystic fibrosis and congenital heart disease: learning from their parents', *Psychology of Sport and Exercise*. 12(6):599–608. doi: 10.1016/j.psychsport.2011.07.001.

Moola, F.J. and Faulkner, G.E. (2014) 'A tale of two cases: the health, illness, and physical activity stories of two children living with cystic fibrosis', *Clinical Child Psychology and Psychiatry*. 19(1):24–42. doi: 10.1177/1359104512465740.

Moola, F.J., Faulkner, G.E.J. and Schneiderman, J.E. (2012) '"No time to play": perceptions toward physical activity in youth with cystic fibrosis', *Adapted Physical Activity Quarterly*. 29(1):44–62. doi: 10.1123/apaq.29.1.44.

NCT03672058 (2018) 'Steps Ahead: optimising Physical Activity and Health in Adults With Cystic Fibrosis Using Fitness Trackers and Personalised Goal-based Text Messaging Support', https://clinicaltrials.gov/show/nct03672058.

Neder, J. A., Nery, L. E., Silva, A. C., Cabral, A. L., & Fernandes, A. L. (1999) 'Short term effects of aerobic training in the clinical management of moderate to severe asthma in children', *Thorax*. 54(3):202–206. doi: 10.1136/thx.54.3.202.

Nixon, P. A., Orenstein, D. M., Kelsey, S. F., & Doershuk, C. F. (1992) 'The prognostic value of exercise testing in patients with cystic fibrosis', *New England Journal of Medicine*. 327(25):1785–1788. doi: 10.1056/NEJM199212173272504.

Nystad, W., Stigum, H. and Carlsen, K.H. (2001) 'Increased level of bronchial responsiveness in inactive children with asthma', *Respiratory Medicine*. 95(10):806–810. doi: 10.1053/rmed.2001.1149.

O'Donnell, A.E. (2008) 'Bronchiectasis', *Chest*. 134(4):815–823. doi: 10.1378/chest.08-0776.

Orenstein, D. M., Henke, K. G., Costill, D. L., Doershuk, C. F., Lemon, P. J., & Stern, R. C. (1983) 'Exercise and heat stress in cystic fibrosis patients', *Pediatric Research*. 17(4):267–269. doi: 10.1203/00006450-198304000-00007.

Orenstein, D.M., Hovell, M.F., Mulvihill, M., Keating, K.K., Hofstetter, C.R., Kelsey, S., Morris, K. & Nixon, P.A. (2004). 'Strength vs aerobic training in children with cystic fibrosis: a randomized controlled trial', *Chest*. 126(4):1204–1214. doi: 10.1378/chest.126.4.1204.

Orenstein, D.M. and Higgins, L.W. (2005) 'Update on the role of exercise in cystic fibrosis', *Current Opinion in Pulmonary Medicine*. 11(6):519–523. doi: 10.1097/01.mcp.0000181476.92810.07.

Paré, G., Jaana, M. and Sicotte, C. (2007) 'Systematic review of home telemonitoring for chronic diseases: the evidence base', *Journal of the American Medical Informatics Association*. 14(3):269–277. doi: 10.1197/jamia.M2270.

Perrault, H., Coughlan, M., Marcotte, J. E., Drblik, S. P., & Lamarre, A. (1992) 'Comparison of cardiac output determinants in response to upright and supine exercise in patients with cystic fibrosis', *Chest.* 101(1):P42–P51. doi: 10.1378/chest.101.1.42.

Philpott, J., Houghton, K. and Luke, A. (2010) 'Physical activity recommendations for children with specific chronic health conditions: juvenile idiopathic arthritis, hemophilia, asthma and cystic fibrosis', *Paediatrics and Child Health.* 20(3):167–172. doi: 10.1093/pch/15.4.213.

Pianosi, P., LeBlanc, J. and Almudevar, A. (2005) 'Peak oxygen uptake and mortality in children with cystic fibrosis', *Thorax.* 60(1):50–54. doi: 10.1136/thx.2003.008102.

Piazza-Waggoner, C., Ferguson, K. S., Daines, C., Acton, J. D., & Powers, S. W. (2006) 'Case study: providing evidence-based behavioral and nutrition treatment to a toddler with cystic fibrosis and multiple food allergies via telehealth', *Pediatric Pulmonology.* 41(10):1001–1004. doi: 10.1002/ppul.20470.

Pieles, G. E., Horn, R., Williams, C. A., & Stuart, A. G. (2014) 'Paediatric exercise training in prevention and treatment', *Archives of Disease in Childhood.* 99(4):380–385. doi: 10.1136/archdischild-2013-303826.

Piercy, K.L., Troiano, R.P., Ballard, R.M., Carlson, S.A., Fulton, J.E., Galuska, D.A., George, S.M. & Olson, R.D. (2018) 'The physical activity guidelines for Americans', *JAMA - Journal of the American Medical Association.* 320(19):2020–2028. doi: 10.1001/jama.2018.14854.

Polisena, J., Tran, K., Cimon, K., Hutton, B., McGill, S., Palmer, K., & Scott, R. E. (2010) 'Home telehealth for chronic obstructive pulmonary disease: A systematic review and meta-analysis', *Journal of Telemedicine and Telecare.* 16(3):120–127. doi: 10.1258/jtt.2009.090812.

Radtke, T., Nevitt, S. J., Hebestreit, H., & Kriemler, S. (2017) 'Physical exercise training for cystic fibrosis', *Cochrane Database of Systematic Reviews.* 11(11). doi: 10.1002/14651858.CD002768.pub4.

Raitakan, O. T., Porkka, K. V. K., Taimela, S., Telama, R., Räsänen, L., & Vllkari, J. S. (1994) 'Effects of persistent physical activity and inactivity on coronary risk factors in children and young adults the cardiovascular risk in young finns study', *American Journal of Epidemiology.* 140(3):195–205. doi: 10.1093/oxfordjournals.aje.a117239.

Ram, F.S.F., Robinson, S.M. and Black, P.N. (2000) 'Effects of physical training in asthma: a systematic review', *British Journal of Sports Medicine.* 34(3):162–167. doi: 10.1136/bjsm.34.3.162.

Randolph, C. and Weiler, J.M. (2014) 'Exercise-induced bronchoconstriction', *Clinical Asthma: Theory and Practice.* doi: 10.1201/b16468.

Raywood, E., Douglas, H., Kapoor, K., Stott, L., Saul, G., & Main, E. (2019) 'Technical support requirements for remote monitoring of physiotherapy in children with cystic fibrosis', *Journal of Cystic Fibrosis.* 18:S158. doi: 10.1016/s1569-1993(19)30648-4.

Raza, T., Joshi, M., Schapira, R. M., & Agha, Z. (2009) 'Pulmonary telemedicine-A model to access the subspecialist services in underserved rural areas', *International Journal of Medical Informatics.* 78:53–59. doi: 10.1016/j.ijmedinf.2008.07.010.

Riebe, D., Franklin, B. A., Thompson, P. D., Garber, C. E., Whitfield, G. P., Magal, M., & Pescatello, L. S. (2015) 'Updating ACSM's recommendations for exercise preparticipation health screening', *Medicine and Science in Sports and Exercise,* 47(11):2473–2479. doi: 10.1249/MSS.0000000000000664.

Ruf, K., Winkler, B., Hebestreit, A., Gruber, W., & Hebestreit, H. (2010) 'Risks associated with exercise testing and sports participation in cystic fibrosis', *Journal of Cystic Fibrosis.* 9(5):339–345. doi: 10.1016/j.jcf.2010.05.006.

Santana-Sosa, E., Gonzalez-Saiz, L., Groeneveld, I.F., Villa-Asensi, J.R., de Aguero, M.I.B.G., Fleck, S.J., López-Mojares, L.M., Pérez, M. and Lucia, A. (2014) 'Benefits of combining inspiratory muscle with "whole muscle" training in children with cystic fibrosis: a randomised controlled trial', *British Journal of Sports Medicine.* 48:1513–1517. doi: 10.1136/bjsports-2012-091892.

Sarfaraz, S., Sund, Z. and Jarad, N. (2010) 'Real-time, once-daily monitoring of symptoms and FEV^1 in cystic fibrosis patients – a feasibility study using a novel device', *Clinical Respiratory Journal.* 4(2):74–82. doi: 10.1111/j.1752-699X.2009.00147.x.

Schneiderman-Walker, J., Pollock, S. L., Corey, M., Wilkes, D. D., Canny, G. J., Pedder, L., & Reisman, J. J. (2000) 'A randomized controlled trial of a 3-year home exercise program in cystic fibrosis', *Journal of Pediatrics.* 136(3):304–310. doi: 10.1067/mpd.2000.103408.

Seear, M., Wensley, D. and West, N. (2005) 'How accurate is the diagnosis of exercise induced asthma among Vancouver schoolchildren?', *Archives of Disease in Childhood.* 90(9):898–902. doi: 10.1136/adc.2004.063974.

Selvadurai, H. C., Blimkie, C. J., Meyers, N., Mellis, C. M., Cooper, P. J., & Van Asperen, P. P. (2002) 'Randomized controlled study of in-hospital exercise training programs in children with cystic fibrosis', *Pediatric Pulmonology.* 33(3):194–200. doi: 10.1002/ppul.10015.

Shaw, D. K., Heggestad-Hereford, J. R., Southard, D. R., & Sparks, K. E. (2001) 'American Association of Cardiovascular and Pulmonary Rehabilitation Telemedicine position statement', *Journal of Cardiopulmonary Rehabilitation.* 21(5):261–262. doi: 10.1097/00008483-200109000-00002.

Shaw, D.K. (2009) 'Overview of telehealth and its application to cardiopulmonary physical therapy', *Cardiopulmonary Physical Therapy Journal.* 20(2):13–18. doi: 10.1097/01823246-200920020-00003.

Shelley, J., Fairclough, S.J., Knowles, Z.R., Southern, K.W., McCormack, P., Dawson, E.A., Graves, L.E. and Hanlon, C. (2018) 'A formative study exploring perceptions of physical activity and physical activity monitoring among children and young people with cystic fibrosis and health care professionals, *BMC Pediatrics.* 18(1):335. doi: 10.1186/s12887-018-1301-x.

Smith, A. and Gouick, L. (2015) 'WS05.2 30 day challenge – using social media to support adult CF patients to exercise in the adult CF service Dundee', *Journal of Cystic Fibrosis.* 14(1):S9. doi: 10.1016/s1569-1993(15)30028-x.

Smith, S.M., Elkin, S.L. and Partridge, M.R. (2009) 'Technology and its role in respiratory care', *Primary Care Respiratory Journal.* 18(3):159–164. doi: 10.4104/pcrj.2009.00038.

Groeneveld, I.F., Gonzalez-Saiz, L., López-Mojares, L.M., Villa-Asensi, J.R., María I, B.G., Fleck, S.J., Pérez, M. and Lucia, A. (2012) 'Intrahospital weight and aerobic training in children with cystic fibrosis: a randomized controlled trial', *Medicine and Science in Sports and Exercise.* 44(1):2–11. doi: 10.1249/MSS.0b013e318228c302.

Stevens, D., Oades, P. J., Armstrong, N., & Williams, C. A. (2011) 'Exercise metabolism during moderate-intensity exercise in children with cystic fibrosis following heavy-intensity exercise', *Applied Physiology, Nutrition and Metabolism.* 36(6): 920–927. doi: 10.1139/H11-117.

Stevens, D., Oades, P.J. and Williams, C.A. (2015) 'Airflow limitation following cardiopulmonary exercise testing and heavy-intensity intermittent exercise in children with cystic fibrosis', *European Journal of Pediatrics.* 174(2):251–257. doi: 10.1007/s00431-014-2387-2.

Swisher, A.K. and Erickson, M. (2008) 'Perceptions of physical activity in a group of adolescents with cystic fibrosis,' *Cardiopulmonary Physical Therapy Journal*. 19(4):107–113. PMID: 20467507.

Tesse, R., Borrelli, G., Mongelli, G., Mastrorilli, V., & Cardinale, F. (2018) 'Treating pediatric asthma according guidelines', *Frontiers in Pediatrics*. 6:234. doi: 10.3389/fped.2018.00234.

Tomporowski, P.D., Lambourne, K. and Okumura, M.S. (2011) 'Physical activity interventions and children's mental function: an introduction and overview', *Preventive Medicine*. 52(1):S3–S9. doi: 10.1016/j.ypmed.2011.01.028.

Tremblay, M. S., Warburton, D. E. R., Janssen, I., Paterson, D. H., Latimer, A. E., & Rhodes, R. E. (2011) 'New Canadian physical activity guidelines', *Applied Physiology, Nutrition and Metabolism*. 36(1):36–46. doi: 10.1139/H11-009.

Tremblay, M.S., Carson, V., Chaput, J.P., Connor Gorber, S., Dinh, T., Duggan, M., Faulkner, G., Gray, C.E., Gruber, R., Janson, K. and Janssen, I. (2016) 'Canadian 24-hour movement guidelines for children and youth: an integration of physical activity, sedentary behaviour, and sleep', *Applied Physiology, Nutrition and Metabolism*. 41(6):S311–S327. doi: 10.1139/apnm-2016-0151.

Tremblay, M.S., Chaput, J.P., Adamo, K.B., Aubert, S., Barnes, J.D., Choquette, L., Duggan, M., Faulkner, G., Goldfield, G.S., Gray, C.E. and Gruber, R. (2017) 'Canadian 24-hour movement guidelines for the early years (0-4 years): An integration of physical activity, sedentary behaviour, and sleep', *BMC Public Health*. 17(5):874. doi: 10.1186/s12889-017-4859-6.

Turchetta, A., Salerno, T., Lucidi, V., Libera, F., Cutrera, R., & Bush, A. (2004) 'Usefulness of a program of hospital-supervised physical training in patients with cystic fibrosis', *Pediatric Pulmonology*. 38(2):115–118. doi: 10.1002/ppul.20073.

Twisk, J. W. R., Kemper, H. C. G., Van Mechelen, W., & Post, G. B. (1997) 'Tracking of risk factors for coronary heart disease over a 14-year period: a comparison between lifestyle and biologic risk factors with data from the Amsterdam growth and health study', *American Journal of Epidemiology*. 145(10):888–898. doi: 10.1093/oxfordjournals.aje.a009048.

Urquhart, D.S., Montgomery, H. and Jaffé, A. (2005) 'Assessment of hypoxia in children with cystic fibrosis', *Archives of Disease in Childhood*. 90(11):1138–1143. doi: 10.1136/adc.2005.071795.

Vahlkvist, S. and Pedersen, S. (2009) 'Fitness, daily activity and body composition in children with newly diagnosed, untreated asthma', *Allergy: European Journal of Allergy and Clinical Immunology*. 64(11):1649–1655. doi: 10.1111/j.1398-9995.2009.02081.x.

Van Doorn, N. (2010) 'Exercise programs for children with cystic fibrosis: a systematic review of randomized controlled trials', *Disability and Rehabilitation*. 32(1):41–49. doi: 10.3109/09638280902991842.

Vallis, M., Piccinini -Vallis, H., Sharma, A. M., & Freedhoff, Y. (2013) 'Modified 5 As: minimal intervention for obesity counseling in primary care,' *Canadian family physician Medecin de famille canadien*. 59(1):27–31. https://www.cfp.ca/content/59/1/27.short.

Welsh, L., Kemp, J.G. and Roberts, R.G.D. (2005) 'Effects of physical conditioning on children and adolescents with asthma', *Sports Medicine*. 35(2):127–141. doi: 10.2165/00007256-200535020-00003.

White, D., Stiller, K. and Haensel, N. (2007) 'Adherence of adult cystic fibrosis patients with airway clearance and exercise regimens', *Journal of Cystic Fibrosis*. 6(3):163–170. doi: 10.1016/j.jcf.2006.06.006.

World Health Organization (2010) 'Global recommendations on physical activity for health', *Geneva: World Health Organization.* doi: 10.1080/11026480410034349.

Wurzel, D.F. and Chang, A.B. (2017) 'An update on pediatric bronchiectasis', *Expert Review of Respiratory Medicine.* 11(7):517–532. doi: 10.1080/17476348.2017.1335197.

Zach, M., Oberwaldner, B. and Hausler, F. (1982) 'Cystic fibrosis: physical exercise versus chest physiotherapy', *Archives of Disease in Childhood.* 57(8):587–589. doi: 10.1136/adc.57.8.587.

Zach, M.S., Purrer, B. and Oberwaldner, B. (1981) 'Effect of swimming on forced expiration and sputum clearance in cystic fibrosis', *The Lancet.* 2(8257):1201–1203. doi: 10.1016/S0140-6736(81)91440-9.

Zeitoun, M. O., Wilk, B. O., Matsuzaka, A., KnOpfli, B. H., Wilson, B. A., & Bar-Or, O. D. (2004) 'Facial cooling enhances exercise-induced bronchoconstriction in asthmatic children', *Medicine and Science in Sports and Exercise,* 36(5):767–771. doi: 10.1249/01.MSS.0000126466.67458.5B.

9 Exercise in Children with Medical Complexity

A Need for Individualised Training

Claudia Astudillo Maggio and Gregory Villarroel Silva

Introduction

Children with medical complexity suffer from a wide range of chronic illnesses that result in frequent hospitalisations, heavy treatment burdens, and an array of physical, cognitive, psychological, emotional, and social disabilities. Amongst this population, there are many causes of cardiopulmonary and mobility impairments. Children who suffer from neuromuscular disease (NMD), cerebral palsy (CP), or specific syndromes (that may have a genetic basis) are frequently afflicted by a combination of problems that align to recognised patterns. Respiratory function may be impaired by skeletal deformity or restricted movement of the thoracic cage and/or weakness of the muscles of respiration that may be a consequence of impaired neurological control or primary muscle disease. Similarly, congenital or acquired lung and upper airway structural abnormalities may impair breathing. Depending on severity, these factors may reduce exercise tolerance, compromise breathing during sleep, and reduce quality of life (QoL) (Joschtel *et al.*, 2018). Furthermore, common comorbidities that have the potential to damage respiratory function further include gastro-oesophageal reflux disease (GORD), unsafe swallow and aspiration, increased predisposition to lower respiratory tract infections (LRTI), due to poor cough and mucus clearance, poor nutrition, and immobility that lead to poor muscle development or deconditioning and reduced bone mineral density (BMD). Associated non-pulmonary barriers to physical activity (PA) include learning disability, cardiovascular, locomotor, and sensory (e.g., visual or auditory) impairments, while nutritional compromise or obesity both impede physical function. International guidelines recommend that healthy children should participate in an average of 60 minutes of moderate to vigorous intensity physical activity (MVPA) per day to achieve health benefits. Establishing a schedule of PA in children with chronic illness is a challenge, yet exercise has the potential to preserve and enhance physical function and QoL by strengthening muscle, improving posture, preserving joint flexibility, and maintaining BMD (Kim *et al.*, 2017; Clutterbuck *et al.*, 2019). There is also evidence from some groups that exercise training can

DOI: 10.4324/9781003020462-9

improve coordination, balance, and day-to-day living skills (Eid *et al.*, 2017; Peungsuwan *et al.*, 2017).

A proportion of children with medical complexity, whose numbers are increasing, have such severe difficulties, that they develop respiratory failure for which support with mechanical ventilation is a therapeutic option (Cohen *et al.*, 2011). The value of PA and adapted forms of exercise is increasingly recognised as an important component of the treatment and rehabilitation of all children with medical complexity.

Inter-relationships between Medical Complexity and Physical Activity – A Spiral of Decline?

Children and adolescents with chronic medical conditions undertake less PA than their healthy peers (Joschtel *et al.*, 2018; West *et al.*, 2019). Physical inactivity and intolerance to exercise is the consequence of many influences including intrinsic disease-specific factors, impaired neuromuscular, locomotor, and cardiopulmonary function, general deconditioning, obesity (or conversely poor nutrition), illness exacerbations including infections and learning difficulties, emotional and psychological problems that undermine understanding and cooperation. Furthermore, extrinsic factors are important and relate to parent and caregiver knowledge, apprehensions and motivation to engage, access to multidisciplinary team support including that of a physiotherapist or personal trainer, institutional (school), and home facility that are all dependent on resources.

Muscle Weakness

Physical capability and exercise performance are dependent on muscle control and function, not only for locomotion, but also for breathing. CP and NMD are associated with reduced cardiopulmonary fitness, exercise capacity, muscle strength, and PA levels that increase the risk of cardiometabolic disease, obesity, and osteoporosis. Such combinations can lead to progressive functional loss over time; potentially fuelling a spiral of decline augmented by physical deconditioning that arises from inactivity, nutritional compromise, and condition-specific pathophysiology. Indeed, in children, mobility restrictions that may be contributed to by support equipment may impede motor skill and physical development (Dumas, 2012).

Cerebral palsy is caused by permanent brain damage due to a number of aetiologies that arise during brain development and affecting 2–3 per 1,000 livebirths. There is a broad spectrum of severity, and clinical patterns for classification are well described (Jonsson *et al.*, 2019). Features and complications of CP overlap with those of NMD although there are distinct differences. In CP, motor control and physical ability are usually the most vulnerable neurological functions affected with relative preservation of higher mental functions except in the most profoundly afflicted children. Features include weakness and selective loss of motor control, typically with limb spasticity, truncal hypotonia, lower muscle mass, poor balance, posture maintenance and coordination, restricted joint movement with contractures. The Gross Motor Function Classification System (GMFCS) grades the severity of disability in CP from I to V (Palisano *et al.*, 2008). Those in groups IV and V are profoundly disabled.

Childhood NMD is an umbrella term for peripheral nerve and muscle disorders, usually with genetic causes leading to either profound early weakness in infancy or to the progressive loss of ambulatory and pulmonary function with age (Dowling *et al.*, 2018). Classifications include disorders of the anterior horn cell (e.g., spinal muscular atrophy, SMA), peripheral nerve (e.g., Charcot–Marie–Tooth disease), the neuromuscular junction (e.g., congenital myasthenic syndrome), and muscle (myopathies and muscular dystrophies, such as Duchenne muscular dystrophy, DMD). Depending on the type of neuromuscular disease (NMD), the pattern of weakness is variable in terms of which muscles are affected, the age of onset, rate of progression, and severity of weakness. These recognised patterns inform systems of sub-classification and aid prognosis, although many now have confirmatory genetic causes, and for some, specific treatments.

Any weakness will have an impact on exercise performance, but those that either selectively involve the muscles of respiration or progress to cause global profound weakness will affect ventilation, initially with shallow breathing and hypoventilation, leading to respiratory failure typically during sleep before when awake. Hypoventilation and an ineffectual cough will predispose to atelectasis (lung segment collapse) and pneumonias, while truncal hypotonia and postural imbalance will lead to thoracic cage deformity such as scoliosis, further compromising breathing.

Non-invasive respiratory support includes both continuous positive airway pressure (CPAP) and non-invasive ventilation (NIV) that may be used in a range of acute and chronic respiratory disorders in children. CPAP may be used when there is adequate respiratory drive, splinting the airways and improving FRC and oxygenation. NIV increases inspiratory volume and respiratory minute volume (VE) improving both CO_2 elimination and oxygenation. Indications, technical difficulties, and safety issues are complex and well summarised in a recent review (Fedor, 2017). NIV can deliver timed, usually pressure limited, or spontaneously triggered insufflations with a backup minimum rate. Triggering may be impaired with muscle weakness, when tidal volumes are low and if there is interface leakage or large dead-space volume. Adapting respiratory support to variability in demand including that of PA and exercise is a challenge. Any mismatch between demand and the level of support and its synchronisation with effort of breathing will reduce efficiency, increase work of breathing, and eventually limit exercise. Neurally adjusted ventilatory assist (NAVA) is one step in technology to address this by detecting electrical diaphragmatic signals that enable the synchronisation of respiratory support to an individual's breathing pattern and is not affected by system leaks. NAVA has been used in infants (Fedor, 2017) and in critically ill adults, it has been shown to facilitate rehabilitation by improving exercise tolerance, through higher work efficiency in relation to oxygen consumption, enhancing training effects to speed recovery (Akoumianaki *et al.*, 2017).

Respiratory Comorbidities and Progressive Lung Disease

Many children with medical complexity, especially when associated with weakness, are prone to suffering significant respiratory complications that contribute to the morbidity and mortality of their condition. Weakness of respiratory muscles and/or thoracic cage deformity lead to shallow breathing, a poor cough, difficulty in clearing secretions, atelectasis at the lung bases, and increased LRTIs (e.g., pneumonia) that precipitate acute decompensation or hamper the weaning of mechanical respiratory support instituted for planned interventions such as surgical scoliosis stabilisation.

GORD is common, carrying a risk of aspiration, particularly when there is abnormal oropharyngeal (bulbar) function compromising swallowing and airway protection reflexes. Upper airway obstruction due to craniofacial dysmorphism, large tonsils or tongue, poor pharyngeal muscle tone, and increased secretions may contribute to respiratory difficulties particularly during sleep, but also during activities.

Respiratory difficulties are worse in children who are or who become non-ambulatory, those with progressive thoracic cage deformity and those who have condition-specific diaphragmatic and/or respiratory muscle weakness. The general clinical features that raise concern about respiratory function in children with NMDs, CP, and genetic syndromes are detailed in Table 9.1 and investigations and interventions utilised and multidisciplinary roles in the diagnosis, monitoring, and management are outlined in Table 9.2.

Deconditioning of Muscles and Exercise Capacity

Apart from primary NMD *per se*, and often co-existing with such conditions, non-specific chronic disease often leads to muscles becoming deconditioned. This is contributed to by inactivity, illness-associated catabolism, and poor nutrition or conversely obesity. Deconditioning is associated with reduction in muscle bulk, strength, and endurance along with a fall in the ventilatory threshold (VT) for working muscle. It has been described in a range of chronic conditions including CP (Verschuren *et al.*, 2016), CF, where more severe illness and poor nutritional status are associated with low aerobic and anaerobic exercise capacity (Wilkes *et al.*, 2009) and children with congenital heart disease (CHD), where poor nutritional status is associated with general and respiratory muscle wasting, a restrictive pattern of pulmonary function and low aerobic capacity (Abassi *et al.*, 2019). Furthermore, respiratory muscles become deconditioned as a result of passive invasive or

Table 9.1 Clinical Features That May Raise Concern about Respiratory Function in Children with Medical Complexity

Medical history	Increased frequency of LRTIs. Worsening ability to cope with respiratory infections. Loss of or declining ability to walk. Conditions known to selectively impair diaphragmatic or respiratory muscle function.
Symptoms	Suggesting SDB: disturbed sleep, headache, daytime somnolence, poor concentration, reduced appetite, and nausea. Difficulty in clearing secretions, dribbling. Choking when eating or difficulty swallowing Reduced exercise tolerance (intensity, duration, frequency), keeping a record of an individual's exercise profile helps to track change.
Signs	Shallow rapid breathing Weak huff or poor demonstrable cough Poor or asymmetrical chest expansion Abnormal findings on chest auscultation: reduced or absent air entry, crackles. Scoliosis and/or chest deformity Hypotonia Obesity or poor nutrition (either may be encountered) Upper airway obstruction: stridor (laryngeal or tracheal narrowing), hoarse voice, stertor (large tonsils, poor pharyngeal tone). Craniofacial dysmorphism: small nasal airway, large tongue, micrognathia, short neck.

Abbreviations: LRTIs = Lower respiratory tract infections, e.g., pneumonia; SDB = sleep disordered breathing, including hypoventilation, apnoea, and obstructive sleep apnoea (OSA).

non-invasive mechanical ventilation, such that weaning off ventilation in those who have a recoverable condition is facilitated by inspiratory muscle training (Martin *et al.*, 2011).

Overweight and Obesity

Overweight may arise in a number of chronic illnesses. Predisposing causes include the imbalance between energy intake and energy expenditure through inactivity, poor motivation or opportunity to undertake PA, overeating, and lack of satiety (e.g., Trisomy 21 and Prader–Willi syndrome), inadvertent delivery of too much energy by enteral tube-feeding (e.g., children dependent on gastrostomy feeding where energy input must take account of activity and desired body composition rather than just a target weight) and endocrine causes such as poorly controlled hypothyroidism or insulin-dependent diabetes without attention to dietary limitations and insulin dosage.

Once established, obesity may affect exercise tolerance through adaptations in the cardiac, respiratory, endocrine, and musculoskeletal systems (West *et al.*, 2019). Cardiovascular changes include increases in cardiac output, blood pressure, and myocardial hypertrophy, compromising physiological reserve needed for PA. Lung function may develop a restrictive

Table 9.2 Investigations and Interventions in Children with Medical Complexity Who Have Compromised Respiratory and Physical Function (Hull *et al.*, 2012)

Investigations	**Lung function** serial data tracks respiratory impairment; predictions based on ulnar length or arm span when height cannot be measured. **VC** (performed slowly; concern when <50% PR) **Cough Peak Flow** (generally from age 12 years; concern when <270 $L{\cdot}min^{-1}$) **Measures of respiratory muscle strength**; MIP, MEP, SNIP **Multidimensional health-related QoL of life questionnaires**. **Overnight oximetry** – at least annually ifVC <60% PR, non-ambulatory, symptoms of SDB and specific conditions known to be associated with OSA, diaphragmatic weakness or rigid spine syndromes. **Capnography** ($TcCO_2$ or $ETCO_2$): to detect hypercapnia during sleep or when awake if more severe. **Polysomnography** – comprehensive physiological sleep study to classify and grade severity of SDB. **Exercise performance** on objective testing, e.g., 6MWT, see Chapter 2. **Video Fluoroscopy Swallow** (liquids and solids) to screen for aspiration. **Oesophageal pH monitoring and impedance** to screen for reflux.
Interventions and the Multi-Disciplinary Team (MDT)	**Medical and nursing:** overview of care, diagnoses, treatments, including **Antibiotics** to treat infection, patient and family education, **Immunisations** (e.g., influenza, pneumococcal). **Physiotherapy**: supervision of exercise testing and training. Deep breathing training, breath stacking, glossopharyngeal breathing in NMD. Methods to help mobilise and expel secretions include: nebulised saline (0.9–3%); Manual cough assist techniques; MI-E devices (very weak children and those with loss of bulbar function); Oscillatory techniques (e.g., high-frequency chest wall oscillation and intrapulmonary percussive ventilation). **Dietetics**: optimise BMI, ensure all necessary nutrients and fluid are provided, especially when enteral tube-feeding is required. **Psychology:** evaluation of child and family to determine anxieties and motivators in relation to treatment adherence, physical activity, and exercise. **Occupational therapy**: postural and mobility supports, living environment adaptations. **Orthopaedics and orthotics**: supportive footwear, joint splints/supports to stabilise joints and posture and prevent injury and pain. Surgery for joint instability or scoliosis stabilisation. **Speech and language therapy**: for advice on safety of swallow. **Medical equipment and electronics technician:** device servicing and support. **Oxygen supplementation:** oxygen alone should not be used for hypoxaemia secondary to hypoventilation, hypercapnia can be made worse.

(*continued*)

Table 9.2 (Continued)

Respiratory support	**Non-invasive Ventilation**: appropriate, once symptomatic night-time hypoventilation or daytime hypercapnia develops, with the aim of reducing breathlessness and fatigue. Early use, especially in conditions with progressive weakness may cause respiratory muscle deconditioning and ventilator dependency. Initially may be used intermittently (via a hand-held mouthpiece in able children), just at night or during acute infections. Device-patient interface problems include leakage, pressure skin injury, and mid-face flattening. Other complications: gastric distension, aspiration, pneumothorax. **Ventilation via a tracheostomy**: once continuous respiratory support is needed. Management requires specialist support. Ethical considerations when consenting for this intervention include the acceptance of care burden, cosmetic consequences, adverse effects on speech, and swallowing which impair QoL. Exercise activity for those on respiratory support increases ventilatory demand, which may be difficult especially if spontaneous triggering is impaired. Synchronising device assistance to increase VE incrementally may be possible with technologies such as NAVA.

Note: Overnight oximetry analysis includes: mean and lowest values, apnoea hypopnoea index (AHI) or desaturation indices (DI > 4% or 3%), and scrutiny of prolonged dips including their relationship to feeding or other events.

Abbreviations: VC = vital capacity; $ETCO_2$ = end-tidal carbon dioxide; M I-E = mechanical insufflation/exsufflation; MIP = maximal inspiratory pressure; MEP = maximal expiratory pressure; NAVA = neurally adjusted ventilatory assist; PR = predicted; QoL = quality of life; SDB = sleep disordered breathing, including hypoventilation, apnoeas, and obstructive sleep apnoea (OSA); SNIP = sniff nasal inspiratory pressure; $TcCO_2$ = transcutaneous carbon dioxide; 6MWT = 6-minute walk test; VE = respiratory minute volume.

pattern with an increased ventilation frequency, and decreased respiratory muscle efficiency adding to metabolic demands in competition for those needed for PA. Overweight increases stress and pain in weight-bearing joints, especially in the lower body. Fat accumulates abnormally within striated muscle fibres of obese children and is linked to impaired phosphorus energy metabolism, insulin resistance, abnormal glucose transport, and abnormal mitochondrial function all of which may compromise muscle function (West *et al.*, 2019).

Osteoporosis

Reduced BMD and osteoporosis is a common complication of NMDs, CP, and other complex medical conditions, contributed to by inactivity, poor nutrition, genetic factors, and low vitamin D levels (dietary, low sun exposure, and anticonvulsant antagonism in children with CP who have epilepsy) (Yaşar *et al.*, 2018). It can contribute to progressive deformity such as scoliosis and painful fractures, compromising activities further.

Multi-system Dysfunction in Children with Medical Complexity

In any child with chronic medical complexity, the multi-system nature of the condition needs to be appreciated so that individual system impairments for targeted treatments can be screened for and the interdependences of systems which contribute to an individual's physical limitation can be recognised. Combined system dysfunction can hasten decline in physical performance as disease progresses, a dramatic example being the development of pulmonary vascular hypertension (PHT) in those with hypoxaemia secondary to severe lung disease. Within the literature however there are numerous examples of how changes in different systems can have a collective negative impact on exercise capacity.

Down syndrome (DS; Trisomy 21) is a common exemplar of a genetic disorder which is associated with a multitude of clinical manifestations including motor developmental delay, hypotonia, balance difficulties with postural sway, weakness in hip abductors and knee extensors, learning difficulties, hypothyroidism, congenital heart disease, upper airway obstructive symptoms, and sleep disordered breathing. Indeed, as is the case in a number of genetic disorders, obesity in DS is a significant problem (Ravel *et al.*, 2020). Exercise may therefore have much to offer children with such a range of problems.

In a study of 834 children, 555 with CHD and 279 controls, CHD was found to be associated with restrictive pulmonary function abnormalities that correlated with a reduction in VO_{2peak} on cardiopulmonary exercise testing (CPET) and a reduced QoL (Abassi *et al.*, 2019). A multivariate analysis to determine factors influencing aerobic capacity (VO_{2max}) on maximal CPET in 496 children CHDs (302 controls), VO_{2max} was significantly lower in the CHD group and the mean VO_{2max} decline per year was significantly higher than in the controls (Amedro *et al.*, 2018). A lower VO_{2max} was associated with increased body mass index (BMI), a lower ventilatory anaerobic threshold (which reflects muscular deconditioning), female sex, a restrictive lung function, right ventricle systolic hypertension, tricuspid regurgitation, and the presence of a genetic anomaly.

Some children born prematurely develop bronchopulmonary dysplasia (BPD) associated with decreased lung function. Ruf *et al.* (2019) concluded, in a cohort of 22 school children with BPD, that it was associated with a reduced exercise capacity (VO_{2peak}) when assessed at school age. However, regardless of BPD, children born prematurely were less physically active and generally more sedentary than controls, indicating that other factors are at play. Exercise capacity in children born prematurely is the subject of Chapter 10 in this book.

Evidence of the Benefits of Exercise Training and Physical Activity in Patients with Chronic Diseases

In healthy children and adolescents, there is consistent evidence of the benefits of exercise: it improves cardiovascular fitness, body composition, musculoskeletal, and mental health (Hosker *et al.*, 2019; Owens *et al.*, 2017) while inactivity in youth is associated with increased cardiometabolic risk in adulthood (Kallio *et al.*, 2021). (PA is essential for the optimal development of physical, psychological, emotional, and social wellbeing. Traditional clinical assessments of children with medical complexity may have focused on symptom control without necessarily promoting a healthy lifestyle. Such a focus that considers individual engagement in physical activities and exercise training has potential to improve cardiorespiratory fitness, muscle mass, and BMD, while reducing adiposity, insulin resistance, cardiometabolic risk, and possibly illness exacerbations. However, disease-specific PA and exercise training recommendations are scarce, especially for children with medical complexity (Joschtel *et al.*, 2018). Short term simple training programs have been studied in children with conditions such as cystic fibrosis and shown to improve cardiopulmonary fitness (Turchetta *et al.*, 2004) but how sustainable such interventions are and how long term disease specific outcomes are modified have yet to be fully ascertained. Exercise training in adults and children with asthma can improve symptoms and so has a place in the comprehensive therapeutic approach to disease control (Francisco *et al.*, 2018). Enthusiasm for this important area of work, however, is growing, but is complicated by the wide variability in patterns and severity of illness manifestations making it difficult to form a consensus viewpoint about optimal training programmes for individuals with specific diseases.

A key outcome for exercise intervention is an improvement in QoL which is achieved through improved fitness and capability to participate in life opportunities open to healthy peers. It is intuitive that the health benefits of exercise training can only be realised by establishing and maintaining activities throughout life and participation in training and its maintenance should be regarded as an outcome for interventions. Exercise performance, training, and assessments in children with CF and asthma are discussed in detail in Chapters 4 and 6, respectively.

The benefits of PA and exercise training in other chronic disease groups have a number of common themes, allowing for some cautious extrapolation of core findings and implications, at least until more work is done in illness-specific groups. Fundamentally, it is active movement that generates a metabolic demand and a physiological response that allows the health benefits of exercise to be accessed. Facilitating this in ambulant or semi-ambulant children with neuromuscular disease or other complex conditions is therefore important but challenging. Difficulties in establishing evidence supporting exercise interventions in CP have been highlighted in a systematic review, identifying that studies tend to have small sample sizes and heterogeneity in the subject population along with considerable uncertainty about the objectivity of outcome measures (Ryan *et al.*, 2017). The review found only limited evidence that aerobic training improved gross motor function with no increase in gait speed. Resistance training was concluded to have no benefit. This and other reviews of exercise intervention in a variety of chronic complex illnesses in children underscore how differences in the format of training (type, intensity, duration, and frequency) are often incomparable, thus making recommendations for PA and exercise prescription problematic.

Individual studies have found that combined gross motor aerobic and resistance training can improve walking ability, functional lower limb strength, and balance in CP (Peungsuwan *et al.*, 2017). A more recent systematic review of seven types of intervention for children with CP in 34 studies determined that gross motor aerobic training combined with resistance exercise and backed up with physiotherapy achieved the best improvement in gross motor function (Clutterbuck *et al.*, 2019). The conclusions in this review emphasised the added value of physiotherapy supervision and support in the training and the need for formal variability in training formats that probably help maintain interest while ensuring there is a comprehensive inclusion of different muscle groups in the training. The review highlighted that '*participation*' as an outcome is frequently overlooked and needs further research with relevance to modified real-world sporting activities. There is also a need to determine whether interventions have any influence on longer term disease complications, for example in CP, whether they deter progressive deformity (e.g., scoliosis) or complications such as painful hip dislocation, both of which lead to further limitation and become a barrier to general care.

Novel interventions utilising computer gaming platforms may promote participation. One small study evaluated the effects of exercising on a gaming 'balance board' (Nintendo Wii®) and found that, following a thrice weekly schedule of activity over 6 weeks, the children with CP had measurable improvement in ankle spasticity and static standing balance (Gatica-Rojas *et al.*, 2017)

Studies investigating the benefits of exercise training in children with NMDs raise a number of important issues. A 12-week pilot study of an arm cycling training programme in 5 children with SMA type II found that cycling distance and duration significantly improved during the programme (Bora *et al.*, 2018). A small study of children aged 4–18 years with a variety of NMDs sequentially evaluated the benefits of an aquatic exercise programme over 10 weeks (Huguet-Rodríguez *et al.*, 2020) and found that both land and water functional skills improved and children under 11 years demonstrated a significant increase in their inspiratory volume, pulse oximetry, and what was considered a clinically, but not statistically significant increase in peak cough flow and inspiratory pressure.

However, uncertainty has been expressed about how well-sustained any benefits of exercise interventions are or whether the longer-term trajectory of decline is affected or even accelerated in certain NMDs (Dahlqvist and Vissing, 2016). A recent review of the role of exercise in muscle and lower motor neurone disease concluded that in general, moderate-intensity aerobic and strength exercises are beneficial for people with muscle disease without causing detrimental exercise-induced muscle damage that could be a consequence of more intense exercise (Sheikh and Vissing, 2019). The same training in motor neurone disease, in adults, appears associated with a disappointing response, although there is some promise of response to high-intensity training in this group. This underscores how diverse conditions within the umbrella of NMD may respond differently to the format of training employed and so much more research is needed especially in those who are already very weak or non-ambulatory.

The emphasis in research investigating exercise training in NMD has centred on functional musculoskeletal and physical capability outcomes rather than cardiopulmonary physiological and fitness outcomes. It would be desirable for interventions to improve or prevent the decline in pulmonary function by increasing the strength and endurance of respiratory muscles, preventing progression of postural deformity, assisting airway clearance and preventing atelectasis, reducing or hastening recovery from LRTIs, and possibly reducing sleep-related hypoventilation. We can hypothesise that improved fitness would be a surrogate for all of these. Longer-term studies are needed to determine whether hospitalisations and measures of cardiopulmonary impairment can be offset or improved by exercise intervention.

Methodologies for the objective assessment of respiratory mechanics and respiratory muscle function have progressed over recent years with attention to their precision, validity and reproducibility (Laveneziana *et al.*, 2019). These promise to help characterise phenotypic features and clinical patterns of different NMDs, particularly in relation to respiratory mechanics and to assess response to treatments as well as predicting prognosis. Techniques include dynamic respiratory muscle imaging (ultrasound, optoelectric, and structured light plethysmography) and respiratory muscle neurophysiology (electromyography, electroencephalography, and transcranial magnetic stimulation) which can be applied at rest and some during exercise when the respiratory muscles are stressed.

Training methods in rehabilitation, where muscles are severely deconditioned, are important. Martin *et al.* (2011) evaluated the progress of 69 adult patients ventilated on intensive care where 35 patients received incremental load inspiratory muscle training and the rest a constant load inspiratory intervention. Participants completed 4 sets of 6–10 breaths, on each of 5 days per week until weaning from mechanical ventilation was achieved or 28 days were completed. The incremental loading was concluded to develop better inspiratory muscle strength and was more successful in weaning patients from support. A systematic review of targeted inspiratory muscle training (IMT) in children and adolescents with neuromuscular disease suggested that inspiratory muscle strength and endurance improved and that early, dose-dependent IMT may slow vital capacity decline, but concluded that there was insufficient evidence to guide clinical IMT practice (Human *et al.*, 2017). In adults with CF, high-intensity IMT was reported to improve inspiratory muscle function, anxiety, and depression scores (Enright *et al.*, 2004), but no benefit was found in a subsequent systematic review of IMT in adults or children with CF (Reid *et al.*, 2008). Outstanding research questions relate to the stage in a specific disease course that it might be worth investing in the cost, time, and effort of IMT and how intense should the training be in order to improve outcomes. Intervention in early or mild disease may not be helpful, while intervention at a late stage may not be successful in salvaging function.

The potential for exercise intervention to prevent or delay the development of osteoporosis is important. Weight-bearing exercises that generate 'ground reaction forces' and active muscle contractions are most likely to optimise osteogenic potential (Gannotti *et al.*, 2016). A recent meta-analysis of specific weight-bearing exercise in children with CP concluded that thigh bone (femur), but not lumber spine BMD, can be improved (Kim *et al.*, 2017). The standardisation of exercise interventions is clearly important in order to understand effects of interventions when applied to specific conditions at specific stages of illness progression.

Conventional physiotherapy was compared with the same plus isokinetic training on 3 days per week for 12 weeks in children aged 9–12 years with DS ($n = 31$) (Eid *et al.*, 2017). Measures of stability and lower limb strength improved in both groups, but this was significantly greater in the training group. A single centre study of toddlers with DS investigated the added benefit of twice weekly sessions of aquatic therapy to their usual physiotherapy over 5 weeks and found that a range of motor parameters, analysed by a motor skills questionnaire improved significantly more when aquatic therapy was included in their schedule (Priya *et al.*, 2019).

Although encouraging, this illustrates how exercise interventions are diverse in terms of intensity, duration, and frequency, as well as how outcomes may lack objectivity, only reflecting change at a specific time window during or following the intervention rather than providing evidence for the desired sustained or long-term benefit. For children with conditions such as DS, evidence for long-term improvement in condition characteristics will intuitively have a general positive impact on general health. A review of the effectiveness of exercise interventions on daily life activities and participation in people with DS used a structured assessment of study quality and outcome measures aligned to the International Classification of Function, Disability and Health (ICF) outcomes and identifies 19 studies (525 participants) that met inclusion criteria (Hardee and Fetters, 2017). Heterogeneity in methodology and the subject population (age 3 to 65 years) precluded a meta-analysis; nevertheless, exercise interventions were concluded to have a positive effect on daily life activities and participation.

The absence of a 'catalogue' of standardised exercise interventions undermines the comparisons between studies and the precision in translating evidence into exercise prescription for specific health conditions. Yet this needs balancing against the difficulties in engaging children in exercise training that does not provide variety of format or allow for individual expression, preference, and personal performance goal setting.

Designing an Individual Activity and Exercise Programme

In children with medical complexity, irrespective of diagnosis numerous factors, in varying degrees, contribute to the impairment of mobility, exercise capacity, and participation. These include cardiopulmonary impairments, muscle weakness or deconditioning, motor control, cognitive impairment, coordination difficulties, visual and auditory disabilities, and reduced range of joint movement and flexibility. Training has been recognised to have a role in rehabilitation as functional impairments worsen during illness exacerbations and when started early, recovery is supported. However, ideally this would be part of a continuum of intervention aiming to secure long-term health benefits by them being incorporated into lifestyle routines that can be modified as illness status fluctuates (Dumas, 2012). The feasibility of engaging children with medical complexity in active exercise depends on the severity of their established disability, their understanding, and cooperation as well as the availability of facility, equipment, and experienced staff.

Learning from the World Health Organisation and the American College of Sports Medicine, guidance for exercise activity in healthy children, it is encouraging that efforts have been made to produce consensus and evidence-based recommendations for people with CP, which will help guide healthcare professionals and standardise practice (Verschuren *et al.*, 2016). These disease-specific recommendations are based on published evidence for benefit from exercise interventions in people with CP, combined with expert opinion and experience that recognise the practicalities and challenges involved with implementation. Contrary to former views, spasticity in cerebral palsy does not increase with exercise training and targeted strength training may be beneficial in terms of maintaining function.

West *et al.* (2019) embraces the same initiative, recognising that exercise intolerance is a prevalent feature of most chronic diseases in childhood, and has proposed formats that can be adapted to individuals across the main groups of chronic respiratory, congenital cardiac, metabolic, systemic inflammatory, and cancer diseases.

At the outset, barriers to PA need identifying, including details of individual physical attributes and limitations and psychological resistance in order to direct changes in behaviour and lifestyle. Individual, family, or carer understanding and motivation are crucial in order to ensure participation, so stresses and anxieties need to be addressed. Implementation depends on resources with access to facility, equipment, and an enthusiastic multidisciplinary team.

Many researchers in this field refer to the dose-dependent effect of PA on health, but that this response is non-linear as health risks are reduced to a greater extent by the initial increments in a progressive activity programme. Additionally, greater 'doses' of activity are needed to increase fitness when compared to the activity needed to maintain established fitness adaptations.

Interventions formats need to be defined; type is classified into aerobic, anaerobic, strength (resistance), and flexibility training for which the intensity, duration, and frequency are planned. However, the programme needs to be aligned to the individual's medical and physical profile and fitness, with the aim of targeting as many muscle groups as is feasible, including the respiratory muscles. Hence a variety of formats involving different activities are needed to achieve this.

There is now awareness that spending more time being sedentary, such as sitting still and watching TV, is associated with increased health risks, and that this is a particular issue for children with neuromuscular diseases and cerebral palsy, especially for those who have higher GMFCS levels of disability. The promotion of light or habitual PA to replace sedentary time alone may have a positive influence on health. This is therefore important in parallel to any exercise programme, especially in those whose condition precludes upright strenuous activities. There are very few contraindications to the promotion of PA and exercise as long as regimens are individualised (Tables 9.3 and 9.4).

Outside of hospital settings, there are very few reports examining the integration of children with complex needs into physical recreational activities, but some have been successful including ice skating (Fragala-Pinkham *et al.*, 2009), outdoor activity camps (Dumas, 2012). Participation is countered by psychosocial hardships associated with medical complexity including the time burden and efforts of care, emotional stresses, mental health problems, and financial constraints.

Table 9.3 A Framework for Constructing a Physical Activity and Exercise Plan for Children with Medical Complexity

Essential considerations when embarking on a training program

- Activities tailored to the individual, taking account of their physical attributes and limitations.
- Intervention plans formulated with involvement of and an agreement between child, family carers, and the multidisciplinary team (see Table 9.2).
- Familiarisation with format and setting is important.
- Healthcare equipment must not impede activity or be disrupted or damaged by it.
- Warm-up activity before and cool-down following training.
- Plan an incremental increase in activity, especially in deconditioned/prior sedentary individuals.
- Ensure adequate rest and recovery between bouts of activity.
- Avoid exertional overload or high-impact activities; pain, discomfort, or injury undermine adherence.
- When applying loads across joints or through the spine, ensure that stability is not challenged. Orthoses can help joint alignment/stability; thoracic applications must not restrict ventilation.
- Variety of activity supports adherence.
- Document format (type, intensity, duration, and frequency) of activity to ensure consistency and precision with individualised monitoring and incremental adjustments.

(continued)

Table 9.3 (Continued)

Type of Training	*Features*	*Examples*
Aerobic training (~70% HR_{max} or 40–85% VO_{2peak}) MVPA	2–7 sessions per week, each lasting 20–60 minutes	Running, Cycling, Dance Swimming, Soccer Self-propelled wheelchair circuits 6MWT
Anaerobic training (>75% HR_{max}; 9–10 on RPE) HIIT	2–3 sessions per week, each lasting 10–30 minutes with 20–90 seconds bouts of work, sets of 3–5 bouts repeated 2–5 times in a session. Rest between bouts should be ~3 × exercise duration (>2 minutes) and >5 minutes between sets.	Sprints, Press-ups, Jumps Climbing stairs/uphill Cycle ergometer (upper or lower limb) Sitting/standing repetitions
Resistance/strength training Repetitions = 50–85% of maximal single repetitive load	2–4 sessions per week, each with 1–3 sets of 5–15 repetitions of work that achieve. Quantified by number of repetitions × load.	Loaded single or multi-joint exercises IMT
Flexibility training	Passive and active controlled movements, positioning and postures.	Yoga Stretching protocols Balance and posture exercises
Promotion of habitual activity (1.5–3.0 MET) **and limitation of sedentary time** (<1.5 MET).	Avoidance or limitation of pastimes that promote inactivity, e.g., passively watching TV. Aim for <2 hours per day being sedentary Setting tasks of things to do on a daily basis. Promotion of movement and physical interaction	Pulling or pushing against resistance, gripping, throwing, and kicking. Ball and bean bag games. Manoeuvres, e.g., between bed and chair. Prone and supine activity helps strengthen neck and shoulder girdle movements. Rotational movements promote crawling and ambulatory skills. Social and environmental prompts to encourage activity, including playful interaction, movement to music or following actions in an activity video or computer game. Upright position is good for BMD, social interaction, diaphragmatic breathing and reduces risk of GORD.

Note: This is a practical guide, and not a formal recommendation, and not all modalities of intervention will be possible in individual children.

Abbreviations: HIIT = high-intensity interval training; HR = heart rate; IMT = inspiratory muscle training; MET = metabolic equivalents of task (relative to basic metabolic rate when resting in sitting position); MVPA = moderate to vigorous physical activity; RPE = rate of perceived exertion scale; VO_{2peak} = aerobic capacity (Verschuren *et al.*, 2016; West *et al.*, 2019).

Table 9.4 Set-up, Monitoring, and Safety Precautions Undertaken When Conducting Exercise Testing and Training for Children Who Require Respiratory Support at the Josefina Martinez Hospital, Chile

Contraindications	
Absolute	*Relative*
Current illness exacerbation or unstable condition, e.g., asthma, ischaemic heart disease. Pulmonary oedema, haemoptysis, pneumothorax symptomatic aortic stenosis Uncontrolled cardiac dysrhythmias	Pulmonary hypertension Hypertrophic cardiomyopathy Electrolyte disturbances Orthopaedic impairments that impair exercise performance Behavioural or mental health impairments that undermine cooperation

Resuscitation equipment

Oxygen source, suction device, and catheters

Manual resuscitation bag and for children with a tracheostomy, sized emergency tracheostomy tubes, and heat/moisture exchange filters

Back-up ventilator with humidifier system, power source, and battery

Monitoring and results (baseline; continuously during activity; during recovery): SpO_2 (bluetooth device that screens out motion artefact; note minimum), HR, RR, RPE

6MWT: above plus distance completed, (note: any rest periods are included in timing)

CPET: above plus W_{peak}, VO_{2peak} and VE, or when ventilation and gas-exchange variables not available, W_{peak} recorded when 85% of HR_{max} reached

Serial data from repeat tests enables reliability to be checked as well as changes due to interventions

Patient preparation

Familiarisation with track, turning around cones and rest chair for 6MWT; treadmill, protocol, and monitoring with CPET

Motivation and goal setting

Attention to appropriate positioning and orthotic aids

Unimpeded mobility of respiratory support equipment with adequate tubing length. Ventilators can be carried in backpacks, strollers/pushcart, or by accompanying caregivers

Pre-activity chest physiotherapy to clear secretions, aided by circuit humidification and aspiration of tracheostomy secretions)

Light meal 1–2 hours pre-exercise followed by fast

All usual medications taken as scheduled

Process and safety

Continuous supervision

All care devices and exercise equipment and track for the 6MWT or treadmill for the CPET need to be checked and free from hazards

Care to avoid dislodgement of tubing

Be prepared to stop test if excessive breathlessness, discomfort, or unsteady gait develops

6MWT, patient is instructed to 'walk as fast as possible' rather than 'as far as possible' along the track without running, turning around the cones/marks, but told that resting is allowed on a provided chair along the way

Encouragement instructions given every minute (see Figure 9.1 or ATS standardised protocol)

(*continued*)

Table 9.4 (*Continued*)

Stopping tests
The reason for the cessation must be recorded
Hypoxaemia: saturation <90% or fall by more than 4%, or <80% in children with chronic hypoxemia
Dysrhythmia
Volitional fatigue/patient's decision due to perceived limit of dyspnoea/effort
Dizziness, faintness, mental confusion, loss of coordination/unsteadiness of gait, chest pain, or any other uncomfortable symptom requiring cessation of activity

Abbreviations: CPET = Cardiopulmonary exercise test; HR = heart rate, either from pulse oximetry of 3-lead electrocardiogram (ECG); HR_{max} = 208 − (0.7 × age), (Tanaka, Monahan and Seals, 2001); 6MWT = 6-minute walk test; RPE = rating of perceived exertion and dyspnoea, (e.g. Borg CR10 scale); RR = respiratory rate; SpO_2 = pulse oximetry, estimate of arterial oxygen saturation; VO_{2peak} = peak oxygen consumption (ml·min^{-1}); W_{peak} = peak work (W); see Chapter 2.

How PA and exercise profiles are sustained and their benefits translated into long-term and adult health benefits needs more evaluation which will be supported by structured interventions, tests that have clinimetric validity, multi-dimensional QoL measures, disease specific outcomes, and complication rates, all of which would best incorporated into regional or national registries providing longitudinal data.

A Model of Exercise Training for Children with Complex Medical Needs

The Josefina Martínez Hospital (JMH), Santiago, Chile is a centre for paediatric respiratory medicine including the provision of integrated care for children with special health care needs (CSHCN; Cohen *et al.*, 2011) who are characterised by:

- Multi-system health and developmental needs coordinated between hospital specialist services, community health, social and educational agencies across multiple locations.
- Multiple impairments including significant physical, sensory, and cognitive disabilities.
- Medical fragility requiring significant and sustained nursing care to prevent further disability or death.
- Technology dependence, requiring medical devices to compensate for the loss of vital body functions.

Prolonged periods of hospitalisation impact on the quality of life of patients and their families and unfortunately are a consistent consequence of chronic respiratory and neuromuscular diseases (Mendez and Astudillo, 2020). The JMH established a pathway of care and rehabilitation for CSHNC with severe respiratory diseases in 2008, recognising the importance of exercise training as a core component, but with the tailoring of interventions to the needs of individuals, achieving positive outcomes and a safe track record (Villarroel *et al.*, 2017, 2020). Between 60 and 70 children with severe illness undergo assessments and rehabilitation each year with a diverse case-mix including post-infective lung damage, bronchopulmonary dysplasia, bronchiolitis obliterans, large airway abnormalities, neuromuscular disorders, and a variety of syndromes (e.g., Down syndrome, Pierre Robin sequence, Moebius syndrome, and central hypoventilation syndrome). Typically these children have the most complex medical needs; most being dependent, particularly during sleep, on invasive mechanical ventilation, via a tracheostomy tube (95%) and the rest on non-invasively (NIV) support via an interface mask. Those with invasive ventilatory support are managed using pressure control and volume-targeted pressure support modes. Approximately half of the children manage with continuous positive airway pressure (CPAP) during the day with a few breathing spontaneously when awake and are usually able to increase their minute ventilation (VE) spontaneously to meet the demands of increased activity while others depend on their ability to trigger an increase in their respiratory rate whilst being ventilated. NAVA is not available to our patient population. Around 25% of the cohort have additional inspired oxygen, but support to increase VE is preferred to increasing oxygen delivery when exercising children. Supplemental oxygen can be cautiously increased, in the absence of hypercapnia, to maintain oximetry saturations over 90% during exercise to decrease dyspnoea and improve exercise tolerance (Nici *et al.*, 2006). Many children also have enteral tube feeding systems, postural, and mobility aids. So, for our cohort of CHSNC, functioning in daily life, let alone establishing exercise training, poses considerable challenges and exercise interventions need to navigate and take account of individual disabilities, skills, and technological support needs.

Entry into the pulmonary rehabilitation programme follows a thorough assessment and optimisation of medical and multi-disciplinary support along with the provision of the most reliable and where possible portable equipment. Education of the child and family about their requirements and the value of PA and exercise training help explore strategies for changes in behaviour and motivation that will promote adherence (Spruit *et al.*, 2013). Challenging behaviours, learning, and socialising difficulties may preclude inclusion in training programmes, but where possible participation may be facilitated by psychological and occupational therapy assessments. The design of individual exercise training formats requires some baseline understanding of physical capability, which includes an assessment of mobility, gait, and stability, combined with a review of safety issues in relation to medical factors, equipment, and monitoring requirements. This will precede some initial submaximal exercise activity to allow scrutiny of the child's physiological responses, tolerance, understanding, and engagement. This can then be progressed to formal 6-minute walk tests (6MWTs) or, for those with capability, submaximal or even incremental maximal treadmill tests, which are always accompanied by a trained physiotherapist to provide motivation and to support any device dependency. The 6MWTs are performed according to American Thoracic Society guidelines (Crapo *et al.*, 2002). Children who are able to exercise on a treadmill undergo an initial familiarisation with a submaximal exercise test before progressing to an incremental cardiopulmonary exercise test (CPET) on a treadmill or on a cycle ergometer. CPET can assess their maximum exercise capacity (Vega-Briceño and Zenteno, 2009), which is considered the 'gold standard' for the evaluation of aerobic capacity (Armstrong and Van Mechelen, 2017); useful in establishing the intensity of work that an individual can tolerate in an exercise training programme (Weisman *et al.*, 2003). However, for the cohort of children in this programme, only a minority are able to undertake CPET tests, and the majority have their assessments and training centred around their 6MWT performance. Baseline capnography and measures of respiratory muscle strength are obtained (see below). Results then serve to design and calibrate individual exercise training formats (type, intensity, duration, and frequency). Realistic medical and patient-centred goals need to be defined and formal progress evaluations need scheduling that offer opportunity to adapt formats over time (Torres-Castro, 2016). Considerations that apply to eligibility, preparation, process, and cessation of testing are summarised in Table 9.4. Integrating play and encouragement are essential in order for interventions to be successful and sustained (Figure 9.1).

Key training programme goals are:

Medical:

- Achieve appropriate cardiopulmonary responses to exercise
- Achieve and maintain participation.
- Increase exercise tolerance
- Increase maximal inspiratory pressure
- Increase pulmonary function
- Decrease respiratory exacerbations
- Decrease mechanical ventilation support

Patient-centred:

- To instil a sense of purpose and achievement
- To improve social integration and activity participation, including school attendance
- Decrease respiratory symptoms
- Increase effort tolerance (able to do more without feeling uncomfortable)
- To maintain stability whilst improving joint flexibility and mobility
- Improve the QoL

Children who are unable to ambulate or who are unable to do a 6MWT due to instability or safety concerns will receive a range of therapies including balance and posture exercises, dance therapy, hydrotherapy, stretching

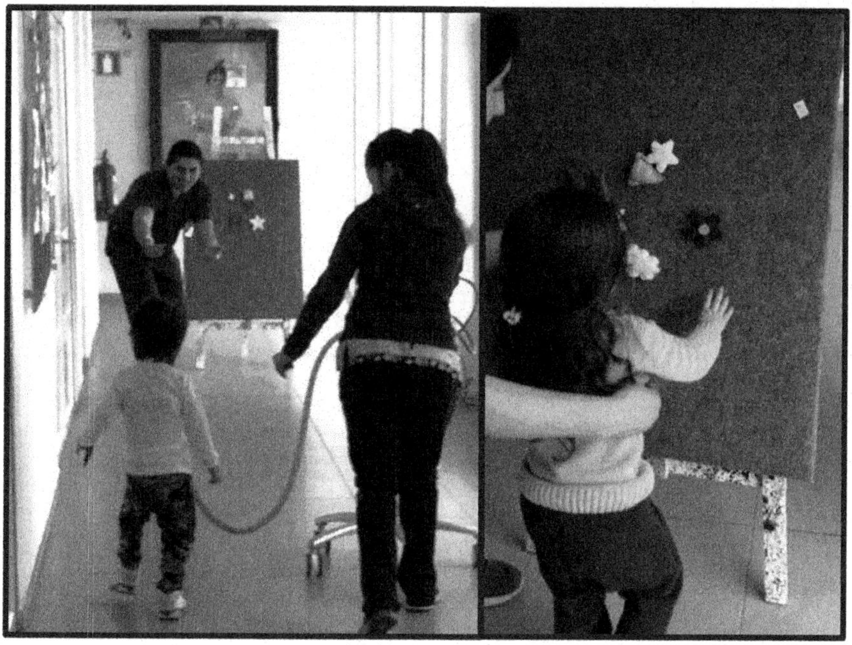

Figure 9.1 Playful stimuli and incentives combined with verbal encouragement are utilised to ensure collaboration and motivate children in order to achieve maximal effort. These need to be age appropriate and individualised. Pre-test familiarisation with the test environment and process helps to prepare children to do their best. The exercise area needs to be free from hazards and obstructions and any medical equipment that the child is attached must be supported and moved so as not to impede progress.

exercises, and workshops of adapted sports which design bespoke activities based on individual abilities.

Training

The majority of ambulatory children in our programme have their aerobic training calibrated and formulated in relation to their 6MWT performance, with a graduated increase in prescribed intensity that aims to achieve a predetermined percentage of the individual's maximal heart rate (HR_{max}), as aligned to their 6MWT speed, for at least 20 minutes. Training sessions are conducted two or ideally three times per week where walking is encouraged to achieve 50–80% HR_{max} in the first 4 sessions, 50–85% HR_{max} for sessions 5–9, and then 50–90% HRmax thereafter (Figure 9.2). These heart rate ranges convey the flexibility in training intensity determined by effort and encouragement. Within our programme, we aim to complete 24 sessions (8–12 weeks). Similar treadmill or cycle ergometry formats can be planned

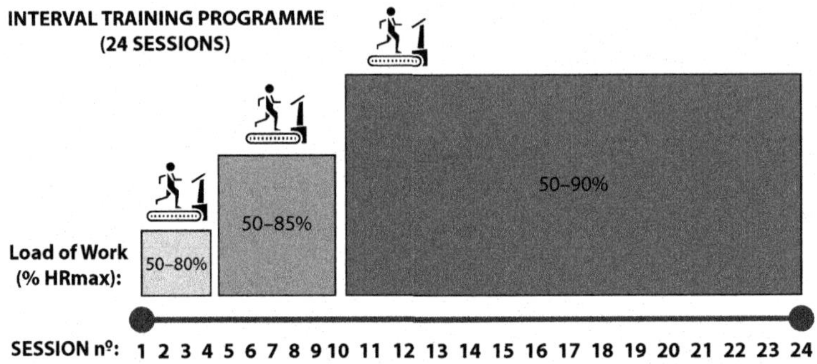

Figure 9.2 Diagramatic outline of a typical aerobic interval training protocol. Following initial familiarisation and calibration testing of the subjects' fitness and ability, regular training sessions are scheduled with a pre-determined duration. The intensity of work is increased incrementally as shown in the step-ups. Variable to increase workload will include speed (level walking or treadmill), incline gradient (treadmill) or resistance (cycle ergometer). At the JMH, training sessions are typically 20 minutes in duration, conducted 2–3 times per week over 8–12 weeks.

for those with capability, which allows for greater precision in monitoring physiology and the amount of work done (Torres-Castro *et al.*, 2016).

During training bouts, continuous monitoring includes heart rate (HR), pulse oximetry, rating of perceived exertion (RPE), and leg fatigue on the modified Borg scale (Gatica *et al.*, 2012). Bluetooth telemonitoring, resistant to motion artefact, is desirable as it avoids wiring becoming an obstacle to progress. On completion of 24 training sessions, formal 6MWT/CPET testing objectively re-evaluates physiological exercise performance.

In our resource-limited setting, further cycles of training may not be possible, but the aim is to facilitate a sustainable plan of exercise and PA for children who are discharged back into the community or to their referring clinicians.

Inspiratory Muscle Training

In patients who can perform maximum inspiratory manoeuvres, maximum inspiratory pressure (MIP) measurement is one method to evaluate respiratory muscle strength at the mouth, as described by Black and Hyatt (1969). Maximal expiratory pressure (MEP) and sniff nasal inspiratory pressures (SNIP) are other techniques for measuring respiratory muscle strength (Hull *et al.*, 2012) as shown in Table 9.5.

In patients with a tracheostomy, MIP can be measured through the mouth as long as the patient can tolerate occlusion of the tube. If the patient cannot tolerate this occlusion, evaluation via the tracheostomy may be performed by inflating the tube cuff until the airway is sealed off with a maximum cuff pressure of 30 cmH_2O to avoid tracheal mucosal injury (Figure 9.3).

Table 9.5 Measurement of Maximal Inspiratory or Expiratory Muscle Strength

Basic Technique in Cooperative Child
MIP
Patient asked to breathe out fully to RV then make a maximal inspiratory effort through an occluded mouthpiece connected to a manometer, reading is taken at 1 second. A small leak in the circuit prevents pressure generation by cheek muscles.
MEP
Patient asked to breathe in fully to TLC then breathe out with maximal effort against an occluded mouthpiece connected to a manometer, reading taken at 1 second. Cheeks are manually supported to prevent distension and a small leak prevents their contribution to the pressure measured.
SNIP
A plug incorporating a catheter connected to a pressure transducer is placed in one nostril and the patient is asked to perform a forceful sniff via the other patent nostril. Cooperation and logistics may be easier than MIP.
MIP in non-collaborative children with tracheostomies
• Preparatory chest physiotherapy and airway clearance including suctioning to clear secretions. • Position upright with an incline of no more than 60 degrees. • Use manual insufflation or 'self-inflating bag' with oxygen to hyper-oxygenate patient • Connect the non-rebreathing T-piece valve to the tracheostomy tube and close the inspiratory entrance for 20 seconds or ten inspirations (see Figure 9.3) • Record the maximal inspiratory pressure obtained • Allow patient to rest for at least 1 minute. • Repeat process up to eight times until three reproducible manoeuvres (<10% variability) are obtained, the highest of which is recorded.

Note: MIP correlates well with SNIP and VC, but may be less good than the latter at predicting respiratory infection frequency, SDB, nocturnal, or daytime hypoventilation (Hull *et al.*, 2012).

Abbreviations: MIP = maximal inspiratory pressure; MEP = maximal expiratory pressure; RV = residual volume; VC = vital capacity; TLC = total lung capacity; SNIP = sniff nasal inspiratory pressure.

Typically, the patient is then asked to expel the air and perform a maximum inspiration measuring the pressure generated with a manometer. In non-co-operative patients, an alternative MIP measuring protocol can be considered (see Table 9.5).

Inspiratory muscle training (IMT) has the potential to improve respiratory function, exercise tolerance, and reduce morbidity during respiratory infections. IMT may be used alone, as it is in some of our non-ambulatory CSHNC, or in conjunction with aerobic or other PA promotion in more physically able children. A key factor that contributes to mechanical ventilation dependency in those recovering from acute major surgical intervention or acute illness decompensation is the deconditioning of inspiratory muscles caused by non-use, catabolism, and inflammatory or metabolic disturbances during the illness or care episode. This impedes the weaning of ventilatory support (Sprague and Hopkins, 2003). The role of the physiotherapist is central in the rehabilitation and discharge planning for children dependent

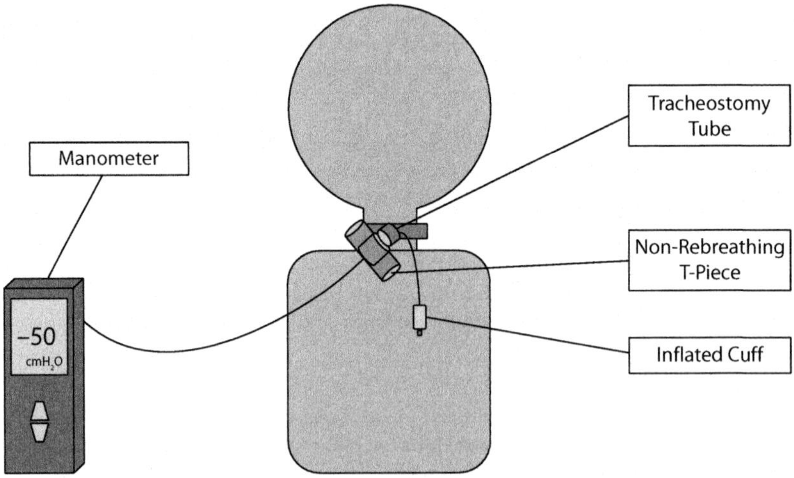

Figure 9.3 Measurement of inspiratory pressure in children with tracheostomies who cannot tolerate breathing through their mouths when their tracheostomy is obstructed. The tube cuff is inflated to prevent breathing around the tube via the upper airway. The non-rebreathing valve obstructs any airflow so that inspiratory effort generates negative pressure which is measured via an enclosed tube circuit connected to a manometer. The procedure can be uncomfortable and so needs to be explained and the subject familiarised with the procedure.

on long-term mechanical ventilation (Jalil *et al.*, 2017). Targeted inspiratory muscle training supervised by a trained physiotherapist offers an intervention that may hasten recovery and even the transition from mechanical ventilation to spontaneous breathing (Blackwood *et al.*, 2014). In our experience, IMT is feasible in many children with tracheostomies including those who are mechanically ventilated. Prior to training, children should undergo respiratory physiotherapy and aspiration of airway secretions. In children with NMD, IMT is initiated with inspiratory valves set at 30% of their MIP. In patients without ventilatory pump problems, it can be increased incrementally according to evaluation and tolerance up to 60% of the MIP. Training session should ideally be conducted twice daily and consist of three bouts of 3 minutes of work (40–50 breaths), each separated by two minutes of rest. In those with a MIP <20 cmH_2O, work series are reduced to 1 minute duration (12–15 breaths) with shorter one-minute periods of rest between (Figure 9.4).

MIP strength evaluations are carried out, for example, at monthly intervals, which inform adjustments to the work intensity. Frequently, MIP increases with training until a 'plateau' is reached, whereupon training time periods are reduced in number, but increased in duration, for example, to two series of 5 minutes of work separated by 2 minutes of rest, which in our experience consolidates progress. The ability to maintain inspiratory airway pressure

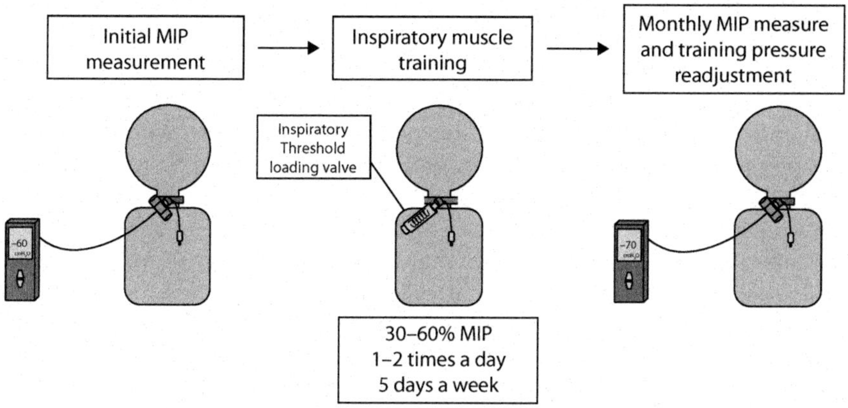

Figure 9.4 Protocol of inspiratory muscle training in tracheostomised children. Bouts of work to generate inspiratory pressure (IP), by breathing through inspiratory valves are regularly scheduled. The target IP is tailored to the individual as a percentage fraction of their MIP and then as training progresses, the valve resistance and so the IP can be incrementally increased.

above −7 cm H_2O serves as an indicator that individuals will tolerate capping of their tracheostomy (Moscoso *et al.*, 2019).

Outcomes Observed in the JMH Model

In our cohort of children following the 6MWT-based intervention, we have observed a mean increase in their walking distance of 17.8% following the 24-session intervention (Villarroel *et al.*, 2020). This increase is favourable when compared to improvements reported by others; 4% in cystic fibrosis (Gruber *et al.*, 2008) and 23.9% in asthma (Latorre-Román, 2014). As discussed above, the benefits of IMT are not well defined in research, changes in MIP are physiological measures and more research is needed to determine the best time and intensity of IMT in specific conditions and to confirm health and functional benefits such as reduced acute exacerbation rates, better exercise tolerance, improved QoL, or a better prognosis. The drop-out rate for children in our 6MWT aerobic training program is less than 10%, and to date we have not encountered any significant adverse events amongst participants. Informal feedback from children and their parents has been positive about our training programme.

Our model is one of rehabilitation and as with all training and exercise programmes, prevention through earlier intervention is a logical path for our wider health community to follow. Follow-up by the JMH service is not currently commissioned in Chile yet ideally, interventions need to be sustained in order to gain the full benefits that we anticipate, and our vision is to establish a wider acceptance and routine of incorporating exercise into the care of CSHNC with prospective longitudinal data on meaningful outcome measures.

Conclusion

At JMH, the clinical team has more than 10 years of experience undertaking exercise and inspiratory pressure training in CSHNC. Despite the challenges of resourcing equipment and sparse data upon which to establish protocols, a personalised rehabilitation programme in a South American hospital has been described and preliminary results have shown promise. However, more research is needed to evaluate the efficacy and effectiveness of the intervention, with broader outcome measures and stratification of intervention formats and exploration of other exercise modalities. Preliminary data showed that once the training begins, the benefits are observable but not easily evaluated. The challenge is to demonstrate the benefits objectively so as to further clinical practice. A pragmatic approach to testing was often required and the 6MWT is one established protocol to evaluate the functional exercise capacity of children with medical complexity. It is an easy test to perform that is well-tolerated and can be adapted for use in patients, who are dependent on technological devices, as both a training modality and an assessment tool. Further research is needed to define the exercise interventions that best improve the health longevity and QoL for children with medical complexity, with an emphasis on prevention of deterioration whilst supporting rehabilitation. An evidence-based intervention catalogue may be needed to truly individualise intervention.

Key Points

- Activity or exercise-related interventions with children with medical complexity is incredibly challenging and a pragmatic approach to its scientific study is required.
- There is a small amount of evidence that exercise offers an important therapeutic intervention for children with medical complexity.
- There are limited reliability, validity, feasibility, and randomised control trials for children with complex medical needs and future studies should focus on establishing the efficacy and effectiveness of exercise for this challenging group of patients.
- Training protocols for children with medical complexity and evaluations need to be individualised and include health and QoL outcomes that are meaningful to the child and their family.
- Interventions require multi-disciplinary involvement and need to be safe, cost-effective, and sustainable.

References

Abassi, H., Gavotto, A., Picot, M.C., Bertet, H., Matecki, S., Guillaumont, S., Moniotte, S., Auquier, P., Moreau, J. and Amedro, P. (2019). Impaired pulmonary function and its association with clinical outcomes, exercise capacity and quality of life in children with congenital heart disease. *International Journal of Cardiology*, 285, 86–92. doi:10.1016/j.ijcard.2019.02.069.

Akoumianaki, E., Dousse, N., Lyazidi, A., Lefebvre, J.C., Graf, S., Cordioli, R.L., Rey, N., Richard, J.C.M. and Brochard, L. (2017). Can proportional ventilation modes facilitate exercise in critically ill patients? A physiological cross-over study. *Annals of Intensive Care*, 7(1), 64. doi:10.1186/s13613-017-0289-y.

Amedro, P., Gavotto, A., Guillaumont, S., Bertet, H., Vincenti, M., De La Villeon, G., Bredy, C., Acar, P., Ovaert, C., Picot, M.C. and Matecki, S. (2018). Cardiopulmonary fitness in children with congenital heart diseases versus healthy children. *Heart*, 104(12), 1026–1036. doi:10.1136/heartjnl-2017-312339.

Armstrong, N. and Van Mechelen, W. (2017). *Oxford Textbook of Children's Sport and Exercise*. Oxford University Press, Oxford, UK.

Black, L.F. and Hyatt, R.E. (1969). Maximal respiratory pressures: normal values and relationships to age and sex. *American Review of Respiratory Diseases*, 99(5), 696–702. doi:10.1164/arrd.1969.99.5.696.

Blackwood, B., Burns, K., Cardwell, C. and O'Halloran, P. (2014). Protocolized versus non-protocolized weaning for reducing the duration of mechanical ventilation in critically ill adult patients. *The Cochrane Database of Systematic Reviews*, 11. doi:10.1002/14651858.CD006904.pub3.

Bora, G., Subaşı-Yıldız, Ş., Yeşbek-Kaymaz, A., Bulut, N., Alemdaroğlu, İ., Tunca-Yılmaz, Ö., Topaloğlu, H., Karaduman, A.A. and Erdem-Yurter, H. (2018). Effects of arm cycling exercise in spinal muscular atrophy type II patients: a pilot study. *Journal of Child Neurology*, 33(3), 209–215. doi:10.1177/0883073817750500.

Clutterbuck, G., Auld, M. and Johnston, L. (2019). Active exercise interventions improve gross motor function of ambulant/semi-ambulant children with cerebral palsy: a systematic review. *Disability and Rehabilitation*, 41(10), 1131–1151. doi:10.1080/09638288.2017.1422035.

Cohen, E., Kuo, D., Agrawal, R., Berry, J., Bhagat, S., Simon, T. and Srivastava, R. (2011). Children with medical complexity: an emerging population for clinical and research initiatives. *Pediatrics*, 127(3): 529–538. doi:10.1542/peds.2010-0910.

Crapo, R.O. Casaburi, R., Coates, A., Enright, P., MacIntyre, N., McKay, R, Johnson, D., Wanger, J. and Zeballos, J. (2002). ATS statement: guidelines for the six-minute walk test. *American Journal of Respiratory and Critical Care Medicine*, 166(1): 111–117. doi:10.1164/ajrccm.166.1.at1102.

Dahlqvist, J.R. and Vissing, J. (2016). Exercise therapy in spinobulbar muscular atrophy and other neuromuscular disorders. *Journal of Molecular Neuroscience*, 58(3), 388–393. doi:10.1007/s12031-015-0686-3.

Dowling, J.J., D. Gonorazky H., Cohn, R.D. and Campbell, C. (2018). Treating pediatric neuromuscular disorders: the future is now. *American Journal of Medical Genetics. Part A*, 176, 804–841. doi:10.1002/ajmg.a.38418.

Dumas, H.M. (2012). Rehabilitation considerations for children dependent on long-term mechanical ventilation. *International Scholarly Research Notices*. doi:10.5402/2012/756103.

Eid, M.A., Aly, S.M., Huneif, M.A. and Ismail, D.K. (2017). Effect of isokinetic training on muscle strength and postural balance in children with Down's syndrome. *International Journal of Rehabilitation Research*, 40(2), 127–133. doi:10.1097/MRR.0000000000000218.

Enright, S., Chatham, K., Ionescu, A.A., Unnithan, V.B. and Shale, D.J. (2004). Inspiratory muscle training improves lung function and exercise capacity in adults with cystic fibrosis. *Chest*, 126(2), 405–411. doi:10.1378/chest.126.2.405.

Fedor, K.L. (2017). Noninvasive respiratory support in infants and children. *Respiratory Care*, 62(6), 699–717. doi:10.4187/respcare.05244.

Fragala-Pinkham, M.A., Dumas, H.M., Boyce, M., Peters, C.Y. and Haley, S.M., 2009. Evaluation of an adaptive ice skating programme for children with disabilities. *Developmental Neurorehabilitation*, 12(4):215–223. doi:10.1080/17518420902980100.

Francisco, C.D.O., Bhatawadekar, S.A., Babineau, J., Reid, W.D. and Yadollahi, A. (2018). Effects of physical exercise training on nocturnal symptoms in asthma: systematic review. *PloS ONE*, 13(10), e0204953. doi:10.1371/journal.pone.0204953.

Gannotti, M.E., Breive, E.L., Miller, K., Mobyed, R. and Cameron, R.A. (2016). Exercise programs designed and dosed to improve bone mineral density in children with cerebral palsy. *Critical Reviews in Physical and Rehabilitation Medicine*, 28(4). doi:10.1615/CritRevPhysRehabilMed.v28.i4.50.

Gatica, D., Puppo, H., Villarroel, G., Martín, I.S., Lagos, R., Montecino, J.J., Lara, C., Zenteno, D. (2012). Valores de referencia test de marcha de seis minutos en niños sanos, *Revista Médica de Chile*, 140, 1014–1021. doi:10.4067/S0034-98872012000800007.

Gatica-Rojas, V., Cartes-Velásquez, R., Méndez-Rebolledo, G., Guzman-Muñoz, E. and Lizama, L.E.C. (2017). Effects of a Nintendo Wii exercise program on spasticity and static standing balance in spastic cerebral palsy. *Developmental Neurorehabilitation*, 20(6), 388–391. doi:10.1080/17518423.2016.1211770.

Gruber, W., Orenstein, D., Braumann, K. and Hüls, G. (2008). Health-related fitness and trainability in children with cystic fibrosis. *Pediatric Pulmonology*, 43(10): 953–64. doi:10.1002/ppul.20881.

Hardee, J.P. and Fetters, L. (2017). The effect of exercise intervention on daily life activities and social participation in individuals with Down syndrome: a systematic review. *Research in Developmental Disabilities*, 62, 81–103. doi:10.1016/j.ridd.2017.01.011.

Hosker, D.K., Elkins, R.M. and Potter, M.P. (2019). Promoting mental health and wellness in youth through physical activity, nutrition, and sleep. *Child and Adolescent Psychiatric Clinics*, 28(2), 171–193. doi:10.1016/j.chc.2018.11.010.

Huguet-Rodríguez, M., Arias-Buría, J.L., Huguet-Rodríguez, B., Blanco-Barrero, R., Braña-Sirgo, D. and Güeita-Rodríguez, J. (2020). Impact of aquatic exercise on respiratory outcomes and functional activities in children with neuromuscular disorders: findings from an open-label and prospective preliminary pilot study. *Brain Sciences*, 10(7), 458. doi:10.3390/brainsci10070458.

Hull, J., Aniapravan, R., Chan, E., Chatwin, M., Forton, J., Gallagher, J., Gibson, N., Gordon, J., Hughes, I., McCulloch, R. and Russell, R.R. (2012). British Thoracic Society guideline for respiratory management of children with neuromuscular weakness. *Thorax*, *67*(Suppl 1), i1–i40. doi:10.1136/thoraxjnl-2012-201964.

Human, A., Corten, L., Jelsma, J. and Morrow, B. (2017). Inspiratory muscle training for children and adolescents with neuromuscular diseases: a systematic review. *Neuromuscular Disorders*, 27(6), 503–517. doi:10.1016/j.nmd.2017.03.009.

Jalil, Y., Villarroel, G., Moscoso, G., Barañao, P., Mendez, M. (2017). Role of respiratory physiotherapists in the discharge process in children with long-term mechanical ventilation. *Neumologia Pediatrica*, 12, 161–168. Accessed March 9 2021: https://www.savalnet.ec/revistas/neumo_ped_octubre_2017/files/assets/basic-html/page-21.html#.

Jonsson, U., Eek, M.N., Sunnerhagen, K.S. and Himmelmann, K., 2019. Cerebral palsy prevalence, subtypes, and associated impairments: a population-based comparison study of adults and children. *Developmental Medicine and Child Neurology*, 61(10), 1162–1167. doi:10.1111/dmcn.14229.

Joschtel, B., Gomersall, S., Tweddy, S., Petsky, H., Chang, A. and Trost S. (2018). Effects of exercise training on physical and psychosocial health in children with chronic respiratory disease: a systematic review and meta-analysis. *BMJ Open Sports and Exercise Medicine,* 4(1):e000409. doi:10.1136/bmjsem-2018-000409.

Kallio, P., Pahkala, K., Heinonen, O.J., Tammelin, T.H., Pälve, K., Hirvensalo, M., Juonala, M., Loo, B.M., Magnussen, C.G., Rovio, S. and Helajärvi, H. (2021). Physical inactivity from youth to adulthood and adult cardiometabolic risk profile. *Preventive Medicine,* 145, 106433.

Kim, S.J., Kim, S.N., Yang, Y.N., Lee, I.S. and Koh, S.E. (2017). Effect of weight bearing exercise to improve bone mineral density in children with cerebral palsy: a meta-analysis. *Journal of musculoskeletal & neuronal interactions,* 17(4), 334. PMC5749042.

Latorre-Román, P.A. (2014). The effectiveness of an indoor intermittent training programme for improving lung function, physical capacity, body composition and quality of life in children with asthma. *Journal of Asthma,* 51, 544–551. doi:10.3109/02770903.2014.888573.

Laveneziana, P., Albuquerque, A., Aliverti, A., Babb, T., Barreiro, E., Dres, M., Dubé, B.P., Fauroux, B., Gea, J., Guenette, J.A. and Hudson, A.L. (2019). ERS statement on respiratory muscle testing at rest and during exercise. *European Respiratory Journal,* 53(6). doi:10.1183/13993003.01214-2018.

Martin, D., Smith, B., Davenport, P., Harman, E., Gonzalez-Rothi, R., Baz, M., Layon, J., Banner, M., Caruso. L., Deoghare, H., Huang, T. and Gabrielli, A. (2011). Inspiratory muscle strength training improves weaning outcome in failure to wean patients: a randomized trial. *Critical Care,* 15, R8. doi:10.1186/cc10081.

Mendez, M. and Astudillo, C. (2020). *Prolonged Hospitalization Due Chronic Respiratory Diseases: From Pediatric Respiratory Diseases. A Comprehensive Textbook.* In Bertrand, P., Sanchez, I. (eds), Springer Nature Switzerland AG., pp. 669–674. doi:10.1007/978-3-030-26961-6.

Moscoso, G., Villarroel, G., Ibañez, N., Astudillo, C. and Jalil, Y. (2019). Maintained inspiratory pressure in pediatric tracheostomized patients as an indicator of tolerance of capped tracheostomy. *Revista Chilena de Enfermedades Respiratorias,* 35(2), 111–115. doi:10.4067/S0717-73482019000200111.

Nici, L., Donner, C., Wouters, E., Zuwallack, R., Ambrosino, N., Bourbeau, J., Carone, M., Celli, B., Engelen, M., Fahy, B., Garvey, C., Goldstein, R., Gosselink, R., Lareau, S., MacIntyre, N., Maltais, F., Morgan, M., O'Donnell, D., Prefault, C., Reardon, J., Rochester, C., Schols, A., Singh, S. and Troosters, T. (2006). American Thoracic Society/European Respiratory Society statement on pulmonary rehabilitation. *American Journal of Respiratory and Critical Care Medicine,* 173(12): 1390–1413. doi:10.1164/rccm.200508-1211ST.

Owens, S., Galloway, R. and Gutin, B. (2017). The case for vigorous physical activity in youth. *American Journal of Lifestyle Medicine,* 11(2), 96–115. doi:10.1177/1559827615594585.

Palisano, R.J., Rosenbaum, P., Bartlett, D. and Livingston, M.H. (2008). Content validity of the expanded and revised gross motor function classification system. *Developmental Medicine and Child Neurology,* 50(10), 744–750. doi:10.1111/j.1469-8749.2008.03089x.

Peungsuwan, P., Parasin, P., Siritaratiwat, W., Prasertnu, J. and Yamauchi, J. (2017). Effects of combined exercise training on functional performance in children with cerebral palsy: a randomized-controlled study. *Pediatric Physical Therapy,* 29(1), 39–46. doi:10.1097/PEP.0000000000000338.

Priya, C., Surekha, R., Srilakshmi, R. and Mithula, V. (2019). Comparative study on aquatic therapy vs. exercise for toddlers with Trisomy 21 (Down's syndrome). *Journal of Down Syndrome and Chromosome Abnormalities*, 5(131), 2472–1115. doi:10.4172/2472-1115.2019.5.131.

Sprague, S.S. and Hopkins,. PD. (2002). Use of inspiratory strength training to wean six patients who were ventilator-dependent. *Physical Therapy*, 82(2), 171–181. doi:10.1093/ptj/83.2.171.

Ravel, A., Mircher, C., Rebillat, A.S., Cieuta-Walti, C. and Megarbane, A. (2020). Feeding problems and gastrointestinal diseases in Down syndrome. *Archives de Pédiatrie*, 27(1), 53–60. doi:10.1016/j.arcped.2019.11.008.

Reid, W.D., Geddes, E.L., O'Brien, K., Brooks, D. and Crowe, J. (2008). Effects of inspiratory muscle training in cystic fibrosis: a systematic review. *Clinical Rehabilitation*, 22(10-11), 1003–1013. doi 10.1177/0269215508090619.

Ruf, K., Thomas, W., Brunner, M., Speer, C.P. and Hebestreit, H. (2019). Diverging effects of premature birth and bronchopulmonary dysplasia on exercise capacity and physical activity–a case control study. *Respiratory Research*, 20(1), 1–9. doi 10.1186/s12931-019-1238-0.

Ryan, J.M., Cassidy, E.E., Noorduyn, S.G. and O'Connell, N.E. (2017). Exercise interventions for cerebral palsy. *Cochrane Database of Systematic Reviews*, (6). doi: 10.1002/14651858.CD011660.pub2.

Sheikh, A.M. and Vissing, J. (2019). Exercise therapy for muscle and lower motor neuron diseases. *Acta Myologica*, 38(4), 215. PMC6955630.

Spruit, M., Singh, S.J, Garvey, C., ZuWallack, R., Nici, L., Rochester, C. et al. (2013). An official American Thoracic Society/European Respiratory Society statement: key concepts and advances in pulmonary rehabilitation *American Journal of Respiratory and Critical Care Medicine*, 188(8), e13–64. doi:10.1164/rccm.201309-1634ST.

Tanaka, H., Monahan, K.D. and Seals, D.R. (2001.) Age-predicted maximal heart rate revisited. *Journal of the American College of Cardiology*, 37(1), 153–156. doi:10.1016/s0735-1097(00)01054-8.

Torres-Castro, R., Zenteno, D., Rodriguez, N.I., Villarroel, G., Alvarez, C., Gatica, D. et al. (2016). Guías De Rehabilitación Respiratoria En Niños Con Enfermedades Respiratorias Crónicas: actualización 2016 Pulmonary Rehabilitation Guidelines in Children With Chronic Respiratory Diseases: 2016 Update. *Neumologia Pediatrica*, 11(3), 114–131. doi:10.4067/S0717-73482020000200109.

Turchetta, A., Salerno, T., Lucidi, V., Libera, F., Cutrera, R. and Bush, A. (2004). Usefulness of a program of hospital-supervised physical training in patients with cystic fibrosis. *Pediatric Pulmonology*, 38, 115–118. doi:10.1002/ppul.20073.

Vega-Briceño, L.E. and Zenteno, D.A. (2009). Clinical Guide for diagnosis and care of children and adolescents with post-infectious bronchiolitis obliterans. *Revista Chilena Enfermedades Respiratorias*, 25, 141–163. doi:10.4067/S0717-73482009000300002.

Verschuren, O., Peterson, M.D., Balemans, A.C. and Hurvitz, E.A. (2016). Exercise and physical activity recommendations for people with cerebral palsy. *Developmental Medicine and Child Neurology*, 58(8), 798–808. doi:10.1111/dmcn.13053.

Villarroel, G. Jalil, Y., Moscoso, G. and Mendez, M. (2017). Evaluacion de la presión inspiratoria máxima en pacientes pediátricos traqueostomizados no colaboradores. *Revista Chilena de Enfermedades Respiratorias*, 33, S59. Accessed March 9 2021 https://serchile.cl/site/docs/suplemento33_2017.pdf.

Villarroel, G., Faúndez, M., Moscoso, G., Jalil, Y. and Astudillo, C. (2020). Entrenamiento sobre cinta rodante en niños con enfermedades respiratorias crónicas. Serie clínica. *Revista Chilena de Enfermedades Respiratorias*, 36(2), 109–114. doi:10.4067/S0717-73482020000200109.

Weisman, I.M. et al. (2003). ATS/ACCP Statement on cardiopulmonary exercise testing. *American Journal of Respiratory and Critical Care Medicine*, 167(2), 211–277. doi: 0.1164/rccm.167.2.211.

West, S., Banls, L., Schneiderman, J.E., Caterini, J.E., Stephens, S., White, G., Dogra, S. and Wells, G. (2019). Physical activity for children with chronic disease; a narrative review and practical aplications, *BMC Pediatrics,* 19, 12. doi:10.1186/s12887-018-1377-3.

Wilkes, D.L., Schneiderman, J.E., Nguyen, T., Heale, L., Moola, F., Ratjen, F., Coates, A.L. and Wells, G.D. (2009). Exercise and physical activity in children with cystic fibrosis. *Paediatric Respiratory Reviews*, 10(3), 105–109. doi:10.1016/j.prrv.2009.04.001.

Yaşar, E., Adigüzel, E., Arslan, M. and Matthews, D.J. (2018). Basics of bone metabolism and osteoporosis in common pediatric neuromuscular disabilities. *European Journal of Paediatric Neurology*, 22(1), 17–26. doi: 10.1016/j.ejpn.2017.08.001.

10 Exercise Capacity in Children Born Early

E. Mark Williams and Sailesh Kotecha

Introduction

The majority of infants are born at term, defined as birth after 37 weeks of gestation, and enter childhood with a healthy cardiopulmonary system. Although considerable growth occurs during the first years of life, the ability to exercise, or more precisely, the ability to be physically active develops quickly. In early infancy, crying and feeding are the most energetic activities, followed by crawling, walking, and running usually by the age of 2 years. By 3 years of age, physical activity involves exploratory play, running, and jumping. As the child's strength and size increases so does their ability to exercise both in intensity and duration. This requires fully functioning cardiovascular and respiratory systems. In some preterm born children (born earlier than 37 weeks of gestation), exercise capacity is reduced. The reasons for this reduction are complex and only just now being reported, however, the principal reason is related to the immaturity of the respiratory system with preterm birth and its clinical treatment. While in the womb lung growth is protected and nurtured, but once born a multitude of problems can impede growth, such as infection, barotrauma from respiratory support, oxygen toxicity due to a high fractional oxygen concentration (FIO_2), and nutritional compromises.

Pre-natal Lung Development

One month after fertilisation, the respiratory system begins developing in the embryo, marking the first of five phases of development (Table 10.1). Starting with the embryonic phase, the primitive larynx, trachea, bronchi, and lungs develop as an endodermal tissue outgrowth from the lining of the developing foregut. This fold gradually pinches off from the primitive pharynx to form the respiratory diverticulum, some of which remains attached (later forming the larynx), while the remainder forms an epithelial lined tube, which becomes the trachea. Initially, this tube is terminated by two lung buds. As gestation progresses, these lungs buds undergo rapid development and growth, and develop into bronchial buds dividing into lobes, two

DOI: 10.4324/9781003020462-10

Table 10.1 Phases of Prenatal Lung Development (Cousins *et al.*, 2018)

Phases		*Duration and Structures Formed*
Embryonic period	Embryonic	3–9 weeks Formation of major airways and pulmonary blood vessels
Organogenesis	Pseudoglandular	5–17 weeks. Smaller airways developing
Foetal period	Canalicular	16–26 weeks air–blood barrier formed. Breathing movements occur.
Differentiation	Saccular[a]	24–38 weeks expansion of airway, surfactant excretion begins. Gas-exchanging tissue develops.
	Alveolar	36 weeks onwards alveoli maturation begins. Able to support gas exchange.

[a]Foetus can survive outside the womb.

in the left lung and three in the right lung. Further dichotomous divisions occur resulting in the formation of thousands of smaller and smaller airways terminating in millions of alveoli, the anatomical structures where gas exchange occurs. The lungs are unnecessary for intrauterine existence, but they must be developed enough for immediate use following birth, they do play a role in supporting the pregnancy and from the canicular phase onwards are an important source of amniotic fluid secreting around 15 $mL \cdot kg^{-1}$ body mass daily into the foetal airways which remain fluid-filled until birth. After birth, when the lungs are filled with air, airway surface fluid is maintained by a balance of absorption and secretion, supporting mucociliary clearance and maintaining ideal conditions for gas transfer and exchange with the blood.

The majority of the development that determines airway function and calibre in later life occurs during the latter half of pregnancy, in the second and third trimesters, during the saccular and alveolar phases (Table 10.1). This phased development occurs throughout gestation and continues after birth until at least 2 years of age (Narayanan *et al.*, 2012). This later phasing allows the differentiation of structure along the airways between those tissues involved in mucus secretion to the delicate alveoli where gas exchange occurs. After 6–7 months of gestation, the mucus secreting respiratory epithelium of the airways begins to form. The thinning of this epithelium at the terminal of the airways is required before functional gas exchange can occur satisfactorily. Next, the formation of functioning type II alveolar cells ensures that surfactant, a mixture of phospholipids and proteins, can be produced. Surfactant is important as its secretion into the alveoli reduces alveolar surface tension, preventing their collapse when they become air-filled at birth and thereafter. Most of the post-natal alveolar growth continues until at least 2 years and possibly beyond (Narayanan *et al.*, 2012; Bush, 2016; McGrath-Morrow and Collaco, 2019; Shen-Hao *et al.*, 2020).

Post-natal Lung Development

Throughout childhood and early adulthood, the lungs continue to enlarge. This is a crucial stage and in children lung function and airway hyper-responsiveness follow that achieved at birth. Lung growth tracks throughout life, thus impaired lung function established by the end of normal growth is unlikely to recover for the rest of an individual's life, although catch-up growth may show some potential for lung function gain with time (Kotecha *et al.*, 2010, 2012, 2013). The physical size and growth of the lungs track skeletal growth, with the two lungs filling the space encompassed within the upper thorax, bounded by the ribcage and the diaphragm inferiorly. It is not until the early twenties that lung function reaches its peak, and the lungs cease to grow (Figure 10.1). This means that tall adults with a "broad-chest" will have large volume lungs and vice versa for shorter people. This gives a direct relationship between lung volume, age, height, and gender in adults. Consequently, males who tend to have a broader chest than females of the same height will have larger lung volumes.

In 2012, the Global Lung Initiative (GLI) group collected lung function data from 97,759 healthy subjects from 33 countries ranging between 2.5 and 95 years of age (Quanjer *et al.*, 2012). The child data shows a linear increase in volume with age, except during puberty when the scaling relationship between body size and lung size is temporarily lost, altering the ratio between lung volume, measured as the forced vital capacity (FVC) and

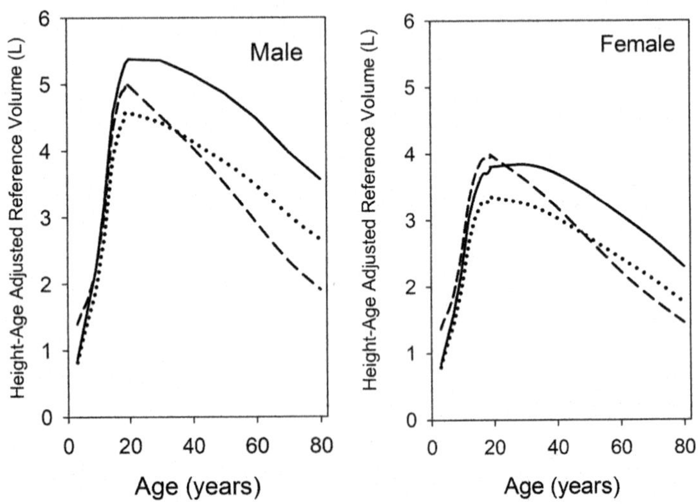

Figure 10.1 Normal values for forced vital capacity (FVC), forced expiratory volume in 1 second (FEV_1), and forced expiratory flow 25–75% (FEF 25–75%). Y-axis is expressed in litres for FVC and FEV_1, and in L sec^{-1} for FEF 25–75%.

Source: Stanojevic *et al.*, (2008).

airway patency, measured as the forced expired volume in one second ($FEV_{1)}$ as shown in Figure 10.2.

Beyond puberty, the increase in lung volume with age is proportional to the increase in the calibre of the airways until growth is complete. This results in the mechanical function of the lungs mirroring growth as well, as the ratio of lung volume to airway circumference remains steady. Unobstructed airways offer the least resistance to airflow thus allowing efficient breathing and larger tidal volumes to be inhaled during inspiration. As a result, maximal expiratory airflow, measured at rest by spirometry as the FEV_1, remains proportional to age, height, and gender (Figures 10.1 and 10.2). It is not only the calibre and volume of the airways that dictate function, but also the area and thickness of the gas exchanging alveolar surface and the matching of ventilation and perfusion that determines the efficiency of gas exchange. The

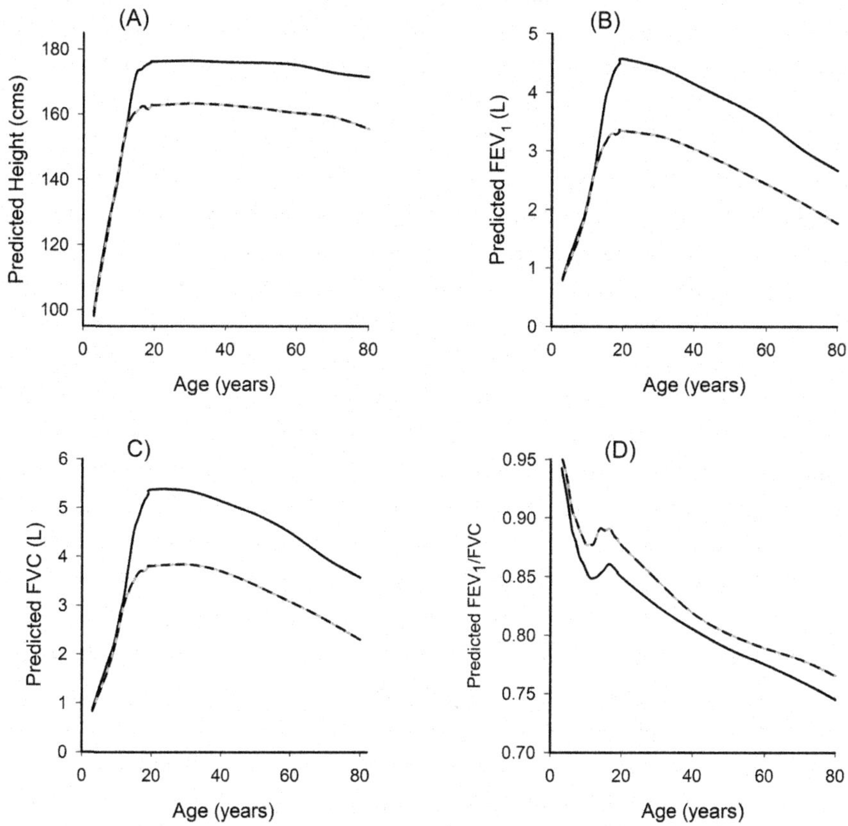

Figure 10.2 Age-specific predictions of height (A), forced expiratory volume in second (FEV_1) (B), forced vital capacity (FVC) (C), and FEV_1/FVC ratio (D), for males (solid line) and females (dashed line), respectively.

Source: Zhang, Hu and Shan, (2017).

alveolarisation of the lungs after birth is very important in development. Poor post-natal alveolarisation in preterm-born babies who are born at an early stage of lung development will therefore compromise gas exchange, limiting oxygen uptake and causing carbon dioxide retention, a consequence of which can be impaired exercise performance and physical activity in later life.

From the age of the mid-twenties onwards, lung function progressively declines as an inevitable consequence of aging (Figure 10.1). In the presence of chronic lung disease or exposure to noxious agents including tobacco smoke or air pollution, this decline can accelerate leading to premature development of chronic obstructive pulmonary disease (COPD). Both physical activity and the ability to exercise are affected by such decline.

Preterm Birth

The lungs are one of the last systems to develop, so when early birth occurs (before 37 weeks of gestation) in around 10% of pregnancies worldwide, the lungs are at an early stage of development. The more premature a neonate is, the more likely is the need for intervention to support their breathing. In those born extremely preterm, before 26 weeks of gestation, the lungs are still in the saccular phase of lung development with the alveoli yet to develop so gas exchange occurs inefficiently and ineffectively across the saccules. Birth before 28 weeks gestation often requires respiratory support with invasive mechanical ventilation or continuous positive airway pressure, exogenous surfactant administration, and often high concentrations of supplemental inspired oxygen to enhance the oxygen gradient between air and blood. The infant is maintained in a temperature-controlled incubator, monitored for infections, and receives intragastric or intravenous nutritional support. Management continues until the baby is able to breathe independently without any support. Extubation from invasive ventilation may be facilitated by treatment with post-natal corticosteroids. However, non-invasive respiratory support and supplemental oxygen may still be required and respiratory stimulants such as caffeine are established to promote control of breathing (Kumar and Lipshultz, 2019). In some countries, inhaled bronchodilators and/or inhaled corticosteroids are used empirically to reduce the work of breathing and dampen airway inflammation, respectively.

Chronic lung disease of prematurity (CLD), also called bronchopulmonary dysplasia (BPD), is diagnosed if the baby remains dependent on supplemental oxygen at either 28 days of age or 36 weeks of corrected gestation (Jobe and Bancalari, 2017). BPD results from parenchymal and airway oxidant, proteolytic and inflammatory injury following the respiratory support measures used in preterm infants delivered at an early stage of lung development. BPD is associated with increased hospitalisation in infancy particularly with viral infections and is associated with long-term reduced lung function and exercise tolerance (Taylor *et al.*, 2014). BPD was first described by Northway in 1967, in relatively mature preterm-born infants who required high-oxygen concentration therapy and high positive pressure mechanical ventilation for their neonatal respiratory distress syndrome (RDS) (Northway *et al.*, 1967). Although the use of mechanical ventilation in RDS improved survival beyond 4 days of age, BPD was so called because of the cycle of injury and repair (dysplasia) to the airway tissue, and alveoli during the period of neonatal intensive care (Northway, 1992). The total number of days on positive-pressure ventilation are the major determinants of lung function in later infancy (Shen-Hao *et al.*, 2020). In RDS surfactant secretion is reduced from the alveolar type II cells. This form of BPD is now termed 'old' BPD as aetiological factors have been modified by modern interventions including the routine administration of antenatal maternal corticosteroids to promote antioxidant and surfactant production in the foetus, routine use of exogenous surfactant and gentler forms of largely non-invasive respiratory support. Mortality and morbidity in preterm-born neonates have greatly improved with gestational viability decreasing to around 23 weeks of gestation. BPD arising nowadays in babies receiving these interventions during their neonatal intensive care course has different characteristics. This 'new' BPD exhibits abnormal alveolar-capillary development (Voynow, 2017). This results in a reduced surface area for gas exchange with fewer, enlarged alveoli (Lai *et al.*, 2019).

In both the new and old forms of BPD (CLD), lung function is impaired including a reduction in FEV_1 and FVC; the impairment appears not to improve with age and lasts throughout childhood and later life (Urs *et al.*, 2018; Cardoen *et al.*, 2019). Intrauterine growth restriction (IUGR) is common in preterm-born infants reflecting stress and or placental dysfunction impacting on foetal growth. Together with other risk factors such as depravation and maternal smoking during and after pregnancy, IUGR is likely to be a contributory factor to adverse future lung function but specific data are scarce (Källén *et al.*, 2013; Stocks and Sonnappa, 2013; Arigliani *et al.*, 2018). Survivors of neonatal intensive care who develop BPD are at the lower end of the lung function trajectory curve thus are now increasingly considered to be at risk of premature development of chronic obstructive pulmonary disease, COPD (McGarth-Morrow and Collaco, 2019).

Attempts to decrease BPD rates include the routine use of antenatal corticosteroids administration to the mother when preterm delivery is anticipated; antenatal corticosteroids promote surfactant synthesis and anti-oxidant enzyme induction in the foetus resulting in decreased incidence of development of RDS in the newborn preterm infant. Prophylactic bovine or porcine-derived exogenous surfactant is routinely administrated prophylactically to the lungs of the at-risk preterm born baby via an endotracheal tube or directly with a catheter shortly after birth, this aims to address the lack of surfactant production in these babies who are at risk of developing neonatal respiratory distress syndrome (RDS).

Preventing the development of BPD is important as, once established, treatments are lacking in evidence with focus instead on preventing further lung injury such as the use of Palivizumab to prevent respiratory syncytial virus (RSV) infection and on ensuring all the nutrients are in place to promote lung growth. Since the infants may have increased pulmonary arterial pressures and may develop pulmonary hypertension, oxygen supplementation is optimised, avoiding hypoxia or hyperoxia (the arterial blood oxygen saturation (SaO_2) being maintained between 90 and 95% at <36 weeks' gestation) to prevent increases in pulmonary arterial pressures, thus the cardiovascular system is closely monitored (Poon, Edwards and Kotecha, 2013).

A comparison of 150 thousand (n = 154,233) neonates born very preterm (<32 weeks gestation) or very low birth weight (<1500 g), in 11 high-income countries, between two epochs, 2007–2011 and 2012–2017, noted that mortality rates had fallen (Lui *et al.*, 2019). The same study shows that the rate of BPD in the very premature born continues to rise in seven of the countries including the U.K. due to improved survival rates. Studies have shown that those born moderately late preterm (between 32 and 36 weeks of gestation) did not show any differences in respiratory health, and physical activity levels were comparable to those born at term (after 37 weeks' gestation) at 13–14 years of age (Vrijlandt *et al.*, 2018). While others have shown that preterm born children have increased respiratory symptoms, inhaler use and doctor-diagnosed asthma (Joshi *et al.*, 2013).

Exercise and Lung Function

In children and adults, the ability to exercise depends on a well-balanced cardiorespiratory system, with both the heart and lungs circulating enough blood and oxygen around the body to ensure that there is sufficient transport and delivery of oxygen especially to the exercising muscles, heart, and tissues, complimented with removal of excess metabolic carbon dioxide from the body. Oxygen uptake via the lungs depends on the integrity of many of its structural and functional features, some of which may be affected by preterm delivery and by the interventions that may have been instituted to maintain life. Young children breathe relatively more air than adults meaning they are disproportionately more affected by lung dysfunction. A term born 1 year old will breathe approximately 25 $L{\cdot}kg^{-1}{\cdot}hour^{-1}$, reducing to 18 $L{\cdot}kg^{-1}{\cdot}hour^{-1}$ for a four old, to 12 $L{\cdot}kg^{-1}{\cdot}hour^{-1}$ at 12, and 4–6 $L{\cdot}kg^{-1}{\cdot}hour^{-1}$ in adulthood.

In health, during exercise, the ability to draw more air into the lungs increases in a linear fashion with exercise intensity. The minute ventilation (VE), a measure of ventilation rate, is metered by the breathing rate and tidal volume (VT) and dead space (VD). In young infants born early, ventilation is increased with a higher respiratory rate and larger relative tidal volumes than term born peers (Pickerd *et al.*, 2013). As the early born child grows with lungs that have had their development impeded, their ability to ventilate remains impaired, and typically they have a higher breathing rate but smaller

VT, which during exercise results in a lower VE, than in those born at term (Joshi *et al.*, 2013; Ruf *et al.*, 2019).

Drawing air into the lungs requires the generation of negative airway pressure in the airways and thorax sufficient to overcome airway resistance. Mid-airway diameter is the main determinant of this resistance so restricted lung growth in early born children, and especially in those with frequent airway inflammation, as in those with asthma will find the work of breathing increased at rest and even more pronounced whilst exercising. A significant risk of exercise-induced bronchoconstriction (EIB) has been reported in premature children (Joshi *et al.*, 2013).

Fresh air reaching the alveoli ensures that the alveolar oxygen tension is higher than that found in the blood, favouring diffusion or transfer across the thin respiratory epithelium into the blood (with carbon dioxide diffusing in the opposite direction). The integrity of this thin respiratory membrane, consisting largely of type I cells, is important. If it thickens, then diffusion is impaired and slowed, which limits the rate of oxygen uptake. In most children at rest, a reduced diffusion rate would not be noticeable but during physical activity would reduce exercise capacity, general everyday physical activity, and play. Evidence of an anatomically reduced airway size has been found in young early born adults, having a smaller dysanaptic ratio than a term born group, and those with a diagnosis of BPD group showing the greatest reduction (Duke *et al.*, 2018). Impaired gas diffusion across the alveolar membrane has been observed in early born children (Ruf *et al.*, 2019).

Right ventricular cardiac output passes through the lungs via an extensive low pressure pulmonary circulation. Apart from blood volume, haemodynamics play an important role in determining exercise capacity and performance. During exercise when cardiac output increases, the blood transit time through the pulmonary circulation and exposure to the alveolar membrane shortens. This has the potential to lower the supply of oxygen, by reducing the systemic arterial blood haemoglobin oxygen content. In preterm born children who had BPD in infancy, pulmonary arterial hypertension (PAH), may evolve through the formation of dysmorphic pulmonary vasculature and compromised angiogenesis during gestation, especially when exposed to hyperoxia in the neonatal period (Abman, 2001). This BPD-associated pulmonary hypertension is present at birth. As the child develops, the PAH resolves usually within a year of birth but a study in young children aged around 7 years with BPD, it was found that around 29% of the study cohort had raised pulmonary blood pressure and was associated with subclinical right ventricular dysfunction (Kwon *et al.*, 2016). The influence on exercise performance has yet to be defined.

Most of the available information regarding exercise capacity in early born children has been gathered from graded exercise performed under laboratory conditions using treadmills and ergometers, where comparisons with healthy age-matched term born children are usually made.

Exercise Capacity and Physical Activity

To measure the integrated physiological response to physical activity requires sophisticated exercise testing equipment. These devices can measure in real-time and simultaneously many cardiopulmonary parameters during a bout of graded exercise for example running on a treadmill or cycling on a fixed bicycle (ergometer) to exhaustion. Exercise assessment requires cooperation of the participant especially when asked to exercise at maximal exertion, all in a confined laboratory setting. In school-age children (aged six and older), this presents further problems due to the need for smaller-sized exercise equipment and sometimes by their limited ability to understand what is required of them during the exercise period (Takken, Ulu and Hulzebos, 2020).

Having dysfunctional lungs, we would expect children born early to exhibit a lower maximal rate of oxygen consumption during maximal exercise (VO_{2max}; $mL \cdot min^{-1} \cdot kg^{-1}$) and a lower maximal ventilation rate, VE_{max}, but some early authors proposed that children, even those who had BPD in their infancy, would perform physically as well as their peers (Baraldi, 2000). To date physical activity studies in young children born at term or early and reported by Lowe *et al.* (2015, 2016, 2017) have found little difference in activity, with there being no difference in activity between girls. This is despite differences in oxygen consumption when exercising. Edwards *et al.* (2015) reviewing 20 studies on exercise capacity in preterm born children born with and without BPD in infancy found small differences in VO_{2max} when corrected for body mass (Figures 10.3 and 10.4).

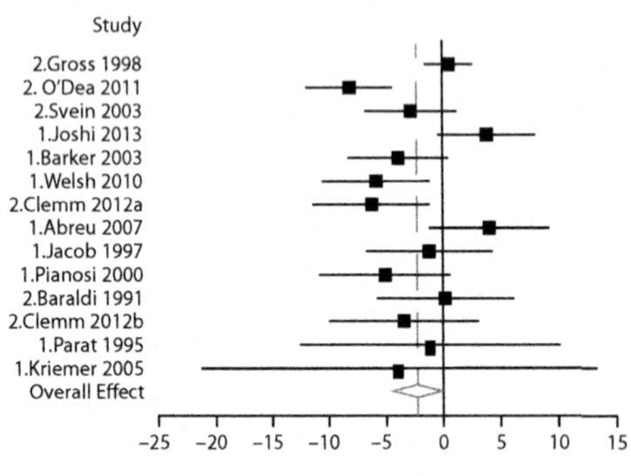

Study	*Preterms (No BPD)*			*Term Controls*		
	Mean	SD	Total	Mean	SD	Total
2.Gross 1998	43.7	5.4	53	43.2	8.6	108
2. O'Dea 2011	42.2	7.8	25	50.3	5.9	28
2.Svein 2003	39.8	7.3	22	42.6	6.5	22
1.Joshi 2013	35.0	7.2	26	31.1	8.4	26
1.Barker 2003	36.9	5.1	12	40.8	6.2	13
1.Welsh 2010	35.3	8.3	15	41.1	6.9	38
2.Clemm 2012a	39.5	7.2	9	45.7	6.7	35
1.Abreu 2007	39.0	6.7	10	34.9	6.1	14
1.Jacob 1997	36.7	9.2	15	37.9	5.3	13
1.Pianosi 2000	41.0	8.0	15	46.0	6.0	15
2.Baraldi 1991	42.9	9.1	15	42.7	9.9	26
2.Clemm 2012b	46.5	9.1	10	49.9	10.3	40
1.Parat 1995	40.0	9.0	5	41.0	9.0	5
1.Kriemer 2005	29.0	9.7	14	32.8	40.7	24

Heterogeneity: $Tau^2 = 9.75$: $Chi^2 = 35.3$, df = 13 (P = 0.0007); I2 = 63%.
Test for overall effect : Z = 2.02 (P = 0.04)

Figure 10.3 A Forest plot comparison of 14 studies reporting VO_{2max} ($mL \cdot kg^{-1} \cdot min^{-1}$) between children born early and born at term. 1. Cycle ergometry, 2. Treadmill. Mean, mean value of VO_{2max} for participants studied; SD, standard deviation of mean; Total, total number of subjects; Weight, overall weight for a study towards total mean difference; 95% CI, 95% confidence interval.

Source: Redrawn from Edwards *et al.*, (2015).

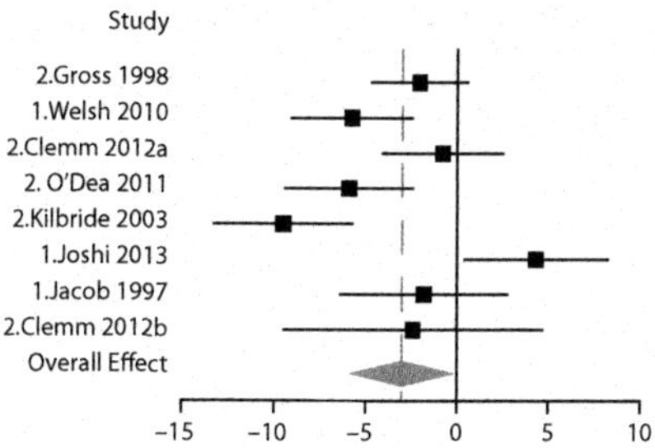

Study	BPD Preterms			Term Controls		
	Mean	SD	Total	Mean	SD	Total
2.Gross 1998	41.1	7.5	43	43.2	8.6	108
1. Welsh 2010	35.3	6.3	23	41.1	6.9	38
2. Clemm 2012a	44.9	4.6	12	45.7	6.7	35
2. O'Dea 2011	44.4	7.4	29	50.3	5.9	28
2.Kilbride 2003	29.0	5.9	13	38.5	5.2	25
1.Joshi 2013	35.4	5.5	24	31.1	8.4	26
1.Jacob 1997	36.1	7.0	15	37.9	5.3	13
2.Clemm 2012b	47.5	11.0	12	49.9	10.3	40

Heterogeneity: $Tau^2 = 13.0$: $Chi^2 = 32.2$, $df = 7$ ($P < 0.0001$); $I^2 = 78\%$. Test for overall effect : $Z = 2.08$ ($P = 0.04$)

Figure 10.4 A Forest plot comparison of eight studies reporting VO_{2max} ($mL \cdot kg^{-1} \cdot min^{-1}$) between children born early with BPD, and term. 1. Cycle ergometry, 2. Treadmill. Mean, mean value of VO_2max for participants studied; SD, standard deviation of mean; Total, total number of subjects; Weight, overall weight for a study towards total mean difference; 95% CI, 95% confidence interval.

Source: Redrawn from Edwards *et al.*, (2015).

A recent study of 8–12-year-old early born children, which included a small group of post-BPD children, reported a 10% reduction in predicted peak oxygen uptake (VO_{2peak}), a reduced FEV_1 and transfer factor for carbon monoxide (TLco) when compared to term born controls (Ruf *et al.*, 2019). The VO_{2peak} was lower in the early born BPD children at 1,292 ± 343 $mL \cdot min^{-1}$ or 83 ± 11% predicted, compared to 1,649 ± 388 $mL \cdot min^{-1}$, or 91 ± 8% in early born children without BPD. A small control group of children born at term had a VO_{2peak} of 94 ± 9% predicted and 1,508 $mL \cdot min^{-1}$. Lung function in the BPD children was the most impaired, although within the normal range, they exhibited a reduced FEV_1 (83 ± 22 vs 105 ± 8% pred), and FVC (95 ± 17 and 106 ± 7% pred). Alveolar diffusion was reduced in both early born groups. This group also assessed physical activity using accelerometers and found that being born early was linked to reduced moderate to vigorous activity (MVPA). The early born children only undertook around half that of the term born children (around 17 vs 35 minutes, respectively). The same study reported prolonged sedentary activity in the early born groups. The reasons for this reduced activity were not identified but could be respiratory in nature due to avoidance of dyspnoea, poor muscle strength, conditioning and coordination, neurodevelopmental, cognitive differences, or behavioural in nature.

It is more likely to be a combination of these factors, and further prospective controlled trials are needed to pin-point which are the principle factors and how they lead to the diverse differences in lifestyle and health observed in those born early (Proulx *et al.*, 2017).

The Swedish study by Svedenkrans *et al.*, (2013) of adults reported exercise capacity of a national cohort of male military conscripts at recruitment at a

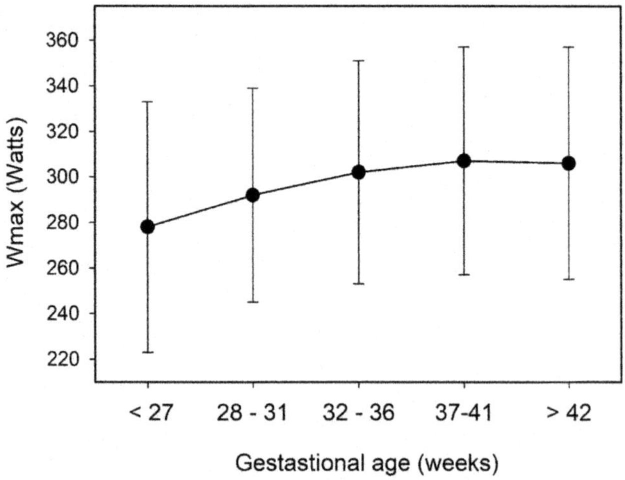

Figure 10.5 Swedish cohort study of male military conscripts (median age 18 years, range 18–26 years). Maximal exercise capacity by gestational age. Mean ± SD shown, ANOVA, overall $p < 0.001$. GA (weeks): ≤27, n = 56; 28–31, n = 726; 32–36, n = 9,930; 37–41, n = 182,490; >42, n = 25,618.

Source: Modified from Svedenkrans *et al.*, (2013).

median age of 18 years (range 18–26, born between 1973 and 1983). From the original population of 428,092, a cohort of 218,820 men provided data, including maximal work rate (W_{max}; watts), assessed by cycle ergometry. The study noted a strong link with gestational age; W_{max} decreased with gestational age. Those born at term (up to 42 weeks of gestation) had a W_{max} of around 300 W, while in those born early at ≤27 weeks of gestation was lower at 278 W (Figure 10.5). These authors extended their study to show that low exercise capacity is also associated with the lower cognitive function (Svedenkrans *et al.*, 2016).

Studies also suggest that children born early and of low birth weight have reduced muscle strength but not mass, which manifests itself as a low grip strength (Dodds *et al.*, 2012, Ahlqvist *et al.*, 2019). All of these studies suggest that overall, low birth weight, and preterm birth impinge on cardiorespiratory fitness and ability to exercise in children (Ahlqvist *et al.*, 2020).

Physical activity in children is influenced by many factors both physiological and psychological but can still be quantified and compared in groups of children under similar conditions. Given that lung function and exercise capacity is reduced in some children born early, we would expect that physical activity would also be less in these children (Tsopanoglou *et al.*, 2014).

A group of young early born children aged 4–6 years were given a 4-week exercise programme with three blocks of interval training each lasting 30–50 minutes per week (Mestre *et al.*, 2018). Despite little difference in lung function, the early born group showed significant improvements in the performance of a 6-minute walk test, an incremental shuttle walk test and a modified sit and reach test in comparison to those born at term. This study providing evidence that increased physical activity in these children may lead to improvements in exercise capacity.

In another study, extremely early born children (<28 weeks, gestation) with extremely low birth weights (ELBW; birthweight of <1,000 g) were found at to be less active than their control term born peers at age 11 (Egan *et al.*, 2020). In this Norwegian cohort, the early born children exercised less, had lower exercise endurance and sports proficiency, and did not engage in team sports. This reduced physical activity had been predictable at age 5 years in an earlier study of the same cohort (Egan *et al.*, 2020). Early born children have been shown to exhibit less regulated temperaments as well as differing physical activity, with lower attention scores (Cassiano *et al.*, 2020). Such children when older could potentially benefit from behavioural change programmes to engage them in beneficial training and healthy exercise (Glen Aylward, 2014).

The long-term implications of being born early and a reduced level of exercise capacity in children and the subsequent consequences on adult life have yet to be explored in future. In particular how these permanent deficiencies in cardiopulmonary dysfunction manifest themselves in a child's activity and future expectations when playing or exercising. Further intervention studies are required to see if this dysfunction can be improved by specific sporting activities which favour improved lung function such as swimming or whether physical activity *per se* is beneficial.

Conclusion

Neonatal pulmonary development continues late into gestation, so children born before term, may require respiratory support and close meticulous, comprehensive clinical management in the weeks and months after birth to nurture the ex-utero lung development and minimise acquired lung injury. Children surviving preterm birth will often exhibit reduced lung function, decreased cardiorespiratory fitness, and be physically less active in comparison to children born at term. This leads to a reduced capacity to exercise and limited physical activity. Many observational studies have been performed, providing greater clarity on the differences between early born and term born children. Fewer studies have addressed the issue of prevention or investigated whether exercise-based interventional studies in early childhood can improve these deficiencies.

Key Points

- The functional development of the prenatal respiratory system to prepare for post-natal life occurs largely during the third trimester. Being born early (<37 weeks of gestation) can interrupt this development.

- Early birth can be associated with low birthweight and complications including bronchopulmonary dysplasia leading to poor lung growth and function in later childhood, reflected in reduced exercise capacity.
- Children born early may often exhibit reduced ability to exercise which can manifest itself as reduced physical activity or less willingness to join in physical activity with other children.
- Evidence suggests that cognitive, neurodevelopmental, and behavioural comorbidities, linked to being born early, may contribute to the decreased physical activity observed in these children.
- Whether physical activity profiles in children born early can be improved by exercise programmes has been poorly investigated but such interventions are likely to result in improvements as observed in other respiratory diseases.

References

Abman, S.H. (2001). Bronchopulmonary dysplasia: "a vascular hypothesis". *American Journal of Respiratory and Critical Care Medicine*, 164, 1755–1756. Doi 10.1164/ajrccm.164.10.2109111c.

Ahlqvist, V.H., Persson, M., Ortega, F.B., Tynelius, P., Magnusson, C., Berglind, D. (2019). Birth weight and grip strength in young Swedish males: a longitudinal matched sibling analysis and across all body mass index ranges. *Scientific Reports*, 9, 9719. Doi 10.1038/s41598-019-46200-0.

Ahlqvist, V.H., Persson, M., Ortega, F.B., Tynelius, P., Magnusson, C., Berglind, D. (2020). Birth weight and cardiorespiratory fitness among young men born at term: the role of genetic and environmental factors. *Journal of the American Heart Association*, 9, e014920. Doi 10.1161/JAHA 119.014290.

Arigliani, M., Spinelli, A.M., Liguoro, I., Cogo, P. (2018). Nutrition and lung growth. *Nutrients, 10*, 919. Doi 10.3390/nu10070919.

Baraldi, E. (2000). Chronic respiratory diseases and sport in children. *International journal of sports medicine*, 21(Supp. 2), 103–105. Doi 10.1055/s-2000-8499.

Bush, A. (2016). Lung development and aging. *Annals of American Thoracic Society*, 13, S438–S446. Doi 10.1513/AnnalsATS.201602-112AW.

Cardoen, F., Vermeulen, F., Proesmans, M., Moens, M., De Boeck, K. (2019). Lung function evolution with old and new type bronchopulmonary dysplasia: a retrospective cohort analysis. *European Journal of Pediatrics*, 178, 1859–1866. Doi 10.1007/s00431-019-03453-1.

Cassiano, R.G.M., Provenzi, L., Linhares, M.B.M., Gaspardo, C.M., Montirosso, R. (2020). Does preterm birth affect child temperament? A meta-analytic study. *Infant Behavior and Development*, 58, 10147. Doi 10.1016/j.infbeh.2019.101417.

Cousins, M., Hart, K., Gallacher, D., Palomino, M.A., Kotecha, S. (2018). Long-term respiratory outcomes following preterm birth. *Revista Médica Clínica Las Condes*, 29(1), 87–97. Doi 10.1016/j.rmclc.2018.02.002

Dodds, R., Denison, H.J., Ntani, G., Cooper, R., Cooper, C., Sayer, A.A., Baird, J. (2012). Birth weight and muscle strength: a systematic review and meta-analysis. *Journal of Nutrition Health and Aging*, 16, 609–615. Doi 10.1007/s12603-012-0053-9.

Duke J.W., Gladstone, I.M., Sheel, A.W., and Lovering, A.T. (2018). Premature birth affects the degree of airway dysanapsis and mechanical ventilatory constraints. *Experimental Physiology*, 103, 261–275. Doi 10.1113/EP086588.

Edwards, M.O., Kotecha, S.J., Lowe, J., Watkins, W.J., Henderson, A.J., Kotecha, S. (2015). Effect of preterm birth on exercise capacity: a systematic review and meta-analysis. *Pediatric Pulmonology*, 50, 293–301. Doi 10.1002/ppul.23117.

Egan, M., Engesth, M.S., Fevang, S., Vollsaeter, M., Eide, G.E., Røksund, O.D., Halvorsen, T., Clemm, H. (2020). Predicting physical activity in a national cohort of children born extremely preterm. *Early Human Development*. Doi 10.1016/j.earlhumdev.2020.105037.

Glen Aylward, P. (2014). Neurodevelopmental outcomes of infants born prematurely. *Journal of Developmental and Behavioural Pediatrics*, 35, 394–407. Doi: 10.1097/01.DBP.0000452240.39511.d4.

Jobe, A.H., Bancalari, E.H. (2017). Controversies about the definition of bronchopulmonary dysplasia at 50 years. *Acta Paediatrica (Oslo, Norway: 1992)*, 106(5), 692–693. Doi 10.1111/apa.13775.

Joshi, S., Powell, T., Watkins, W.J., Drayton, M., Williams, E.M., Kotecha, S. (2013). Exercise-induced bronchoconstriction in school-aged children who had chronic lung disease in infancy. *The Journal of Pediatrics*, 162, 813–818. Doi 10.1016/j.peds.2012.09.040.

Källén, B., Finnström, O., Nygren, K.G., Olausson, P.O. (2013). Association between preterm birth and intrauterine growth retardation and child asthma. *European Respiratory Journal*, 41, 671–676. Doi. 10.1183/09031936.00041912.

Kotecha, S.J., Watkins, W.J., Heron, J., Henderson, J., Dunstan, F.D., Kotecha, S. (2010). Spirometric lung function in school-age children. Effect of intrauterine growth reduction and catch-up growth. *American Journal of Respiratory and Critical Care Medicine*, 181, 969–974. Doi 10.1164/rccm.200906-08970C.

Kotecha, S.J., Watkins, W.J., Paranjothy, S., Dunstan, F.D., Henderson, A.J., Kotecha, S. (2012). Effect of late preterm birth on longitudinal lung spirometry in school age children and adolescents. *Thorax*, *67*, 54–61. Doi 10.1136/thoraxjnl-2011-200329.

Kotecha, S.J., Edwards, M.O., Watkins, W.J., Henderson, A.J., Paranjothy, S., Dunstan, F.D. Kotecha, S. (2013). Effect of preterm birth on later FEV1: a systematic review and meta-analysis. *Thorax*, *68*, 760–766. Doi 10.1136/thoraxjnl-2012-203079.

Kumar, V.H.S., Lipshultz, S. (2019). Caffeine and clinical outcomes in premature neonates. *Children*, 24, 118. Doi 10.3390/children6110118.

Kwon, H.W., Kim, H.S., An, H.S., Kwon, B.S., Kim, G.B., Shin, S.H., Kim, E.K., Bae, E.J., Noh, C.I., Choi, J.H. (2016). Long-term outcomes of pulmonary hypertension in preterm infants with bronchopulmonary dysplasia. *Neonatology*, 110(3), 181–189. Doi 10.1159/000445476.

Lai, P.Y., Jing, X., Michalkiewicz, T., Entringer, B., Ke, X., Majnik, A., Kriegel, A.J., Liu, P., Lane, R.H., Konduri, G.G. (2019). Adverse early-life environment impairs postnatal lung development in mice. *Physiological genomics*, 51(9), 462–470. Doi 10.1152/physiolgenomics.00016.2019.

Lowe, J., Watkins, W.J., Kotecha, S., Edwards, M.O., Henderson, A.J., Kotecha, S. (2015). Physical activity in school-age children born preterm. *The Journal of Pediatrics*, 166, 877–883. Doi 10.1016/j.jpeds.2014.12.013.

Lowe, J., Watkins, W.J., Kotecha, S.J., Kotecha, S. (2016). Physical activity and sedentary behaviour in preterm-born 7-year-old children. *PLoS ONE*, 11, e0155229, 1–14. Doi 10.1371/journal.pone.0155229.

Lowe. J., Cousins, M., Kotecha, S.J., Kotecha, S. (2017). Physical activity outcomes following preterm birth. *Paediatric Respiratory Reviews*, 22, 76–82. Doi 10.1016/j.prrv.2016.08.012.

Lui, K., Lee, S.K., Kusuda, S., Adams, M., Vento, M., Reichman, B., Darlow, B.A., Lehtonen, L., Modi, N., Norman, M., Håkansson, S., Bassler, D., Rusconi, F., Lodha, A., Yang, J., Shah, P.S. (2019). Trends in outcome for neonates born very preterm and low birth weight in 11 high-income countries. *The Journal of Pediatrics*, 215, 32–40. Doi 10.1016/j.jpeds.2019.08.020.

McGrath-Morrow, S.A., Collaco, J.M. (2019). Bronchopulmonary dysplasia: what are its links to COPD? *Therapeutic Advances in Respiratory Disease*, 13, 1–15. Doi 10.1177/175346661989492.

Mestre, N.M., Papaleo, A., Hidalgo, V.M., Caty, G. (2018). Physical activity program improves functional exercise capacity and flexibility in extremely preterm children with bronchopulmonary dysplasia aged 4-6 years: a randomized controlled trial. *Archivos de Bronchoneumogia*, 54, 607–613. Doi 10.1016/j.arbres.2018.05.001.

Narayanan, M., Owers-Bradley, J., Beardsmore, C.S., Mada, M., Ball, I., Garipov, R., Panesar, K.S., Kuehni, C.E., Spycher, B.D., Williams, S.E., Silverman, M. (2012). Alveolarization continues during childhood and adolescence: new evidence from helium-3 magnetic resonance. *American Journal of Respiratory and Critical Care Medicine*, 185(2), 186–191. Doi 10.1164/rccm.201107-1348OC.

Northway Jr, W.H., Rosan, R.C., Porter, D.Y. (1967). Pulmonary disease following respiratory therapy of hyaline-membrane disease: bronchopulmonary dysplasia. *New England Journal of Medicine, 276*, 357–368. Doi 10.1056/NEJM196702162760701.

Northway Jr, W.H. (1992). Bronchopulmonary dysplasia: twenty-five years later. *Pediatrics,* 89, 969–973. ISSN 1098-4275.

Pickerd, N., Williams, E.M., Kotecha, S. (2013). Electromagnetic inductance plethysmography to measure tidal breathing in preterm and term infants. *Pediatric Pulmonology,* 48, 160–167. Doi 10.1002/ppul.22584.

Poon, C.Y., Edwards, M.O., Kotecha, S. (2013). Long term cardiovascular consequences of chronic lung disease of prematurity. *Paediatric Respiratory Reviews*, 14, 242–249. Doi 10.1016/j.prrv.2012.08.003.

Proulx, K., Majnemer, A., Dahan-Oliel, N., Mazer, B., Nadeau, L., Vanier, K., Maltais, D.B. (2017). Factors associated with moderate to vigorous physical activity in adolescents born preterm. *Pediatric Exercise Science*, 29(2), 260–267. Doi 10.1123/pes.2016-0164.

Quanjer, P.H., Stanojevic, S., Cole, T.J., Baur, X., Hall, G.L., Culver, B.H., Enright, P.L. (2012). ERS Global Lung Function Initiative. Multi-ethnic reference values for spirometry for the 3–95-yr age range: the global lung function 2012 equations. *European Respiratory Journal*, 40, 1324–1343. Doi 10.1183/09031936.00080312.

Ruf, K., Thomas, W., Brunner, M., Speer, C.P., Hebestreit, H. (2019). Diverging effects of premature birth and bronchopulmonary dysplasia on exercise capacity and physical activity – a case control study. *Respiratory Research*, 20, 260. Doi 10.1186/s12931-019-1238-0.

Shen-Hao, L., Chiang, M.C., Chu, S.M., Hsu, J.F., Yao, T.C., Tsai, M.H., Hua, M.C., Chiu, C.Y., Yeh, K.W., Huang, J.L., Liao, S.L. (2020). Evolution and determinants of lung function until late infancy among infants born preterm. *Scientific Reports*, 10, 490. Doi 10.1038/s41598-019-57359

Stanojevic, S., Wade, A., Stocks, J., Hankinson, J., Coates, A.L., Pan, H., Rosenthal, M., Corey, M., Lebecque, P., Cole, T.J. (2008). Reference ranges for spirometry across all ages: a new approach. *American Journal of Respiratory and Critical Care Medicine*, 177, 253–260. Doi 10.1164/rccm.200708-1248OC.

Stocks, J., Sonnappa, S. (2013). Early life influences on the development of chronic pulmonary disease. *Therapeutic advances in respiratory disease.* 7, 161–173. Doi 10.1177/1753456813479428.

Svedenkrans, J., Henckel, E., Kowalski, J., Norman, M., Bohlin, K. (2013). Long-term impact of preterm birth on exercise capacity in healthy young men: a national population-based cohort study. *PLoS ONE*, 8(12), e80869. Doi 10.1371/journal.pone.008069.

Svedenkrans, J., Kowalski, J., Norman, M., Bohlin, K. (2016). Low exercise capacity increases the risk of low cognitive function in healthy young men born preterm: a population-based cohort study. *PLoS ONE*, 11(8), e0161314. Doi 10.1371/journal.pone.0161314.

Takken, T., Ulu, H.S., Hulzebos, H.J. (2020). Clinical recommendations for cardiopulmonary exercise testing in children with respiratory diseases. *Expert Review of Respiratory Medicine.* Doi 10.1080/17476348.2020.1752195.

Taylor, J. B., Nyp, M.F., Norberg, M., Dai, H., Escobar, H., Ellerbeck, E., Truog, W.E. (2014). Impact of intercurrent respiratory infections on lung health in infants born <29 weeks with bronchopulmonary dysplasia. *Journal of Perinatology, 34*, 223–228. Doi 10.1038/jp.2013.152.

Tsopanoglou, S.P., Davidson, J., Goulart, A.L., de Moraes Barros, M.C., dos Santos, A.M.N. (2014). Functional capacity during exercise in very low birth weight premature children. *Pediatric Pulmonology*, 49, 91–98. Doi 10.1002/pplu.22754.

Urs, R., Kotecha, S., Hall, G.L., Simpson, S.J. (2018). Persistent and progressive long-term lung disease in survivors of preterm birth. *Paediatric Respiratory Reviews*, 28, 87–94. Doi 10.1016/j.prrv.2018.04.001.

Vrijlandt, E.J.L.E., Reijneveld, S.A., Aris-Meijer, J.L., Bos, A.F (2018). Respiratory health in adolescents born moderately-late preterm in a community-based cohort. *The Journal of Pediatrics*, 203, 429–236. Doi 10.1016/j.jpeds.2018.07.03.

Voynow, J.A. (2017). "New" bronchopulmonary dysplasia and chronic lung disease. *Paediatric Respiratory Reviews*, 24, 17–18. Doi 10.1016/j.prrv.2017.06.006.

Zhang, J., Hu, X., Shan, G. (2017). Spirometry reference values for population aged 7-80 years in China. *Respirology*, 22, 1630–1636. Doi 10.1111/resp.13118.

Index

Italicized and **bold** pages refer to figures and tables respectively.

Acceptance and Commitment Therapy (ACT) 63
ACSM *see* American College of Sports Medicine (ACSM)
ActiGraph 88
ActionPACT **161**
ACT *see* Acceptance and Commitment Therapy (ACT); Asthma Control Test (ACT)
ACTIVATE-CF **161**
aerobic exercise, for asthma 152
aerobic fitness 11; for bronchiectasis 79–82
age, and physical activity 99–100
AHA *see* American Heart Association (AHA)
Air Quality Indices (AQI) 133
airway injury 130–131
allergens 134
allergic rhinitis 135–137
'Allergic rhinitis and its impact on Asthma' study (ARIA) 136
allergic sensitisation 131–132
American Academy of Paediatricians 15
American College and Sports Medicine Association 12
American College of Sports Medicine (ACSM) 118, 150, 186
American Heart Association (AHA) 78
American Physiological Society 38
anaerobic exercise, for asthma 153
anaerobic fitness, for bronchiectasis 82
anaerobic threshold (AT) 87
AQI *see* Air Quality Indices (AQI)
AS *see* Asthma Score (AS)
ASS *see* Asthma Severity Score (ASS)
asthma 55, 58, 59, 111–122, 149; competitive sports and 134–135; exercise-induced 114–117, *116*, 134–135, **135**; exercise training for 117–120; bronchial hyperresponsiveness 119–120; control 118; fitness 118; quality of life 119; resting spirometric lung function 119–120; obesity and 113–114; overweight and 113; physical activity for 112–114, 151–153; swimming and 120–121
Asthma Control Test (ACT) 116
Asthma Score (AS) 56
Asthma Severity Score (ASS) 56
AT *see* anaerobic threshold (AT)
attitudes, and physical activity 101–102
autonomic nervous system activity, and lung function 131

behaviour change 96–107; habits and physical activity 99; physical activity among people with CF, determinants of: age and gender 99–100; attitudes 101–102; beliefs 101–102; environment 103–104; health 100; motivations 101–102; social influences 102–103; physical activity for CF, interventions targeting 104–106; theoretical perspectives of 97–99
beliefs, and physical activity 101–102
bench step test 12
benzodiazepines 64
BHR *see* bronchial hyper-responsiveness (BHR)
BMD *see* bone mineral density (BMD)
BMI *see* body mass index (BMI)
body mass index (BMI) 6, 12, 22, 112, 181
bone mineral density (BMD) 174, 182, 185

Borg CR-10, 54
Borg Rating of Perceived Exertion 54
Borg scale 54
born early children, exercise capacity in 204–216; exercise and lung function 210–211; physical activity 212–216, *212–214*; post-natal lung development 206–208, *206*, *207*; pre-natal lung development 204–205, **205**; preterm birth 208–210
BPD *see* bronchopulmonary dysplasia (BPD)
Bratteby Walk Test 36
breakthrough exercise-induced asthma (BT-EIA) 116
breathing: dysfunctional 53–54; exercises 61–62; mechanics of 49–50; neurology of 49; pattern disorders 53; techniques 61–62
Breathing Freely 61
breathlessness 48–65; assessment of: objective measures 56–57, *56*; subjective measures 54–55; in children 50–54; dysfunctional breathing 53–54; exercise limitation 51; respiratory illness 51–53, **52**; definition of 48; future research of 64–65; mechanisms of 49–50; perception of: breathing exercises 61–62; breathing techniques 61–62; cognitive 57–58; developmental 59; emotional 58–59; pharmacological intervention 64; physical training 60; positioning 61–62, *62*; psychological interventions 62–64, *63*; respiratory support measures 64; social 58; therapeutic approaches 59–60; *see also* dyspnoea
British Thoracic Society (BTS) 27
bronchial hyper-responsiveness (BHR) 117–120, 131
bronchiectasis 72–89; aerobic fitness for: cardiopulmonary exercise testing 79–81, *81*; field tests 81–82; anaerobic fitness for 82; exercise testing for 73–76, *74*, *75*; motivation and volition during 78; reporting 86–88; risks of 78; habitual physical (in)activity and 88–89; impaired physical function in: additional mediators 78; cardiovascular contributors 77; muscular contributors 76–77; pulmonary contributors 76; localised muscle function testing for: peripheral muscle testing 83–85, *84*; respiratory muscle testing 85–86, *84*; physical activity for 153–159
bronchoconstriction, exercise-induced 114–117, *116*, 134–136, 138, 151; pharmacological treatment for **136**; treatment goals for **135**
bronchodilators 64
bronchopulmonary dysplasia (BPD) 181, 208–213
Bruce protocol 37
BT-EIA *see* breakthrough exercise-induced asthma (BT-EIA)
BTS *see* British Thoracic Society (BTS)
Buteyko 61

CAES-2 *see* Clinical Asthma Evaluation Score 2 (CAES-2)
Canadian Society for Exercise Physiology (CSEP) 150
cardiopulmonary exercise testing (CPET) 11, 12, 33, 35–38, *37*, 192, 194; for paediatric bronchiectasis 74, 75, *75*, 77, 79–81, *81*, 86, 87
cardiovascular contributors to impaired physical function 77
CC16 *see* Clara cell secretory protein (CC16)
CF *see* cystic fibrosis (CF)
CFRD *see* CF-related diabetes (CFRD)
CF-related diabetes (CFRD) 73, 78
CFTR *see* cystic fibrosis transmembrane conductance regulator (CFTR)
CHD *see* congenital heart disease (CHD)
Chester Step Test (CST) 81–82
children: breathlessness in 50–54; dysfunctional breathing 53–54; exercise limitation 51; respiratory illness 51–53, **52**; with chronic health conditions: physical activity in 8–10, *10*; physical fitness in 10–12; healthy, physical activity of 4–8, *5*; with medical complexity, exercise in 174–198; *see also individual entries*
children with special health care needs (CSHCN): model of exercise training for 190–193, *193*; non-ambulatory 195
chronic lung disease of prematurity (CLD) *see* bronchopulmonary dysplasia (BPD)
chronic medical conditions: children/young people with, physical activity in 8–10, *10*; classification System of **3**; definition of 2, *4*; holistic approach to 12–13; medical approach to 12–13; prevalence of 2, 4

chronic obstructive pulmonary disease (COPD) 208
Clara cell secretory protein (CC16) 131, 132
CLD *see* chronic lung disease of prematurity (CLD)
CLE *see* continuous laryngoscopy during exercise (CLE)
Clinical Asthma Evaluation Score 2 (CAES-2) 56
Cognitive Behaviour Therapy (CBT) 63, *63*
cognitive perception of breathlessness 57–58
cold air 134
competitive sports and respiratory illness 128–142; aetiology 129–130; allergic rhinitis 135–137; asthma 134–135; cough 134; exercised-associated inducible laryngeal obstruction 137–139; external or environmental factors: allergens 134; cold air 134; pollution 133–134; swimming pool disinfectants 132–133; future research 140; gastro-oesophageal reflux disease 139; initial considerations 128–129; internal or functional factors: airway injury 130–131; allergic sensitisation 131–132; autonomic nervous system activity and lung function 131; endocrine effects 132; non-allergic rhinitis 135–137; non-pharmacological interventions for 139; pathogenesis 129–130
congenital heart disease: barriers to physical activity in 13
congenital heart disease (CHD) 177
continuous laryngoscopy during exercise (CLE) 138
continuous positive airway pressure (CPAP) 64, 176, 191
COPD *see* chronic obstructive pulmonary disease (COPD)
coping strategies: 'active' *versus* 'passive' 102; functional 102
cough 134
CPAP *see* continuous positive airway pressure (CPAP)
CPET *see* cardiopulmonary exercise testing (CPET)
CSEP *see* Canadian Society for Exercise Physiology (CSEP)
CSHCN *see* children with special health care needs (CSHCN)
CST *see* Chester Step Test (CST)
cycle ergometry tests 37, *37*
cystic fibrosis (CF) 65, 149; barriers to physical activity in 13; behaviour change and 96–107; cardiopulmonary exercise testing for 36–37; exercise testing for 35; field tests for 35, 36; physical activity among people with, determinants of: age and gender 99–100; attitudes 101–102; beliefs 101–102; environment 103–104; health 100–101; motivations 101–102; social influences 102–103; physical activity for 153–159, 182; interventions targeting 104–106; physical fitness and 12; physical training for 60; randomised controlled exercise interventions in **154–156**; spirometry tests for 30; survival rates of 4; in young people 72–89; aerobic fitness for 79–82; anaerobic fitness for 82; exercise testing for 73–76, *74*, *75*; field tests for 81–82; habitual physical (in)activity 88–89; impaired physical function in 76–78; localised muscle function testing for 83–86; motivation and volition during exercise testing 78; reporting of exercise test 86–88; risks of exercise testing 78
cystic fibrosis transmembrane conductance regulator (CFTR) 73

Dalhousie Dyspnoea scale 55
DBPs *see* disinfection by-products (DBPs)
developmental perception of breathlessness 59
Diagnostic and Statistical Manual of Mental Disorders (DSM-5) 58
DigiWalker pedometer 89
disinfection by-products (DBPs) 120, 121, 132
Down syndrome (DS; Trisomy 21) 181, 185
DS *see* Down syndrome (DS; Trisomy 21)
DSM-5 *see* Diagnostic and Statistical Manual of Mental Disorders (DSM-5)
dysfunctional breathing 53–54
dyspnoea 48; definition of 48; exercise testing for 33; *see also* breathlessness

EIAH *see* exercise-induced arterial hypoxemia (EIAH)
EIA *see* exercise-induced asthma (EIA)

EIB *see* exercise-induced bronchoconstriction (EIB)
EILO *see* exercise-induced laryngeal obstruction (EILO)
EIM *see* *Exercise is Medicine©* (EIM)
ELBW *see* extremely low birth weight (ELBW)
emotional perception of breathlessness 58–59
endocrine effects 132
environment, and physical activity 103–104
ERS *see* European Respiratory Society (ERS)
eucapnic voluntary hyperpnoea (EVH) 115, 135
European CF Society 37
European Respiratory Society (ERS) 37, 75
EVH *see* eucapnic voluntary hyperpnoea (EVH)
exercise: capacity, in children born early 204–216; exercise and lung function 210–211; post-natal lung development 206–208, *206*, *207*; pre-natal lung development 204–205, **205**; preterm birth 208–210; in children with medical complexity 174–198; in healthy children 4–8, *5*; limitation, for breathlessness 51; programme, designing 186–190, **187–188**, **189–190**; in young people 4–8, *5*
exercise-induced arterial hypoxemia (EIAH) 117
exercise-induced asthma (EIA) 114–117, *116*, 134–135; breakthrough 116; pharmacological treatment for **136**; treatment goals for **115**
exercise-induced bronchoconstriction (EIB) 114–117, *116*, 134–136, **135**, 138, 151; pharmacological treatment for **136**; in premature children 211; treatment goals for **115**
exercise-induced laryngeal obstruction (EILO) 54, 117, 121, 137–139
Exercise is Medicine© (EIM) 12–13, 159
exercise testing: for bronchiectasis 73–76, *74*, *75*; for pulmonary function 33–35, **34**; technical considerations 38–39
exercise training: for asthma 117–120; model of 190–193, *193*; in patients with chronic diseases, benefits of 181–185
ExerciseWorks© 12
extremely low birth weight (ELBW) 215

fat-free mass (FFM) 22
FEV_1 *see* forced expiratory volume in one second (FEV_1)
FFM *see* fat-free mass (FFM)
Fick equation 11
field tests: for paediatric bronchiectasis 81–82; for pulmonary function 33, 35–36, 39
FIO_2 *see* fractional oxygen concentration (FIO_2)
fitness, and asthma 118
'5 As' 159, **159**
forced expiratory volume in one second (FEV_1) 24, 27–29, 31, 115, 119, 120, 157, *206*, 207, *207*, 209, 213
forced vital capacity (FVC) 27, 29, 206, *206*, *207*, 209
fractional oxygen concentration (FIO_2) 204
functional neuroimaging 57–58
FVC *see* forced vital capacity (FVC)

gas diffusion techniques 31–33
gas dilution techniques 31–33
gas exchange threshold (GET) 87
gastro-oesophageal reflux disease (GORD) 139, 177
gender and physical activity 99–100
GET *see* gas exchange threshold (GET)
GLI *see* Global Lung Function Initiative (GLI)
Global DRO *see* Global Drug Reference Online (Global DRO)
Global Drug Reference Online (Global DRO) 140
Global Initiative for Asthma guidelines 152
Global Lung Function Initiative (GLI) 29, 30, 206
GMFCS *see* Gross Motor Function Classification System (GMFCS)
Godfrey protocol 37
GORD *see* gastro-oesophageal reflux disease (GORD)
Gross Motor Function Classification System (GMFCS) 176, 187

habits, and physical activity 99
Habitual Activity Estimation Scale (HAES) 89
habitual physical (in)activity, and bronchiectasis 88–89
HAES *see* Habitual Activity Estimation Scale (HAES)

health, and physical activity 100–101
healthy children: physical activity and exercise in 4–8, *5*
heat-and-moisture-exchanging devices (HMEs) 139
HMEs *see* heat-and-moisture-exchanging devices (HMEs)
holistic approach to chronic medical conditions 12–13
hyperventilation 51, 53, 55, 58, 61, 80, 114, 117
hypoglycaemia 9
hypoventilation 176, 184

ICF *see* International Classification of Function, Disability and Health (ICF)
ILO *see* inducible laryngeal obstruction (ILO)
IL-6 *see* interleukin 6 (IL-6)
IL-10 *see* interleukin 10 (IL-10)
impulsive system 99
IMT *see* inspiratory muscle training (IMT)
incremental shuttle walk test (ISWT) 35
individual activity, designing 186–190, **187–188**, **189–190**
inducible laryngeal obstruction (ILO) 54; exercise-induced 54
inspiratory muscle training (IMT) 61–62, 184–185, 194–197
interleukin 6 (IL-6) 114, 115, 131
interleukin 10 (IL-10) 131
International Classification of Function, Disability and Health (ICF) 185
International Society of Physical Activity and Health (ISPAH) 13
International Sport Federations 129
International Tennis Federation (ITF) 129
intrauterine growth restriction (IUGR) 209
ISPAH *see* International Society of Physical Activity and Health (ISPAH)
iStep test 36, 81
ISWT *see* incremental shuttle walk test (ISWT)
ITF *see* International Tennis Federation (ITF)
IUGR *see* intrauterine growth restriction (IUGR)

JMH *see* Josefina Martínez Hospital (JMH), Santiago, Chile
Josefina Martínez Hospital (JMH), Santiago, Chile 190, 197, 198

laryngeal disorders 53–54
LCI *see* lung clearance index (LCI)
leukotriene receptor antagonists (LTRAs) 117
localised muscle function testing, for bronchiectasis: peripheral muscle testing 83–85, *84*; respiratory muscle testing 85–86, *84*
lower respiratory tract infections (LRTI) 174, 177, 184
LRTI *see* lower respiratory tract infections (LRTI)
LTRAs *see* leukotriene receptor antagonists (LTRAs)
lung clearance index (LCI) 23, 31, 33, 39

maximal expiratory pressure (MEP) 85, 194, **195**
maximal oxygen uptake (VO_2) 11, 12
maximal voluntary ventilation (MVV) 87
maximum inspiratory pressure (MIP) 85, 194–196, **195**, *196*, *197*; in non-collaborative children with tracheostomies **195**
MBW *see* multiple breath inert gas washout (MBW)
MCP 1 *see* monocyte chemotactic protein 1 (MCP 1)
medical approach to chronic medical conditions 12–13
medical complexity, exercise in children with 174–198; exercise training, model of 190–193, *193*; individual activity and exercise programme, designing 186–190, **187–188**, **189–190**; relationship with physical activity: multi-system dysfunction 181; muscles and exercise capacity, deconditioning 177–178; muscle weakness 175–177; obesity 178, 180; osteoporosis 180; overweight 178, 180; respiratory comorbidities and progressive lung disease 177, **178**, **179–180**; training 193–197, *194*; inspiratory muscle training 194–197; outcomes observed in JMH model 197
MEP *see* maximal expiratory pressure (MEP)
metabolic equivalents (METs) 6, 9
METs *see* metabolic equivalents (METs)
MI *see* Motivational Interviewing (MI)
MIP *see* maximum inspiratory pressure (MIP)
moderate to vigorous intensity physical activity (MVPA) 174, 213
modified shuttle walk test (MSWT) 35, 36
monocyte chemotactic protein 1 (MCP 1) 115

Motivational Interviewing (MI) 63, 105
motivations: and physical activity 101–102; Self-Determination Theory 97–98
MSWT *see* modified shuttle walk test (MSWT)
multiple breath inert gas washout (MBW) 23, 31
multi-system dysfunction, in children with medical complexity 181
muscle weakness 175–177
muscular contributors to impaired physical function 76–77
MVPA *see* moderate to vigorous intensity physical activity (MVPA)
MVV *see* maximal voluntary ventilation (MVV)

National Asthma Education and Prevention Guidelines for the Diagnosis and Management of Asthma 152
National Survey of Children's Health (2007) 2
'National Youth Fitness Survey, The' 113
NAVA *see* neurally adjusted ventilatory assist (NAVA)
neurally adjusted ventilatory assist (NAVA) 176–177, 191
neuromuscular disease (NMD) 175–177, 180, 183, 184, 196
new digital technologies 160–162
Nijmegen Questionnaire (NQ) 55
Nintendo Wii® 183
NIV *see* non-invasive ventilation (NIV)
NMD *see* neuromuscular disease (NMD)
non-allergic rhinitis 135–137
non-communicable diseases 1, 51, 149
non-invasive ventilation (NIV) 176
NQ *see* Nijmegen Questionnaire (NQ)

obesity: and asthma 113–114; and physical activity 178, 180
OMNI scale 55
1-minute sit-to-stand test (STS1) 36, 82
osmotic theory 115
osteoporosis 180
overweight: and asthma 113; and physical activity 178, 180

Paediatric Early Warning Systems (PEWS) 57
Paediatric Respiratory Assessment Measure (PRAM) 56
paediatric respiratory illness, and breathlessness 51–53, **52**
PAH *see* pulmonary arterial hypertension (PAH)
Papworth Method 61
PAQLQ *see* Pediatric Asthma Quality of Life Questionnaire (PAQLQ)
PA *see* physical activity (PA)
pathological breathlessness 53
peak expiratory flow (PEF) 27
peak oxygen uptake (VO_{2peak}) 24, 33, 35–37, 80, 81, 86, 87, 181
peak work-rate (WR_{peak}) 37
Pediatric Asthma Quality of Life Questionnaire (PAQLQ) 119
PEF *see* peak expiratory flow (PEF)
Perceived Exertion scale 54, 55
peripheral muscle testing, for bronchiectasis 83–85, *84*
PEWS *see* Paediatric Early Warning Systems (PEWS)
pharmacological intervention for breathlessness 64
PHT *see* pulmonary vascular hypertension (PHT)
physical activity (PA) 149–164; among people with CF, determinants of: age and gender 99–100; attitudes 101–102; beliefs 101–102; environment 103–104; health 100–101; motivations 101–102; social influences 102–103; and asthma 112–114; barriers to 159–160; for CF, interventions targeting 104–106; of children born early 212–216, *214–216*; in children with chronic health conditions 8–10, *10*; facilitators 159–160; habits and 99; of healthy children 4–8, *5*; implications of 13–14; moderate to vigorous intensity 174; in patients with chronic diseases, benefits of 181–185; relationship with medical complexity: multi-system dysfunction 181; muscles and exercise capacity, deconditioning 177–178; muscle weakness 175–177; obesity 178, 180; osteoporosis 180; overweight 178, 180; respiratory comorbidities and progressive lung disease 177, **178**, **179–180**; of young people 4–8, *5*; with chronic health conditions 8–10, *10*
physical fitness: and bronchiectasis 79; in children with chronic health conditions 10–12; in young with chronic health conditions 10–12

physical training for breathlessness 60
plethysmography 33
pollution 133–134
post-natal lung development 206–208, *206*, *207*
pre-natal lung development 204–205, **205**
preterm birth 208–210
progressive lung disease, respiratory comorbidities and 177
Project Fizzyo **161**
psychological interventions for breathlessness 62–64, *63*
pulmonary arterial hypertension (PAH) 211
pulmonary contributors to impaired physical function 76
pulmonary function tests 21–39, **24–25**; cardiopulmonary exercise testing 35–38, *37*; exercise testing 33–35, **34**; technical considerations 38–39; field tests 33, 35–36, 38; gas diffusion techniques 31; gas dilution techniques 31; growth 21–22; laboratory tests 33; maturation 21–22; monitoring in clinical practice 22–23; peak expiratory flow 27; plethysmography 33; reasons for 23–24, *24*; spirometry 27–31, **25–26**, *28*, *29*, **32**
pulmonary vascular hypertension (PHT) 181

QoL *see* quality of life (QoL)
quality of life (QoL) 23, 35, 39, 150, 174, 182, 197; and asthma 118, 119

'ramp-incremental' protocol 37
rapid shallow breathing (RSB) 61
rating of perceived exertion (RPE) 194
RDS *see* respiratory distress syndrome (RDS)
reflective system 99
resistance training 182
respiratory comorbidities, and progressive lung disease 177
respiratory distress syndrome (RDS) 209
respiratory muscle endurance (RME) 85–86
respiratory muscle testing, for bronchiectasis 85–86, *84*
respiratory syncytial virus (RSV) infection 210
resting spirometric lung function 119–120
RME *see* respiratory muscle endurance (RME)
RPE *see* rating of perceived exertion (RPE)
RSB *see* rapid shallow breathing (RSB)
RSV *see* respiratory syncytial virus (RSV) infection

SABA *see* short-acting Beta2-agonists (SABA)
sedentary behaviours and health, relationship between 7
Self-Determination Theory 97–98
self-efficacy 98–99, 103, 105
short-acting Beta2-agonists (SABA) 117
6-minute walk test (6MWT) 12, 36, 38, 191–194, 197, 198
6MWT *see* 6-minute walk test (6MWT)
sniff nasal inspiratory pressures (SNIP) 194, **195**
SNIP *see* sniff nasal inspiratory pressures (SNIP)
Social Good Fund 106
social influences, on physical activity behaviour 102–103
social perception of breathlessness 58
socioeconomic status 100
spirometry 22–23, 27–31; abnormal flow-volume loops *29*; comprehensive assessment **32**; flow volume loops during moderate/intensive exercise *28*; normal resting maximal flow-volume loop *28*
Spirotiger® *84*
SRT *see* Steep Ramp Test (SRT)
Steep Ramp Test (SRT) 80–81
Steps Ahead: Optimising Physical Activity and Health in Adults with Cystic Fibrosis **161**
STS1 *see* 1-minute sit-to-stand test (STS1)
swimming, and asthma 120–121
swimming pool disinfectants 132–133

telehealth/medicine 160–162
therapeutic approaches to breathlessness 59–60
Therapeutic Use Exemption (TUE) 140

thermic theory 115
'This Girl Can' campaign 100
three-minute step test 36
TLC *see* total lung capacity (TLC)
total lung capacity (TLC) 21
tracking 5–6
TUE *see* Therapeutic Use Exemption (TUE)
type 1 diabetes 9; barriers to physical activity in 13

U.S. Maternal and Child Health Bureau: chronic medical condition, definition of 2
U.S. National Survey of Children's Health 2007 149

VAS *see* Visual Analogue Scales (VAS)
VAT *see* ventilatory anaerobic threshold (VAT)
VC *see* vital capacity (VC) manoeuvres
ventilation 49–50; hyperventilation 51, 53, 55, 58, 61, 80, 114, 117; hypoventilation 176, 184
ventilatory anaerobic threshold (VAT) 177
ventilatory threshold 87
Visual Analogue Scales (VAS) 55
vital capacity (VC) manoeuvres 27
VO_{2peak} *see* peak oxygen uptake (VO_{2peak})

WADA *see* World Anti-doping Agency (WADA)
'We Are Undefeatable' campaign 100
Wingate testing 82
World Anti-doping Agency (WADA) 140, **141**
World Health Organization 150, 186
WR_{peak} *see* peak work-rate (WR_{peak})

Yoga 61
young people: with chronic health conditions: physical activity in 8–10, *10*; physical fitness in 10–12; cystic fibrosis/bronchiectasis in 72–89; aerobic fitness 79–82; anaerobic fitness 82; exercise testing for 73–76, *74*, *75*; field tests 81–82; habitual physical (in)activity 88–89; impaired physical function 76–78; localised muscle function testing 83–86; motivation and volition during exercise testing 78; reporting of exercise test 86–88; risks of exercise testing 78; physical activity and exercise in 4–8, *5*
Youth Olympic Games 2010 129
Youth Olympic Games 2018 129